PHYSICAL AGENTS FOR PHYSICAL THERAPISTS

PHYSICAL AGENTS FOR PHYSICAL THERAPISTS

Second Edition

By

JAMES E. GRIFFIN, Ph.D.

Director, Program in Physical Therapy
Professor of Physiology and Health Science
Ball State University
Muncie, Indiana

and

TERENCE C. KARSELIS, M.S.

Associate Professor of Medical Technology
School of Allied Health Professions
Medical College of Virginia
Virginia Commonwealth University
Richmond, Virginia

With a Contribution by

Dean P. Currier, Ph.D.

Professor of Physical Therapy
University of Kentucky
Lexington, Kentucky

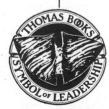

CHARLES C THOMAS • PUBLISHER
Springfield • Illinois • U.S.A.

Published and Distributed Throughout the World by
CHARLES C THOMAS • PUBLISHER
2600 South First Street
Springfield, Illinois 62717, U.S.A.

© *1978 and 1982, by* CHARLES C THOMAS • PUBLISHER

ISBN 0-398-04579-8

Library of Congress Catalog Card Number: 81-8986

With THOMAS BOOKS careful attention is given to all details of manufacturing and design. It is the Publisher's desire to present books that are satisfactory as to their physical qualities and artistic possibilities and appropriate for their particular use. THOMAS BOOKS will be true to those laws of quality that assure a good name and good will.

First Edition, 1978
Second Edition, 1982

Library of Congress Cataloging in Publication Data

Griffin, James E.
  Physical agents for physical therapists.

  Includes bibliographical references and
index.
  1. Physical therapy. 2. Physical therapy —
Equipment and supplies. I. Karselis, Terence.
II. Currier, Dean P. III. Title.
RM701.G75 1981   615.8'2   81-8986
ISBN 0-398-04579-8   AACR2

Printed in the United States of America
C-1

PREFACE

THIS BOOK deals with the clinical application of physical agents. It is intended as a text for the baccalaureate- and graduate-level physical therapy student. It is assumed that the student has a reasonable background in undergraduate-level biology, chemistry, pathology, and physics and that the material contained herein will be supplemented by appropriate lectures and demonstrations.

The reason for writing the book is that nowhere in recent years has any physical therapist made an attempt to bring together and apply the advances in physiology and electronics that have evolved from clinical or laboratory research. These advances permit more logical use of cold, heat, nerve and muscle stimulating currents, diathermy, and ultraviolet and ultrasonic energy in helping the patient to be relieved of pain and to regain independence in activities of daily living.

In the Second Edition there has been major rewrite and expansion of the chapters on pain, and on nerve and muscle stimulating currents, as well as moderate revision of all other chapters, with the objective of making the book more useful to the clinical therapist. Special emphasis has been placed on providing the therapist with documentation for trying new treatments and equipment when initial treatments did not provide the desired short- or long-term goals.

A wealth of material has been reported in various journals within the last several decades. The literature cited in the book is in no way complete or exhaustive. It has been chosen as representative of developing new concepts of disease and treatment, or as confirming older concepts that have withstood the test of time.

Sections of the various chapters dealing with treatment tech-

v

nics do not spell out details that are more effectively learned within practice classes. Technics are given in detail when the described procedure can lead to improved patient care.

Chapters on electronic instrumentation design, hazards, and safety requirements reflect the major changes in federal regulations that became effective in 1979. Conceptual knowledge of modern apparatus design and of advances in physiological rationale for choice of physical agent to alleviate a problem should minimize the occasion for the physical therapist to become involved in malpractice suits because of use of defective equipment or because of misapplication of good equipment and/or technics.

The authors are indebted to Doctor Dean P. Currier for his new section within Chapter 3, discussing EMG, nerve conduction velocity, and biofeedback, and to Doctor Duncan T. Kennedy for his excellent new illustrations pertinent to clinical neuroanatomy.

J.E.G.
T.C.K.

CONTENTS

PHYSICAL AGENTS
FOR PHYSICAL
THERAPISTS

Chapter 1

PAIN

Perhaps the simplest definition of pain is that "it is a hurt that we feel."[1] The standard medical dictionary definition of pain is that it is a more or less localized sensation of discomfort, distress, or agony, resulting from the stimulation of specialized nerve endings.[2]

If a physical therapist wishes to be useful in the relief of pain, he needs to know as much as possible about the biophysical effects of physical agents. If a patient is limited in his activities of daily living because of pain, or because he perceives his pain as a major factor during his waking hours, it is unlikely that he will make much progress in regaining control over range of motion, use of assistive devices, or gaining in strength until such time as the pain has been relieved, or at least reduced to a tolerable level.

Regular administration of the appropriate physical agent can be highly effective in relieving pain in properly selected patients. Physical agents may also be used in conjunction with medication and/or postsurgically. Frequently, the patient will derive greater benefit from therapeutic exercise if the exercise is preceded by a carefully selected physical agent.

CAUSES OF PAIN

Causes of pain are myriad. Quite often there will be abnormal activity of muscle, peripheral circulation, and/or the nervous system, either as a cause or the result of the patient's perception of pain.

Spasm may be defined as an abnormal and continuing hyperactivity of any type of contractile tissue, such as skeletal, smooth, or cardiac muscle. Although far less common than spasm in either skeletal or smooth muscle, the cardiac muscle spasm, which is a dominant feature in true angina pectoris, is one of the most severe forms of pain. If this abnormal cardiac muscle contraction can be relaxed, the accompanying pain will be diminished.

When pain is present, there is often concomitant local circulatory impairment. One known cause of such impairment is skeletal muscle spasm, which can significantly limit venous return. Such flow deficit can give rise to additional pain because the deficit leads to inadequate local removal of metabolic waste products.

Vasospasm is the abnormal continuing hyperactivity of smooth muscles in the walls of blood vessels. It is of particular importance in arterial vessels with a diameter of a few millimeters. The ratio of muscle to other tissues is especially high in arterial vessels of small diameter. Vasospasm can be triggered by peripheral or central irritation of sympathetic nerves, or by edema formation. (The role of the parasympathetic nervous system in response to pain is less well delineated.) In all cases, vasospasm leads to the reduction or cessation of arterial flow. Significant reduction gives rise to pain, and in extreme cases to irreversible damage, in the tissues supplied by the malfunctioning vessels. Organic occlusive peripheral vascular diseases can cause severe chronic impairment of circulation and and give rise to steadily increasing pain over weeks and months.

Furthermore, diminished circulation, either arterial or venous, can give rise to skeletal or cardiac muscle spasm because of inadequate local nutrition or ineffective removal of waste products from the local area served by the malfunctioning vessels.

The nervous system can also play a major role in pain production. The sensory portions of the nervous system must be functioning and have functioning connections to the spinal cord and on up to higher (cortical) levels before the patient can be aware of noxious stimuli. The rare infant with a congenital lesion such that he cannot perceive pain seldom survives his infancy. He dies as a consequence of injury or disease of which no one is aware. Skeletal muscle hyperactivity, vasospasm, and nervous system malfunction can all occur without the patient feeling pain if pain pathways to the cortex are interrupted by trauma or disease.

The abnormal activity without pain can be just as much or more of a handicap to activities of daily living. Abnormal muscular hyperactivity without pain is commonly seen in the chronic phase of the traumatic paraplegic or quadriplegic patient. In such patients, the primary lesion is usually in the spinal cord; more rarely, it occurs within the cranial vault. Usually, the peripheral nervous system remains largely intact, but because of edema, anatomical cord severance, or other lesion in the cord, pain pathways are interrupted. Because of neuroanatomical relationships within the spinal cord, pain and other sensation is more apt to be lost than is motor nerve control over skeletal muscle or sympathetic nerve control over smooth muscle in blood vessel walls.

CLASSIFICATION OF PAIN

The clinical physician usually classifies pain into three major categories. One type is often called a fast-onset, pricking type of pain. A second category is frequently described as of slow onset, leading to a burning sensation. The third type is commonly pictured as a deep, dull ache. This ache is frequently remote from the causal site and usually is due to the dysfunction of some portion of the viscera. Bishop[3] has done an outstanding job in reviewing what has evolved over the last several decades in our knowledge of the anatomy, physiology, and management of pain. This review has exhaustively documented what is understood about pain that is amenable to physical therapy procedures.

It now appears certain that the fast, pricking pain is most often transmitted from the periphery into the central nervous system by delta axons, which are 4 to 6 microns in diameter, whereas the smaller, unmyelinated C fibers normally transmit pain stimuli leading to a burning sensation. It is this latter type of pain with which the physical therapist is most often concerned, pain of slow onset, great persistence, and accompanied by powerful responses, both physiological and psychological. The third general category of pain awareness, visceral or aching pain, is more apt to be a life-threatening indicator and is not often amenable to physical therapy procedures.

Abnormal functioning of local areas of skeletal muscle, circulation, and the nervous system are very much interrelated. Each abnormality can be a cause of pain; each can be the result of noxious stimuli. Each can be a part of the vicious cycle of pain — spasm — more pain — more spasm. Under some circumstances, appropriate administration of the most suitable physical agent can be the best means to interrupt that vicious cycle and thereby achieve cumulative, lasting pain relief.

The psychological aspects of pain are somewhat more elusive and controversial than the physiological components. The psychological aspects can be conveniently considered on the basis of the importance that the subject attaches to his pain. Sternbach[1] expressed these variables quite well when he wrote,

> It is not pain which is mental or physical, functional or organic, psychic or somatic, but our ways of thinking about pain and the systems of terms we use to describe pain which may be so dichotomized. All pain can be described in both languages, the psychological and the physiological. Pain itself is not one or the other. But because pain can be described in both mental or physical terms, pain is a truly psychosomatic concept. From this point of view, all pain is real; and all pain is also psychosomatic since both mental and physical descriptions are possible.

The key to how intense or how minimal is an individual's response to pain is probably previous conditioning plus present distraction. Either can serve to increase or decrease anxiety and thus to increase or decrease pain. There is no reliable objective measure of pain intensity.

THEORIES OF PAIN AWARENESS

A moment's reflection will allow you to recall that our peripheral receptors are constantly bombarded by various stimuli — sound, light, touch, body segment position, and so forth. It has been demonstrable for years that sensory and motor impulse propagation[1] triggered by any of the wide variety of sensory receptor stimuli have identical physiological characteristics, yet the normal individual has no problem discerning whether a propagated impulse volley is sending a message about change in temperature, pressure, etc. Therefore, the impulses transmitted by any sensory axon must eventually impinge upon some portion of the central nervous system. Only then are we consciously aware of the change in our environment and the degree of change. Further reflection will allow you to agree that at any point in time we are acutely aware of only one or possibly two different kinds of stimuli.

There have been many theories published about possible mechanisms and pathways for pain perception and pain relief. Possibly the one that comes the nearest to affording a reasonable working hypothesis in accounting for all presently known aspects of pain and pain relief is that presented by Melzack and Wall[4] in 1965. Their gate control theory proposed a neural mechanism in the spinal cord, which can increase or decrease the flow of pain impulses from the periphery to the brain. When other sensory input is minimal, pain awareness is great. When other sensory input is equal to or greater than pain input, awareness of the latter is diminished. This gate control theory can well account for the concept of counterirritation, which is very useful in attempting to explain why judicious intermittent use of heat, cold, ultrasound, and nerve stimulating currents can relieve pain. By 1974, Melzack[5] was able to state and defend the hypothesis that the neospinothalamic system selects and modulates sensory input in such a fashion as to permit the discriminative dimension of pain. He further stated that activation of reticular and limbic structures through the paramedical ascending system underlies the motivational drive and unpleasant affect that trigger the organism into action. Lastly, Melzack presented evidence that neocortical or higher central nervous system processes (suggestion, anxiety, and attention) exert control over activity in both discriminative and motivational systems (Fig. 1-1).

There have been many favorable as well as dissident criticisms of the original gate control concept. One result of much additional research was a major restatement of the concept in 1978. According to Wall,[6] the brain becomes aware of pain by way of a gate in the spinal cord, which reacts to injury response, other afferent impulses, and to descending control; these factors modify the impulse flow, which passes through the gate and which then proceeds to the many neuronal structures that modify sensory awareness. Currently it appears that the concept of

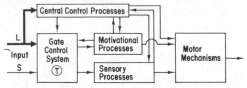

Figure 1-1. Schema for demonstrating the gate control theory of pain. L — large, fast-transmitting axons. S — small, slow-transmitting axons. T — transmission cephalad from spinal cord after sorting. Motivational processes include central intensity monitoring. Sensory processes include spatiotemporal analysis. From International Symposium on Pain (Advances in Neurology, Volume 4), p. 526. Editor, John J. Bonica. © 1974 by Raven Press, New York.

spinal cord gate control over peripheral sensory input to awareness centers is well accepted. Further, as originally proposed by Melzack and Wall,[4] the most likely region within the cord for location of the gate is the substantia gelatinosa. The mechanism(s) by which the gate operates will continue to be under study for a long period of time.

During the 1970s an additional factor in pain perception and pain relief came to the forefront, namely that many populations of neurones within the central and peripheral nervous system are capable of producing opiates, which, upon demand, are transmitted to synapses or other specific cell binding sites (Fig. 1-2). Evidence is strong that there are many such receptor sites

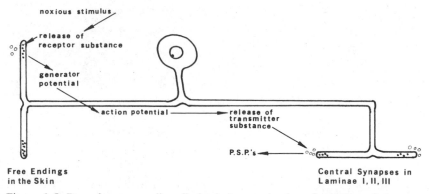

Figure 1-2. Dorsal root ganglia cell, depicting projections from the soft tissues, mostly skin, and going to central synapses in the dorsal horn area of the spinal cord. Courtesy of Dr. Duncan T. Kennedy, Muncie, Indiana.

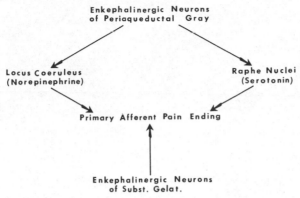

Figure 1-3. Schema of known concentrations of receptor sites within the CNS, and probable major transmitters and messengers in the respective areas.[3, 7, 21] Courtesy of Dr. Duncan T. Kennedy, Muncie, Indiana.

within the anterior spinothalamic (paleospinothalamic, containing mostly C fiber axons and synapses) pathway, within major components of the limbic system, and in the substantia gelatinosa.[7, 21]

It is now generally accepted that there are significant concentrations of opiate receptors in the following locations:

1. amygdala
2. hypothalamus
3. periaqueductal gray matter (PAG)
4. medial thalamus

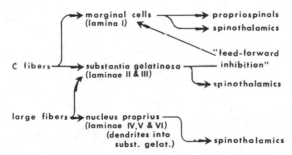

Figure 1-4. Schema of probable linkages of peripheral sensory neurones and relationships to tracts within the cord and thalamus. Courtesy of Dr. Duncan T. Kennedy, Muncie, Indiana.

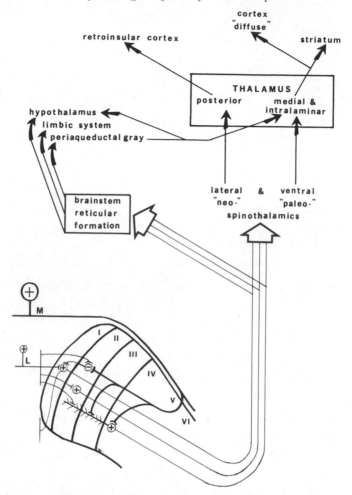

Figure 1-5. CNS areas and tracts that are known to respond to peripheral sensory input, especially pain. Courtesy of Dr. Duncan T. Kennedy, Muncie, Indiana. I-VI = Rexed's laminae in the dorsal horn; M = medial division of the dorsal root; L = lateral division of the dorsal root; plus = excitatory neurone; minus = inhibitory neuron.

    5. solitary nuclei

    6. dorsal horn of spinal cord (laminae I, II, III)

See Figures 1-5 and 1-6 for the anatomical interrelations. Receptors are usually thought to be localized on afferent and primary afferent preterminal and terminal fibers; hence the notion that the mechanism of receptor function is most likely to be pre-synaptic inhibition.

Enkephalinergic interneurones are frequently localized in the same areas as the opiate receptors. There is some evidence for axoaxonic synapse within the substantia gelatinosa between enkephalinergic neurones and the primary afferent pain terminals.[3, 7, 21] It is known that serotonin is localized in the raphe nuclei, norepinephrine in the locus coeruleus, and gamma-aminobutyric acid is a major neurotransmitter among interneurones. All three have been shown to inhibit the release of Substance P from sensory neurones in tissue culture experiments. (*See* Figs. 1-3, 1-4, 1-5, and 1-6 for detail of anatomical interrelationships.)

Most of the presently known endogenous opiates are classified as endorphins (enkephalins) and are known to have a direct effect on pain awareness and on emotional behavior. It is also well established that many of them function as synaptic neurotransmitters, probably by modifying the movement of sodium (and potassium) across limiting membranes. The oldest known endorphin is called Substance P (for peptide). It was discovered in the early 1930s, but its function was not known until the 1950s. Its structure was not identified until 1970.[8] Substance P is now well recognized as a major neurotransmitter for impulses carried by alpha and possibly delta sized axons going from the periphery into the dorsal horn of the spinal cord.[3] Several investigators have shown independently that Substance P is released from presynaptic terminals when peripheral nerves are stimulated electrically.[8] Some evidence has been reported that the mechanism by which the gate control operates is the amount of Substance P released in and around the region of the substantia gelatinosa.[8, 9] (*See* Figs. 1-2, 1-3, and 1-4 for anatomical detail and interrelationships.)

As physical therapists, our primary concern with pain and pain relief is to add sufficient energy to the patient to provide sufficient increase in nonpainful sensory input to override or counterbalance the painful sensory input, or to transiently diminish the ability of axons to conduct. The problem frequently is how to drive a physiologically acceptable quantity of energy to the needed depth without damaging intervening tissues.

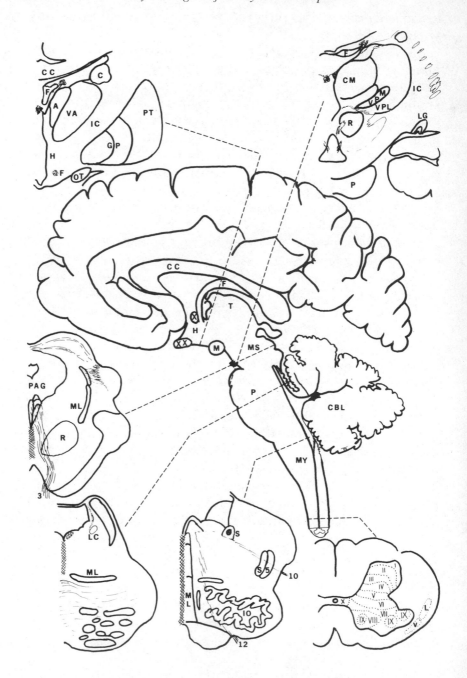

KNOWN EFFECTS OF CLINICALLY APPLICABLE
HEAT AND COLD

When cold is applied to a patient for the purpose of relieving pain, the objective is to lower tissue temperature within physiological limits. Fortunately, altering the temperature of cutaneous nerves can do much to reduce hyperactivity of underlying contractile tissue. Miglietta[10] showed that application of cold to the skin can bring about significant reduction of deep muscle spasm within one minute. However, Wolf and Basmajian[11] have demonstrated that even when intense cold is applied to a small area of skin, it takes an application time of at least

---

←

Figure 1-6. Schema of a midsagittal section of the CNS, with detailed enlargements of areas known to influence subject perception of pain. Courtesy of Dr. Duncan T. Kennedy, Muncie, Indiana. Redrawn from *Atlas of Cross Section Anatomy of the Brain* by Emil Villiger. Copyright © 1951 McGraw-Hill Book Company. Used with the permission of McGraw-Hill Book Company.

A = anterior nucleus of thalamus
C = caudate nucleus
CBL = cerebellum
CC = corpus callosum
CM = centromedian (an intralaminar) nucleus
F = fornix
GP = globus pallidus
H = hypothalamus
IC = internal capsule
L = lateral spinothalamic tract
LC = locus coeruleus
LG = lateral geniculate
M = mammilary body
ML = medial lemniscus
MS = mesencephalon (midbrain)
MY = myelencephalon (medulla)
OT = optic tract
P = pons
PAG = periaqueductal gray matter
PT = putamen
R = red nucleus
S = nucleus and tractus solitarius
S5 = spinal nucleus and tract of the fifth (trigeminal) cranial nerve
T = thalamus
V = ventral spinothalamic tract
VA = ventral anterior nucleus of thalamus
VPL = ventroposterior lateral nucleus of the thalamus
VPM = ventroposterior medial nucleus of the thalamus
X = anterior commissure
XX = optic chiasm
3 = third (oculomotor) cranial nerve
10 = tenth (vagus) cranial nerve
12 = twelfth (hypoglossal) cranial nerve
I — X = Rexed's laminae
X adjacent to spinal canal = nuclei of the raphe

five minutes before there will be a 1°C reduction in muscle temperature at a depth of 5 cm. In earlier experiments more nearly approaching standard clinical application of cold to a local area, Bierman[12] demonstrated that cold must be applied for thirty minutes before there is a similar drop in deep muscle temperature. Abramson et al.[13] have published evidence that there is always vasoconstriction with a drop in muscle temperature.

Reviews of clinical cryotherapy[14, 15] and of the physiological effects of heat and cold[16] indicate that much of the measurable effect of conductive and/or radiant heating and of conductive cooling is an indirect response due to the stimulation of cutaneous nerves. Effects of these agents on skeletal muscle and subcutaneous circulation are due more to such indirect effects than to primary energy absorption or release by subcutaneous tissues.

Voluminous literature has developed over the years demonstrating that when cutaneous thermal receptors are stimulated by heat, there is an increase in nerve conduction velocity, an increase in cutaneous circulation brought about by local cutaneous release of histamine (a potent vasodilator) or histaminelike substances, and a further increase in cutaneous circulation as warmed blood reaches the vasomotor regulators within the central nervous system. There is also reduction of skeletal muscle tension as motor nerve *impulses* diminish in number in response to prolonged steady-state cutaneous thermal stimulation.

When cold is applied to the skin, with techniques suitable for relieving pain, there is reduction in cutaneous nerve conduction velocity, vasodilation followed by vasoconstriction, and reduction in skeletal muscle tension. It is interesting to note that both increase and decrease in sensory nerve conduction velocity, as well as both cutaneous vasodilation and vasoconstriction, can lead to relaxation of underlying muscle. Any standard text on electromyographic techniques[17, 18] will give ample data indicating that both sensory and motor nerve conduction velocity shift in direct proportion to temperature change in those tissues.

When heat is applied locally, one anticipates transient local vasodilation, rise in tissue temperature, and an increase in nerve conduction velocity and muscle relaxation. When cold is applied in a similar fashion, the effects are the opposite, except that cutaneously applied cold, like heat, leads to muscle relaxation. Both heat and cold are effective in relieving pain. Heat appears more useful in the chronic phase of most pathologies, with the notable exception of lesions resulting in central nervous system induced spasticity. Cold appears to be more useful in the acute phase of the pathology and/or where skeletal muscle hyperactivity is quite severe.

Both heat and cold are useful in reduction of edema, with and without concomitant pain. Again, heat is likely to be more useful in the chronic phase, i.e. when residual edema is still present more than forty-eight hours after the trauma resulting in edema has occurred. With any soft tissue or bone trauma, blood vessels are usually disrupted, allowing fluid to leak out. Normal repair processes seal off the torn vessels within minutes. Larger vessels require longer than small vessels. When there is no evidence of any continuing edema formation, heat may be safely applied to increase capillary permeability and thus aid in the resorption of the extravastated fluid and dissolution of the organized hematoma which is a necessary part of the sealing procedure. Heat should not be applied if the local area is still hemorrhaging, since the subsequent increase in capillary permeability will prevent adequate sealing of torn blood vessels.

On the other hand, application of cold induces vasoconstriction, decreases capillary permeability, and so tends to slow continued fluid leakage from ruptured vessels. This is usually desirable for forty-eight to seventy-two hours after trauma.

One must be sure that edema present is due to local trauma rather than due to cardiac, pulmonary, and/or renal pathology before using either heat or cold. Vigorous application of either heat or cold in the presence of any such lesion is hazardous. If both trauma and such major life-threatening lesions are present, use of heat or cold should be much gentler.

Application of short wave or microwave diathermy, or ultrasound, will all cause a greater temperature rise in deeper tissue than will the application of any form of conductive heat (hot packs, paraffin bath, whirlpool) or radiant heat (infrared lamps and bakers).[19] Conversely, the diathermies and ultrasonic energy will not cause as much of a rise in skin temperature or have as much effect on cutaneous nerves or circulation. There is good evidence that when these more deeply penetrating physical agents are properly utilized, the increased depth of penetration is in large part dependent upon the frequency of the energy delivered to the patient.[19, 20]

In the 1960s and 1970s there has been a marked increase in the clinical use of nerve and muscle stimulating currents for the relief of pain. At least three procedures have come into widespread use, namely to —

1. induce intermittent skeletal muscle contraction and relaxation in order to minimize circulatory stasis and/or muscle hyper- or hypotonicity.
2. induce transcutaneous nerve stimulation, which appears to alter peripheral axon input through the spinal cord gate, with subsequent modification of impulse volley flow to pain awareness centers, and
3. induce patient awareness of what he feels (or sees or hears) when the patient is voluntarily attempting to increase or decrease skeletal muscle tension in a more nearly functionally adequate fashion (often called biofeedback).

When using any of the above electrical stimulating techniques, there is no intention or expectation of inducing a significant tissue temperature rise. The addition of energy is intended to stimulate the cutaneous sensory nervous system and/or the peripheral motor nerve supply, and/or the skeletal muscle fibers directly. The objective of these techniques is to, either passively or concomitant with patient attempts at active contraction, alter the degree of skeletal muscle tension.

If muscle hyper- or hypotonicity is a factor in the patient's pain, the use of nerve and muscle stimulating currents is a viable treatment option that merits consideration when thinking of ways to relieve pain in a particular patient.

In general, application of cold (withdrawal of thermal energy) is the treatment of choice in patients with acute trauma or severe spasticity. Application of conductive heat or induction of a tissue temperature rise by magnetic or electric field effects (the diathermies) seems most effective in subacute or chronic traumatic or disease problems. Electrical stimulation for pain relief is most commonly reserved for patients with long-standing chronic pain.

The wide range of operating frequencies available to the physical therapist is discussed in some detail in the chapter dealing specifically with the biophysical effects of the electromagnetic and acoustic spectra (*see* Chapter 2).

REFERENCES

1. Sternbach, Richard A.: *Pain: A Psychophysiological Approach.* New York, Acad Pr, 1968.
2. *Dorland's Illustrated Medical Dictionary*, 24th ed. Philadelphia, Saunders, 1965.
3. Bishop, Beverly P.: Pain: Its physiology and rationale for management. *Phys Ther, 60:*13-27, 1980.
4. Melzack, R. and Wall, P. D.: Pain mechanisms: A new theory. *Science, 150:*971-79, 1965.
5. Melzack, R.: Control mechanisms: Psychological aspects. In Bonica, J. (Ed.): *Advances in Neurology,* Vol. 4. New York, Raven, 1974, pp 275-80.
6. Wall, P. D.: The gate control theory of pain mechanisms: Reexamination and restatement. *Brain, 101:*1-18, 1978.
7. Snyder, S. H.: Opiate receptors and internal opiates. *N Engl J Med, 296(5):*266-79, 1977.
8. Marx, J. L.: Is Substance P a transmitter of pain signals? *Science, 205:*886-89, 1979.
9. Marx, J. L.: Analgesia: How the body inhibits pain perception. *Science, 195:*471-73, 1977.
10. Miglietta, O.: Action of cold on spasticity. *Am J Phys Med, 52:*198-204, 1973.
11. Wolf, S. L. and Basmajian, J. V.: Intramuscular temperatures deep to localized cold stimulation. *Phys Ther, 53:*1284-88, 1973.
12. Bierman, W.: Therapeutic use of cold. *JAMA, 157:*189-92, 1955.
13. Abramson, D. I. et al.: Vascular basis for pain due to cold. *Arch Phys Med Rehabil, 47:*300-305, 1966.
14. Olson, J. E. and Stravino, V. D.: A review of cryotherapy. *Phys Ther, 52:*840-53, 1972.
15. Rocks, J. A.: Intrinsic shoulder pain syndrome. *Phys Ther. 59:*153-59, 1979.
16. Downey, J. A.: Physiological effects of heat and cold. *Phys Ther, 44:*713-17, 1964.

17. Licht, S. (Ed.): *Electrodiagnosis and Electromyography,* 3rd ed. New Haven, Licht, 1971.
18. Goodgold, Joseph and Eberstein, Arthur: *Electrodiagnosis of Neuromuscular Diseases.* Baltimore, Williams & Wilkins, 1972.
19. Licht, S. (Ed.): *Therapeutic Heat and Cold,* 2nd ed. New Haven, Licht, 1965, Chapters 5, 8, 9, 11.
20. Goldman, D. E. and Heuter, T. F.: Tabular data on velocity and absorption of high frequency sound in mammalian tissues. *J Acoust Soc Am, 28:*35-37, 1956.
21. Snyder, S. H.: Brain peptides as neurotransmitters. *Science, 209:*976-983, 1980.

Chapter 2

INTRODUCTION TO THE ELECTROMAGNETIC AND ACOUSTIC SPECTRA

THE PHYSICAL AGENTS that are the domain of the physical therapist include heat, cold, water, ultrasonic energy, nerve and muscle stimulating currents, ultraviolet light, and massage. Massage is not included in this book because it neither adds to nor takes away a significant amount of energy from the patient. When pain is relieved by any of the other physical agents, a major mechanism of pain relief is absorption or removal of energy, with subsequent effects. There is no question that massage can benefit properly selected patients, but there is more question as to the mechanisms involved than there is with the other physical agents.

INFRARED OR THERMAL ENERGY

Perhaps the most widely used physical agent is some type of energy that causes a local transient tissue temperature rise. The source will usually be producing some form of infrared energy. It is clinically applicable in many convenient forms. Hot packs are probably the most widely used form of infrared energy. They are normally stored in water kept at temperatures of 70° to 88°C. Properly applied, hot packs are very efficient at raising skin temperature to the upper limit of safety, 45°C. The paraffin bath is equally efficient. It is frequently used when it is desirable to raise the temperature of skin and subcutaneous tissues of the digits, especially of the upper extremities. The paraffin bath is commonly kept at temperatures of 52° to 57°C for use with the upper extremities. If the bath is intended for use with the lower extremities, the temperature is usually kept lower, at about 42°

19

to 50°C, because even in the normal subject, circulation is less efficient, especially in the distal lower extremity.

Infrared lamps and bakers are another source of infrared energy, now rarely used in the physical therapy clinic. Depending upon the type of heating unit used, the source temperature could range from about 400° to more than 3,000°C. Consequently, the lamp is never placed close to the skin. Depending upon intensity of output, the lamp or baker would be positioned 10 to 65 cm away from the skin. Like the hot pack and the paraffin bath, lamps and bakers can raise skin temperature to the upper limit of safety within a matter of minutes.

In the late 1970s a new form of dry heat came onto the clinical marketplace, with the trade name of Fluidotherapy®.* Some evidence has been presented that raising superficial tissue temperatures by means of exposure to a heated powder kept in constant motion by blowing air through it is at least as effective as the paraffin bath or whirlpool in the management of chronic pain due to musculoskeletal disorders. (*See* Chapter 5 for details and references.)

The whirlpool and the Hubbard tank are widely used sources of infrared energy. Depending upon whether heating or cooling of the skin is desired, the area to be treated is immersed in water at temperatures ranging from 42° to 30°C, and sometimes lower in selected patients. Normal skin temperature approaches 37°C in the head, neck, and trunk and gradually decreases to about 32° in the distal portion of the extremities. It is then obvious that one would not expect as great a skin temperature rise with the whirlpool or Hubbard tank as compared to the hot pack or paraffin bath. However, hydrotherapy is commonly used to treat much larger segments of the patient.

In both the moist and dry forms of infrared used to raise skin temperature, thermal energy is generated and then transmitted to the patient with the intent of causing a beneficial reaction via the cutaneous nervous system and/or the cutaneous circulation. Body reaction to the absorption of a stimulating quantity of any form of infrared usually includes transient local skeletal muscle relaxation. The relaxation can be measured objectively by use of

* Fluidotherapy Corporation Therapy Devices, Houston, Texas 77081.

electromyography before and after treatment[1, 2] or subjectively by palpation.

It is well established that no form of infrared energy can have primary penetration deeper than 1 cm[3]. Hence the muscle relaxation is rarely due to direct absorption of the infrared energy but rather to direct effect on cutaneous nerve receptors and on cutaneous blood vessels, with a later reduction of motor nerve impulse flow. If the energy is absorbed over a long enough time, there *may* also be an increase in blood flow to underlying muscle. Any and all of these changes can lead to pain relief if the pain was due to muscle hyperactivity.

The gate control theory of pain and pain relief (*see* Chapter 1) could account for the reduction in motor nerve impulse outflow, since the cutaneous nervous system is now being flooded with less noxious stimuli. If this more pleasant stimulus is kept at a steady state for a period of time (minutes), additional steady-state energy addition may no longer be preceived as stimulus but rather as a new environment, with less need for muscle response. One of the net effects of steady-state stimulus is muscle relaxation.[3] It is also possible, if infrared energy is absorbed over a long period of time and in sufficient quantity, that the thermal receptors, which were originally stimulated by exposure to change in temperature, gradually accommodate to the new temperature and gradually diminish in activity.

Another reaction that is known to take place when skin is absorbing infrared energy or when heat is being withdrawn from the skin is the release of histamine by dermal cells. The histamine release causes capillary dilation. This change is perceived in lightly pigmented skin as hyperemia, a reddening of the skin. This reddening of the skin normally disappears within less than thirty minutes after the intense source of thermal energy has been removed.

At the same time that cutaneous thermal receptors and the skin itself is being stimulated, cutaneous blood temperature is being raised. If blood in the local area is warmed enough so that the temperature of all the circulating blood is raised as little as 0.1°C, the hypothalamus (a major vasomotor regulatory center within the central nervous system) responds by causing vasodilation in deeper tissues underlying the area of exposure to intense heat. Since blood to fill the newly dilated capillaries has to come from somewhere within the body, and since underlying muscle is nearby, there is frequently a small drop in muscle temperature in the local area for the first few minutes.[4] Then, when the hypothalamus is triggered by change in blood temperature, vasodilation may also occur in the underlying muscle. Additional blood to supply the underlying muscle is likely to come from the normal blood reservoirs, i.e. spleen, gut, or muscle not in the area absorbing energy. If energy absorption by the skin continues over a twenty- to thirty-minute period, the underlying muscle temperature may also rise slightly, but never as much as the skin temperature if the source of energy is infrared.[4]

Cold, as used clinically, is also a form of infrared energy, since any object has a temperature above $0°K$ ($-273°C$) is radiating thermal energy. Cold is frequently applied to a local area of a patient in the form of cold packs, commonly stored at $0°C$ ± $10°C$. Such application causes rapid reduction of skin temperature. Underlying skin temperature will frequently decrease by $5°$ to $10°C$ within the standard ten-minute treatment. When this occurs, skin and deeper-lying tissues lose energy (heat) in proportion to the temperature differential between the cold pack and the skin.

In procedures where cold is applied, as was the case with the "hot" form of infrared, there is a marked reaction by the cutaneous nerves and the circulation of the skin. There is a lesser reaction by deeper tissues. If the temperature differential is great and prolonged, the reactions will tend to be extensive. The final effect, as is the case when the "hot" form of infrared is applied, is likely to be muscle relaxation, but through different mechanisms. Known mechanisms for responses to application of heat and cold are discussed in Chapter 5.

One should remember that the human eye cannot see infrared wavelengths. In the case of luminous sources of infrared radiation, one does see the visible light that is generated concomitantly.

THE DIATHERMIES

In addition to the various ways of generating clinically useful thermal energy and transmitting it to the patient with the intent of causing a local tissue temperature rise (TTR), the TTR can also be achieved upon absorption of high frequency electric and/or magnetic field energy. Absorbing tissues will convert part of the absorbed energy into heat. Thus, the diathermies may be referred to as conversive heating. The common clinical sources for this technic are designated as short wave and microwave diathermy. With proper application, these wavelengths can penetrate more deeply than any form of infrared. Consequently, the diathermies are frequently referred to as "deep heat." When applied improperly or with lack of consideration for variation in response among the various tissues that lie deep to the skin, absorption of energy of diathermy wavelengths can be hazardous. This is in large part true because there are far fewer thermal receptors beneath the skin until energy penetrates to the periosteum. Hence, it is easy to raise the temperature of subcutaneous fat and muscle to destructive levels (above 45°C) without anyone being aware of it at the time of treatment.

The therapist must be very conscious of how much subcutaneous fat overlies the tissues in which a significant rise in temperature is desired. Almost equally important is the realization of the proximity of bone to the surface where the diathermy is applied. It is easy to cause a pathological tissue temperature rise in either of these tissues when they are exposed to energy of wavelengths classified as diathermy. The mechanisms for hazard are different for fat as compared to bone. These mechanisms are discussed in Chapter 4.

NERVE AND MUSCLE STIMULATING CURRENTS

When electrical energy of frequencies appropriate to stimulate peripheral nerve or muscle is absorbed, the ensuing tissue temperature rise should be insignificant and certainly well below a hazardous level. This is because stimulating currents are not used in continuous modulation for prolonged periods of time, i.e. minutes, but rather with some form of surge or interruption; hence, energy is transmitted to the patient intermittently. Duration of the individual stimulus is usually less than one second, with a pause of one or more seconds between each stimulus.

Nerve and muscle stimulating currents are not used with the intent of causing a tissue temperature rise. They are used with the intent of causing intermittent skeletal muscle contraction and relaxation, or with the intent of flooding the cutaneous sensory nervous system with relatively pleasant stimuli in order to relieve pain (*see* gate control theory, Chapter 1). The frequency and other stimulus parameters needed to produce the desired response will vary, depending upon the extent and severity of the lesion and whether the muscle to be stimulated is hypertonic or hypotonic. Reasons for needing wide variation in stimulus characteristics are discussed in Chapter 3.

ULTRAVIOLET LIGHT

When electromagnetic energy of the frequency range classified as "ultraviolet" is used, the intent is not to cause a tissue temperature rise but rather to cause one or more chemical reactions within the absorbing tissue. If the dose is heavy, a readily measurable temperature rise will occur, but only as a delayed reaction. The delay will be on the order of several hours. This temperature rise is secondary to the chemical stimulation. Ultraviolet treatment time is of much shorter duration (seconds) as compared to the usual treatment time when any form of energy is used with the intent of causing a tissue temperature rise. This is because ultraviolet energy does not penetrate. Most of it is absorbed within the first millimeter and all within the second millimeter of absorbing skin or other tissue. Hence, there is essentially no volume absorption as there is with all forms of energy used to cause a tissue temperature rise.

Individual treatment time will depend upon the output characteristics of the source of ultraviolet light and upon the reaction desired. Just as is the case with infrared energy, the human eye does not see ultraviolet wavelengths. What is seen is the visible light that all clinical ultraviolet (UV) sources produce at the same time they are producing the shorter UV wavelengths.

Treatment techniques and rationale for use are discussed in Chapter 6.

ULTRASONIC ENERGY

When ultrasonic energy is utilized, for either thermal or nonthermal effects, treatment time is longer than with ultraviolet light but shorter than when any form of infrared or diathermy is used. Even though it is well established that clinical ultrasonic energy penetrates more deeply than any other form of energy that physical therapists use, the net tissue temperature rise may be greater than that achieved with the diathermies or infrared energy. Presumably this is in large part due to the much greater efficiency of transmission of ultrasonic energy from the source into the patient.

Of special importance is the fact that there is a lesser rise in temperature of subcutaneous fat as compared to that of under-lying muscle and bone. Rise in fat temperature can be a real obstacle to adequate rise in muscle temperature when the di-athermies are used. There are additional thermal and non-thermal effects of absorption of ultrasonic energy which are unique to ultrasound. This form of energy is discussed in detail in Chapter 7.

RELATIONSHIPS OF WAVELENGTH, FREQUENCY, AND DEPTH OF PENETRATION

When considering which type of energy should be applied to a given patient, the first factor that should be considered is wavelength. Among the energy forms available to physical ther-apists, the longer the wavelength, the deeper the penetration. Wavelength is standardly defined as the distance between the top of one wave and the identical phase of the succeeding wave.[5] Frequency is the reciprocal of wavelength and is standardly defined as the number of oscillations or vibrations per second.[5]

Nerve and muscle stimulating currents have the longest wavelengths, and hence the lowest frequencies, of any energy that physical therapists use. These wavelengths are usually ex-pressed as kilometers. The clinical frequency range is on the order of 0.5 to 2,000 Hertz (Hz) or cycles per second (c.p.s.). Since stimulating currents are a part of the electromagnetic spectrum, their velocity approximates that of the speed of light in a vacuum (about 300,000,000 meters per second.). At sea level, the speed of light is a little slower, about 296,700,000 m/s. Since velocity equals wavelength times frequency ($c = \lambda \times f$), a current having a frequency of 20 Hertz (Hz) has a wavelength of 15,000,000 in a vacuum and about 14,835,000 m at sea level.

These wavelengths are equal to 15,000 and 14,835 kilometers (km) respectively. Since stimulating currents have the longest wavelengths of any energy that physical therapists use, *if all other factors are equal,* their depth of penetration will be the greatest.

Diathermy wavelengths are usually expressed as meters or centimeters. Short-wave diathermy has a wavelength range of 30 to 3 m since the frequency range is 10 million to 100 million Hertz (MHz). Microwave diathermy has a wavelength range of 3 m to 3 cm since it has a frequency range of 100 to 10,000 MHz. These ranges are based on the velocity of electromagnetic energy in a vacuum. At atmospheric pressure, the wavelengths are a little shorter since the velocity is slightly lower.

Infrared and ultraviolet wavelengths are much shorter and their frequencies much higher than those for stimulating currents or the diathermies. It is well established that their depth of penetration is significantly less. Infrared (IR) and ultraviolet (UV) wavelengths are commonly expressed as nanometers (nm) or Angstrom units (Å). One billion nm = 1 meter. An older term, the millimicron, is equivalent to the nanometer. Both are equal to 10^{-9} meter. One Å = 10^{-10} m. Both the nanometer and the Angstrom are very small units of linear measure. The corresponding frequencies are so high that the only practical way to enumerate them is by use of the powers of ten. When one considers that clinical IR sources may range in temperature from below zero to more than 3,000°C, there is consequently a frequency range of 2×10^{12} to 4×10^{13} Hz. The theoretical IR wavelength range that may be used clinically is 15,000 to 750 nm (150,000 to 7,500 Å) for source temperatures ranging from −80 to 3,000°C, respectively.[3]

IR and UV wavelengths are temperature dependent.[3] Table 2-I lists selected temperatures, corresponding wavelengths, and clinical uses. The lower the temperature, the longer the wavelength. A cold pack stored at 0°C (273°K) will have a wavelength of about 10,570 nm or 105,714 Å. If the temperature of an IR lamp averages 3,000°C, the wavelength average will be about 851 nm or 8,510 Å. When one considers UV frequencies, which are higher than those of the hottest infrared source, their wavelengths are shorter still. The average UV source tempera-

TABLE 2-I

CONVERSION TABLE FOR KELVIN, CENTIGRADE, AND FAHRENHEIT TEMPERATURES AND THEIR WAVELENGTHS IN THE INFRARED AND ULTRAVIOLET SPECTRA

Kelvin	Centigrade (Celsius)	Fahrenheit (to nearest whole number)	Wavelength (in Angstrom Units)	Clinical Example
190	—83	—118	151,895	Not used clinically — too cold. Is "Far Infrared"
250	—23	—10	115,440	Extreme storage of cold pack
260	—13	8	111,000	Usual storage of cold pack
280	7	45	103,072	Usual storage of cold pack
290	17	63	99,517	Very cold Whirlpool (WP)
300	27	81	96,200	Cold WP & Hubbard Tank (HT)
310	37	99	93,097	Neutral WP & usual HT
				Upper limit HT is 40°C
				Upper limit WP is 42°C
320	47	117	90,187	Low temperature paraffin bath
330	57	135	87,455	High temperature paraffin bath
340	67	153	84,882	Usual storage hot pack
350	77	171	82,457	Usual storage hot pack
360	87	189	80,167	Upper limit hot pack
370	97	207	78,000	A few degrees less than boiling point of water
700	427	801	41,229	Low temperature Far IR Lamp
1,000	727	1,341	28,860	Medium temperature Far IR Lamp
2,000	1,727	3,140	14,430	Medium temperature Near IR Lamp
3,000	2,727	4,941	9,620	High temperature Near IR Lamp
4,000	3,727	6,766	7,215	Approaching long wavelengths of visible light
5,000	4,727	8,566	5,772	Approaching short wavelengths of visible light
10,000	9,727	17,566	2,886	Within UV spectrum

ture is on the order of 9,700°C. The average UV frequency is on the order of 7×10^{13} to 7×10^{14} Hz. The wavelength range in clinical use is 320 to 185 nm.

Table 2-II places all of the physical agents that are a part of the electromagnetic spectrum in logical order. The reader should bear in mind that ultrasonic energy is not a part of the electromagnetic spectrum (EMS). The most important thing about the

TABLE 2-II
THE ELECTROMAGNETIC SPECTRUM

Category	Theoretical Frequency Range	Theoretical Wavelength Range	Clinically Utilized Frequencies	Clinically Utilized Wavelengths	Clinical Objective
Nerve and Muscle Stimulating Currents	0 to 10,000 Hz (DC or AC)	Infinity to 30 km	0 to 2,000 Hz	Infinity to 150 km	Muscle Contraction. Ion Transfer (DC only)
Commercial and Military Radio and Television Diathermies	10,000 Hz to 10 MHz	30 km to 30 m			
Short wave	10 MHz to 100 MHz	30 m to 3 m	13.56 or 27.12 MHz	22 or 11 m	Tissue Temperature Rise (TTR)
Microwave	100 MHz to 10,000 MHz	3m to 3 cm	915 or 2,450 MHz	33 or 12 cm	TTR
Various Sources of Infrared	2×10^{12} to 7×10^{13} HZ	28,860,000 to 7,500 Å	2×10^{13} to 7×10^{13} Hz	105,000 to 10,000 Å	Tissue Temperature Drop or TTR
Visible Light	7×10^{13} Hz	7,500 to 4,000 Å			
Ultraviolet Light	7×10^{13} Hz	4,000 to 136 Å	7×10^{13} Hz	4,000 to 1,850 Å	Tissue Chemical Change
High Energy Ionizing and Penetrating Radiation (X-ray, alpha, beta, gamma, and cosmic radiation)	10^{16} to Infinity	136 to less than 1 Å			

EMS for the physical therapist is that wavelengths toward the bottom of this table have progressively less depth of penetration. This may at first thought seem paradoxical inasmuch as it is common knowledge that x-rays are very penetrating and produce a clear picture of bone in the intact individual. X-rays and other electromagnetic energy of still shorter wavelengths have a far greater concentration of energy per unit area within the source than is true for the wavelengths used by physical therapists. Thus, energy radiating from sources below UV in Table 2-II have vastly greater driving forces than the energies used by physical therapists.

Only since the 1950s has it been possible to drive EMS energy of longer wavelengths, i.e. infrared, in a manner similar to x-rays. This has resulted in the abiliy to form LASER beams (Light Amplification by Stimulated Emission of Radiation). LASER is beyond the scope of this book and is not in use by physical therapists.

All professional personnel concerned with physical medicine need to remember that hot and cold packs, paraffin baths, whirlpools, and Hubbard tanks are just as much sources of infrared radiation as are IR lamps and bakers. The generating source temperatures are quite different. Consequently, wavelengths and frequencies of their radiation are different. A cold pack stored at $-10°C$ ($263°K$) will have initial radiation with a wavelength of 109,734 Å. If it was stored at 10°C, its initial wavelength will be 101,979 Å.* Practice with calculations of this sort should help in remembering the relationships between wavelength and frequency.

Clinicians are in general agreement, however, that the physiological changes induced by absorption of infrared are the same, regardless of wavelength, if they cause the same temperature rise in a given tissue. Likewise, if energy is withdrawn from the patient (the IR source is of colder temperature than the subject's skin temperature), the physiological effects will be the same regardless of wavelength.[3]

---

* It is known that IR at a temperature of 3,000°K has a wavelength of 9,620 Å. If these values are multiplied together, the result is 28,860,000. If this constant is divided by the Kelvin temperature of a source whose wavelength is unknown, the wavelength for that temperature will appear as the quotient, in Angstrom units.

DIFFERENCES BETWEEN THE ELECTROMAGNETIC
AND ACOUSTIC SPECTRA

Sound and ultrasound are parts of the acoustic spectrum of energies. They are not part of the electromagnetic spectrum. Although previously discussed relationships between wavelength and frequency hold for both spectra, there are numerous physical and biophysical differences.

All EMS wavelengths travel most efficiently through a vacuum, suffer a slight loss of velocity when penetrating a gaseous medium, and exhibit a still greater loss when driven through a liquid. Electromagnetic energy utilized by physical therapists penetrates solids poorly. On the other hand, acoustic (vibrational) energy is not transmitted through a vacuum, travels poorly through gases, and is transmitted quite well through gas-free liquids. Acoustic energy velocity is greatest when penetrating solids of high density.

Irrespective of the medium for transmission, the velocity of all the energies that comprise the EMS is on the order of 300 million meters per second, whereas the velocity of acoustic energy is on the order of a few hundred to a few thousand m/s. With electromagnetic energy, as the density of the transmitting medium increases, velocity decreases because of interfering collisions with the molecules that make up the transmitting medium. Conversely, with acoustic energy, as the density of the medium increases, velocity rises. In biological liquids and soft tissues, clinical ultrasonic energy has a velocity on the order of 1500 meters per second. In cortical bone, the velocity increases to more than 3000 m/s. Acoustic energy is transmitted directly from molecule to molecule.

That portion of the acoustic spectrum which physical therapists use in the treatment of patients has been designated as ultrasound, indicative that these wavelengths are inaudible. For much the same reason, within the EMS, wavelengths close to but longer than those which stimulate the human eye are designated as *infra*red. Those wavelengths which are slightly shorter than those which stimulate the eye are called *ultra*violet.

The term *supersonic* is equivalent to ultrasonic but by convention has been reserved for reference to airplanes that are capable of moving faster than the speed of audible sound.

Because of the significant difference in velocity between electromagnetic and acoustic waves, the relationship between wavelength and frequency is different, even though the formula for expressing the relationship is the same. Velocity equals wavelength times frequency ($c = \lambda \times f$). Thus, for EMS energy having a frequency of one megacycle (1 Mhz), the wavelength would be 300 m in a vacuum and about 297 m in atmosphere at sea level. Ultrasonic energy of the same frequency would have a wavelength of 0.3 mm in atmosphere, about 1.5 mm in soft tissue, and 3.5 mm in cortical bone. Since it takes 1000 mm to equal 1 meter, wavelength differences between EMS and acoustic energy for any given frequency are quite large.

Sound of any wavelength, audible or inaudible, cannot travel through a vacuum. Ultrasound travels very poorly through any gas. However, the human ear can testify thousands of times daily that audible sound travels very well through the atmosphere. The difference between sound and ultrasound in this respect is that the gas molecules that make up the atmosphere, i.e. nitrogen, oxygen, carbon dioxide, absorb almost completely the 1 mm and shorter wavelengths that comprise ultrasound, whereas audible sound (frequencies lower than 20,000 Hz) has wavelengths longer than 1 cm and up to 30 cm. One can only wonder if transmission of vibrational energy is influenced by the ratio of wavelength to molecule size and/or to the relatively vast differences in distance between molecules of a gas as compared to a liquid or a solid.

At any rate, ultrasonic energy, as used clinically, requires the use of a liquid or semisolid (ointment or gel) coupling agent to achieve significant transmission of this form of energy from source to patient.

The majority of ultrasonic generators in clinical use in this country have an operating frequency of 1 Mc and hence a wavelength of about 1.5 mm when penetrating soft tissues. A few generators are in use with operating frequencies as low as 500 Kc and fewer still with frequencies as high as 4 Mc. It is anticipated that the 1980s will also see clinical use of 90 Kc ultrasound in selected patients because its depth of penetration is approximately double that of the standard 1 Mc and the nonthermal effects of 90 Kc seem to be predominant. Reasons for selection of these different frequencies are discussed in Chapter 7.

NATURAL LAWS PERTINENT TO THE USE OF PHYSICAL AGENTS

Some of the relationships between velocity, frequency, and wavelength of energy forms that physical therapists utilize have been discussed. It is now necessary to explore the physical laws that control what one can and cannot do when adding or removing energy from living tissues. These laws were discovered in the latter part of the nineteenth century and are immutable for physical inanimate systems. Later, it will become obvious that some modifications are necessary when these same laws are applied to living tissues.

The Law of Grotthus-Draper

Whenever energy emanates from a source, it is either absorbed, transmitted, reflected, or refracted. The most important law is that the energy must be absorbed before it can have any effect. This fact was demonstrated at about the same time by two investigators, Grotthus and Draper, working independently. Both were studying ultraviolet light. They both established that if energy is not absorbed, it must be transmitted. It follows that the greater the absorption, the less the transmission and hence the less penetration. Therefore, absorption and penetration are reciprocal. If energy is transmitted, it may be in a relatively straight line, or turned away completely from matter with which it collides (reflection), or the angle of transmission within the object with which it collides may be changed (refraction). The classical example of reflection is that of visible light waves striking a mirror. How much of the energy striking the mirror will be absorbed as compared to how much is reflected will depend in part upon the angle at which the light waves strike the mirror. Those waves which strike at a right angle will be largely absorbed. Those waves which strike at other than a right angle will be reflected. The more planar the surface of the mirror, the greater the reflection and thus the more nearly perfect visible image.

Clinically, reflection is a factor that must be taken into consideration when applying luminous infrared, ultraviolet light, or ultrasonic energy. In the case of luminous IR, as the concomitant visible light either strikes the reflector and is thereby aimed toward the patient or radiates directly from the source, some of these eye-stimulating wavelengths will reach the retina. The intensity may be high enough to be irritating to the retina, in which case the patient is apt to move out of position. This problem can be minimized by draping the lamp so that the visible light does not reach the retina in significant quantity.

Ultraviolet lamps usually have highly efficient reflectors. Hence, reflection of the visible output from the lamp can again reach the retina, along with the UV component. In the case of UV, both the visible and UV output can be irritating, and draping the lamp frequently is not an adequate solution. The usual fabric draping materials may re-reflect especially the UV, and almost any lightly colored fabric will reflect more UV than will any darker colored fabric. Hence, some kind of UV-filtering goggles usually are indicated to achieve adequate eye protection. There can also be serious reflection from nearby partition material, onto both the patient and the therapist. To minimize this problem, there should be no cubicle curtains or lightly painted walls within about 150 cm of the UV source.

Reflection of ultrasonic energy becomes a problem when bone is within the limit of penetration of this form of energy. In the standard moving sound head technic, approximately 35 percent of the energy that penetrates to cortical bone will be reflected.[6] Thus, tissues close to absorbing bone are exposed to energy coming from the ultrasonic source plus that reflected by the bone. This will give rise to a greater tissue temperature increase than would otherwise be anticipated. Hence, if bone is close to the surface, source intensity should be less than if there is a large volume of soft tissue in the area under treatment. In part because of reflection of ultrasonic energy by bone, direct contact sonation of skin over bony prominences should be avoided. Painful "hot spots" are apt to occur. Fortunately, the periosteum is richly supplied with thermal sensors. Perception of this thermal pain will cause the patient to move away from the energy source before serious damage occurs. Areas with irregular contour can be treated with other ultrasonic technics. These are discussed in Chapter 7.

Refraction may be considered as a lesser case of reflection. In refraction, the penetrating energy is not turned away completely from the surface of the tissue with which it collides but is partially absorbed and partially transmitted. That portion which is transmitted will change direction of penetration within the transmitting medium. Clinically, refraction is of importance only when ultrasonic energy is being utilized. As long as the tissue that is being penetrated is homogenous, there is no significant refraction. Subcutaneous fat is the most nearly homogenous tissue in the intact human. Negligible refraction takes place here. As the transmitted energy penetrates to underlying muscle, nerve, and blood vessels and to other structures of highly varying density, some refraction is inevitable. The more dense the tissue being penetrated, the greater the refraction. Thus, exposure of tendon or ligament will cause more refraction than exposure of muscle or fascia.

As the energy penetrates from a more dense to a less dense tissue, dispersion of energy will occur. If penetration is from less dense to more dense tissue, there will be shear wave formation. Shear wave formation can lead to concentration of energy in a small volume of tissue and hence to "hot spot" formation. Refraction within tendon plus reflection from adjacent bone can become a major problem in concentration of the ultrasonic energy. If the patient's perception of pain is within normal limits, when this occurs the patient will instinctively move away from the energy source and no harm will be done. If, for whatever reason, the patient's pain perception is not normal, real damage can be done. If any tissue has its temperature raised above 45°C, a burn can occur.

The Arndt-Schultz Principle

The next basic law to be considered is usually referred to as the Arndt-Schultz Principle. It states that (a) if the quantity of energy absorbed is too small to stimulate the absorbing tissue, no significant reaction will take place; (b) if the quantity of energy absorbed per unit time is adequate to stimulate, the absorbing unit of matter will perform its normal function; and (c) if the quantity of energy absorbed per unit time is too great, the absorbing unit of matter will be disrupted and cannot perform its normal function. Such disruption can be reversible or irreversible, depending both on the quantity of energy absorbed and the rate at which it is absorbed.

The physical therapist's objective within the framework of the Arndt-Schultz Principle is to add (or, with application of cold, to withdraw) enough energy to stimulate the absorbing tissues to normal function. In the case of physical agents known to cause a tissue temperature rise, i.e. most of the sources of infrared, the diathermies, and ultrasound, the local tissue temperature should not be elevated to more than 45°C, since tissue destruction is likely to occur if the temperature of that tissue goes higher. When stimulating currents are utilized, the most common objective is to cause intermittent contraction of skeletal muscle. The stimulation should not be so intense that it causes pain, nor should it cause abnormal muscle hyperactivity. When ultraviolet light is applied, an observable reaction is always delayed, on the order of hours. Hence, testing for an individual's reaction to the UV source prior to treatment is almost mandatory. The desired objective is chemical change within the absorbing tissues.

Maxwell's Precept

There is a third general law which has no precise label. It has evolved from Maxwell's work in electrostatics and can be stated as follows: For any unit of matter at rest, there will be a balance of charge between the inside and outside of the limiting membrane; when that unit of matter absorbs energy, there will be an alteration of charge and the unit of matter will not be at rest until the charge balance is restored.

For the purposes of the physical therapist, this law is quite important when considering actions and reactions of excitable membranes, i.e. nerve and muscle, but physiologists are becoming increasingly aware of the importance of charge shift during intracellular metabolism[7] and in living bone reorientation.[8] For the physical therapist, awareness of potential difference (separation of dissimilar charge) between the inside and outside of excitable membranes is important in choosing the best current type and other electrical parameters when applying nerve and muscle stimulating currents in neurological and other disorders.

Other physical laws, not germane to *all* portions of the electromagnetic and acoustic spectra, are discussed in other chapters as needed.

REFERENCES

1. Licht, S. (Ed.): *Electrodiagnosis and Electromyography*, 3rd ed. New Haven, Licht, 1971, Chapters 10 and 18.
2. Goodgold, Joseph and Eberstein, Arthur: *Electrodiagnosis of Neuromuscular Diseases*. Baltimore, Williams & Wilkins, 1972.
3. Licht, S. (Ed.): *Therapeutic Heat and Cold*, 2nd ed. New Haven, Licht, 1965, Chapters 1, 9, and 17.
4. Abramson, D. I.: *Circulation in the Extremities*. New York, Acad Pr, 1967, Chapters 6, 7, 11, and 12.
5. *Dorland's Illustrated Medical Dictionary*, 24th ed. Philadelphia, Saunders, 1965.
6. Lehmann, J. F. and Guy, A. W.: Ultrasound therapy. *Proc Workshop on Interaction of Ultrasound and Biological Tissues*. Washington, D.C., HEW Pub. (FDA 73:8008), Sept., 1972.
7. Jehle, H.: Charge fluctuation forces in biological systems. *Ann NY Acad Sci, 158*:240-55, May 16, 1969.
8. Bourne, G. (Ed.): *The Biochemistry and Physiology of Bone*, 2nd ed., Volume III. New York, Acad Pr, 1971, Chapter 1.

Chapter 3

NERVE AND MUSCLE
STIMULATING CURRENTS

Nerve and muscle stimulating currents can be useful in any disorder in which the patient has lost, or never had (i.e. congenital lesion), adequate voluntary control over skeletal muscle. The lesion may have been the result of trauma or a disease process, or it may have an emotional basis. The deficit may be orthopedic, neurological, vascular, or psychogenic in origin. There is little question that as soon as the patient regains voluntary control over his muscles to a functional degree, active exercise will be both physiologically and psychologically superior to externally applied nerve and muscle stimulating current (NMSC). But until such time as the patient has achieved useful control, it is better to make use of NMSC rather than do nothing or to use only passive exercise. A host of problems secondary to skeletal muscle hyper- or hypoactivity can be minimized with judicious use of NMSC.

Since World War II, rapid improvement in electrical stimulating devices has resulted in greatly increased patient comfort. Partly as a result of improved comfort and partly because many patients with central nervous system lesions continue to have unresolved motor deficits in spite of widespread application of increasingly sophisticated manual therapeutic exercise techniques, use of electrical stimulation has greatly increased. Expanded use has been widely reported for patients with central nervous system lesions[1-14] and for patients with chronic pain.[15-25] Investigators continue to study optimal treatment procedures in peripheral nervous system lesions[26-30] and for patients with peripheral circulatory stasis.[31-34]

37

THE LAW OF DUBOIS REYMOND

There is one law that governs nerve and muscle response to externally applied NMSC, namely the Law of DuBois Reymond. In its simplest form, the law states that it is the variation in current density rather than absolute density at any given instant which acts as a stimulus to nerve or muscle.[35]

To restate this law in a way more useful to the physical therapist, one may say that three criteria must be met in order to stimulate an excitable membrane to normal response:

1. The amplitude of the individual stimulus must be high enough so that depolarization of the membrane will take place.
2. The rate of change of voltage must be sufficiently rapid so that accommodation does not occur.
3. The duration of the individual stimulus must be long enough, i.e. energy must flow long enough in one direction, so that the time course of latent period, action potential, and recovery can take place.

All excitable membranes have a resting potential (separation of charge between the inside and the outside of the membrane), measurable in millivolts.[35] The membrane requires a decrease in potential (depolarization) or an increase (hyperpolarization) before an action potential can occur. Normal human axons require a 15 to 20 mv depolarization before formation of an action potential. An axon will not propagate impulses, nor will a muscle fiber contract, until the action potential is generated by a stimulus.

An excitable membrane is a capacitor. In other words, when the membrane is in its resting state, there is a potential difference between the inside and outside of the membrane, with the membrane itself acting as the dielectric. The capacitance of a normal axon is on the order of 1 to 1.3 microfarads/cm^2. The capacitance of a normal muscle fiber is on the order of 4.6 to 6 mf/cm^2.[35] The larger the capacitance, the *less frequently* a capacitor can discharge. A useful physical analogy is to consider two capacitors, one having plates the size of a dime, the other with plates the size of a half dollar. If equal DC voltages are applied separately to each capacitor, the smaller unit will have reached the limit of its ability to store electrons sooner than the bigger unit. When a capacitor can no longer store incoming energy, it discharges. Hence, if equal quantities of energy are added at an equal rate, the unit with a lesser capacitance will discharge more often.

All normal nerve fibers have a smaller capacitance than any muscle fiber. Variation in the fastest possible rate of discharge is inherent in the individual membrane. The electrical and chemical events within the membrane that are responsible for the variation in rate of discharge are not known at this time. The clinical effect of the difference in capacity between nerve and muscle is that since nerve can respond to a greater number of stimuli per unit time, muscle with an intact nerve supply can respond to a higher frequency (60 Hz and higher) of stimulus than can denervated muscle. Denervated muscle requires frequencies of 40 Hz or lower before it can respond to each stimulus.[36]

The clinical picture is complicated by the fact that in the patient exposed to NMSC, a single axon or muscle fiber is never stimulated, but rather hundreds of axons and thousands of muscle fibers respond to the stimulus. Within a muscle mass, e.g. biceps brachii, some of the muscle fibers may have a normal nerve supply, others a hyperactive nerve supply, and still others a hypoactive nerve supply. Thus, a single stimulus can produce a wide variety of responses, and serial stimulation can cause major change in the mass response.

In general, but with many exceptions, large diameter axons have a small capacity and therefore are capable of responding to each of 1,000 or more stimuli per second. Axons of small diameter and large capacity may not respond to stimuli at a rate of more than fifty per second. If the stimulus amplitude is held constant at a threshold or higher level, the visible response is continuing muscle contraction (tetanic response) until the series of stimuli is stopped, providing the stimulus frequency is approximately 50 Hz or higher. If the stimulus frequency is appreciably lower (40 Hz or less), the visible response takes on the appearance of intermittent contraction and relaxation, even though the peak intensity is constant. If DC with continuous modulation is applied there will be a visible response only at the time of make and, rarely, break of the patient circuit, even though the amplitude is held constant for a matter of seconds. This is termed a twitch response. The reason for the difference in response to this truly constant current is that as long as energy is flowing at a constant amplitude *in one direction,* the excitable membrane cannot recover from its depolarized (or hyperpolarized) state. Having once contracted and relaxed, the muscle cannot contract again until the normal resting potential of the stimulated excitable membranes has been restored. After the single twitch, the muscle remains flaccid until energy flow in one direction has ceased.

A completely denervated muscle mass often requires a stimulus rate as low as ½ to 20 Hz in order to be able to respond to each stimulus. At 20 Hz, the peak (stimulating) amplitude can occur no more than fifty times in one second ($1000 \div 20 = 50$). Hence, the membrane will have at least 20 ms to restore normal resting potential.[36] Axons of smallest capacity require a stimulus of about 0.1 ms duration in order to become depolarized and thus to propagate impulses.

If the intensity is high and current must flow for more than 1 ms before there is an observable muscle response, there is a significant lesion affecting motor nerve supply.[36] Modern clinical apparatus can provide a wide range of stimulus duration and other stimulus parameters with an adequate degree of precision. Since in general the shorter the duration of the individual stimulus, the greater the patient comfort, a part of the therapist's task is to determine what frequency will give the best compromise between desired muscle response and patient comfort. This compromise frequency may vary as the degree of neurological damage fluctuates for better or worse. Hence, it is wise to have available apparatus that permits easy variation in stimulus duration, frequency, and other stimulating current parameters.

CLINICAL SIGNIFICANCE OF THE LAW OF DUBOIS REYMOND

If the time, in milliseconds, required to go from zero to peak amplitude is too slow, an excitable membrane will adjust its ion flow (calcium, sodium, potassium, chloride) across the membrane so as to maintain its resting potential rather than depolarize. This adjustment is called accommodation. No action potential is generated. There is no propagation of impulse and no muscle contraction. Clinically, no axon will depolarize if the time to go from zero to peak amplitude is more than about 10 ms.[36] Consequently, if the stimulus frequency is lower than 40 to 50 Hz, any response is likely to be due to direct stimulation of muscle because axons supplying the muscle will accommodate to the more slowly rising peak amplitudes. The smaller the capacity of the axon, the greater the likelihood that accommodation will take place.

Clinically, the fact of accommodation can be very useful if denervated muscle lies deep to normally innervated muscle. If the rate of rise from zero to peak amplitude is slow, the more superficial but normally functioning axons will not respond, but underlying denervated muscle, having a greater capacitance (greater ability to store energy before discharge), will respond to the slower change in amplitude by depolarization, formation of muscle action potential, and, finally, fiber contraction. Patients with such incomplete denervation patterns usually tolerate slowly rising current peaks better than rapidly rising peaks, since the normally innervated muscle is not likely to contract. The fewer the number of muscle fibers which contract in response to a given stimulus, the greater the patient comfort. This is especially true if the patient's sensory nervous system has remained intact, since sensory as well as motor axons respond by depolarization if stimulus parameters are suitable for axon stimulation.

If a continuous modulation direct current (DC) of threshold or higher intensity is applied to a normally innervated muscle mass, there will be a contractile response only at the instant of completion of the externally applied electrical circuit. While DC is flowing at a uniform rate (no significant voltage rise or fall), there can be *no* nerve or muscle response after the single contraction (immediately followed by relaxation), even though the DC flows for seconds or minutes. Depolarization will have occurred at the instant of circuit completion, *and it is maintained* in axons stimulated by the negative (−) pole. Hyperpolarization will have occurred at the positive pole at that same time, and it likewise is maintained as long as DC flows. The single muscle response that occurs with this type of stimulus is called a twitch response.

On the other hand, if a current of equal intensity but with a frequency of 60 Hz is applied for a matter of seconds to a normally innervated muscle mass, the muscle will contract upon completion of the circuit *and stay contracted* until the circuit is opened. This is called a tetanic response. Obviously, the 60 Hz current has caused a much greater stimulus response in the normally innervated muscle. The greater response is due to the fact that the voltage fluctuated from zero to peak amplitude 120 times each second.

Conversely, if an identical stimulus were applied to a completely denervated muscle, no response would occur. Change in voltage level 120 times per second does not cause depolarization of the higher capacity muscle membrane. If a 10 to 20 Hz stimulus was applied for several seconds to a denervated muscle, a series of twitches would occur. Voltage fluctuations less than about 40 times per second permit energy to flow long enough in one direction so that the denervated muscle membrane can depolarize, generate a muscle action potential, and lead to muscle contraction.

In general, axons require current flow in one direction for 0.1 to 1 ms for depolarization to occur. Muscle fibers, in the absence of a normal motor nerve, must have similar current flow for 2.5 to 3 ms for depolarization to occur.[36] When the muscle has been deprived of its nerve supply for weeks, the necessary duration of current flow increases markedly, so that flow in one direction for up to 10 ms may be needed. The difference in time required of current flow in one direction depends largely on the difference in capacity of the different types of excitable membranes.

SKIN IMPEDANCE

Another major clinical variable is the skin impedance (resistance) to the externally applied stimulus. Sea water has a resistivity of about 20 ohm-cm. Normal skin has an impedance of not less than 200 ohm-cm to all frequencies in clinical use.[27] In various lesions, especially those involving cutaneous nerves, impedance can be many times higher. This is also true for some skin diseases, even though the skin where the electrodes are applied gives no evidence of disease. Patients with psoriasis are the prime example.

The higher the impedance of the skin, the greater the strength of stimulus needed in order that a threshold intensity will reach the underlying motor nerve. When using classical low voltage-milliamperage NMSC, it is generally accepted that no muscle mass with a normal motor nerve supply should require more than 50 volts AC or 80 v DC to elicit a contractile response. For this type of NMSC, skin impedance to DC is almost always higher than that to AC. Electron (and ion) flow in one direction only (DC) leads to chemical reactions in the skin that transiently increase impedance. About 10 percent of patients and/or normal subjects with a normal motor nerve supply will have a skin chemistry that permits an equivalent response with a lower intensity when DC is used as compared to AC.

On the other hand, when the newer high voltage-microamperage generators are used, the output is always DC with a pulse rise time of a few microseconds. Muscle contraction will rarely occur with less than 75 volts; 150 to 200 is required for many normally innervated muscles, and up to 500 peak volts may be needed if impedance is high and/or mass denervation has occurred. The extremely fast voltage fluctuation makes this type of NMSC well tolerated even when maximum voltage is needed. (See the section in this chapter on high voltage stimulation for more detailed information.)

VARIATION IN STIMULUS-RESPONSE
IN THE CLINIC VERSUS THE LABORATORY

If the motor nerve supply to a muscle is intact and skin impedance is within normal limits, but the patient does not have voluntary control over skeletal muscle for other reasons, use of stimulating currents at or above 1000 Hz will usually cause muscle contraction with less discomfort than when lower frequencies are used.

A single motor nerve will supply anywhere from one or two hundred to several thousands of muscle fibers. Furthermore, in ordinary volitional contraction, not all fibers within the muscle mass are contracting simultaneously, even though the mass has developed considerable tension and has undergone shortening in length in response to internal stimulus. If an external stimulus of 50 to 250 Hz is applied, many more muscle fibers may contract simultaneously than if voluntary contraction takes place. The more fibers that contract simultaneously, the more painful the tetanic response will be. Cutaneous axons are also stimulated by the external stimulus. For any given intensity, they are stimulated more than the underlying motor nerves because cutaneous receptors and axons are closer to the source of stimulus; hence, they receive more of a stimulus.

In the laboratory, as opposed to the clinic, anesthetized or isolated denervated muscle preparations can be studied. Under these circumstances, it may be more convenient to increase intensity rather than alter frequency of the stimulating current. Where stimulus intensity can be unlimited, denervated muscle can be stimulated with a 60 Hz or higher current. Patients with intact skin and sensory nervous systems, however, would not tolerate such intensities. In the laboratory, nerve or muscle can be stimulated directly rather than through intervening skin and subcutaneous fat. Therefore, the intensity required for a contractile response will be far less — on the order of one volt — whereas, as stated before, clinically one may need up to 50 v AC or 80 v DC (along with 1 to 80 milliamperes of current) to elicit a contractile response.

If the therapist is using a stimulating current on a patient with an intact peripheral nervous system, the muscle response *always* occurs as a result of depolarization of motor nerves rather than from direct depolarization of the muscle membrane. The smaller the capacity of the membrane, the less amplitude of stimulus required to cause the depolarization.

INFLUENCE OF THE LAW OF DUBOIS REYMOND ON STIMULATOR DESIGN

Many models of nerve and muscle stimulating apparatus have the capability of delivering current to the patient in continuous, or surge, or interrupted modulation. Also, the frequency of the stimulus (AC or DC) can be varied anywhere from zero (DC only) to ½ to 3,000 Hz (AC or DC). The surge or interrupted modulation can be varied in rate from five to sixty times *per minute*. Sophisticated stimulators may also have DC with automatically reversing polarity, with full or half wave rectification, and the capability of simultaneous use of up to ten electrodes. Justification for this wide range of variation in stimulus parameters is the wide variety of peripheral and central neurological lesions, vascular and orthopedic problems, as well as the great range of skin impedance, depending upon the effect of the lesion on axons, receptors, and circulation of the skin in the area to be stimulated. With a wide choice of parameters to draw upon, the therapist should always be able to elicit a contractile response, unless the lesion has been of such long duration that muscle fiber has been replaced by fatty or fibrous tissue. If this has occurred, no stimulus can cause contraction.

The designation *continuous modulation* indicates that the stimulus amplitude does not fluctuate. Figure 3-1a is representative of a continuous AC sine wave. Figure 3-1b illustrates continuous modulation DC. It is clear that continuous modulation DC has no waveform and no rise or fall of voltage at any given intensity, whereas AC sine wave continuous modulation has a constantly fluctuating voltage with a symmetrical pattern. Both are correctly called continuous modulation, but the induced muscle contraction will appear totally different.

An AC sine wave *surge modulation* is pictured in Figure 3-2a. Figure 3-2b diagrams DC *surge modulation*. It can be seen in both cases that there is a gradual fluctuation of amplitude. With an *interrupted modulation* (Figs. 3-3a and 3-3b), there are repeating periods of energy flow and no flow, with *abrupt* shift from zero to a constant peak amplitude. The induced contractile response will vary depending upon current type (AC or DC), modulation used (continuous, surge, interrupted), and, of course, whether or not the peripheral nervous system (motor and/or sensory) is intact.

When applied to a normally innervated muscle, a stimulus having a frequency of about 50 Hz or higher will cause muscle contraction if the intensity of stimulus is great enough to cause

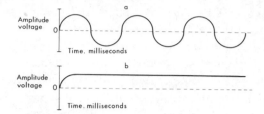

Figure 3-1. (a) Alternating Current (AC), sine waveform, continuous modulation. Note the regular rise and fall in amplitude, with reversal of direction of electron flow once each cycle.
(b) Direct Current (DC), continuous modulation. There is no waveform. Note that the amplitude, at any given intensity, is constant, and that there is no reversal of direction of electron flow.

membrane depolarization. Continuous modulation at threshold or greater intensity will cause a tetanic contraction of the muscle. Enough individual muscle fibers are stimulated, through their motor nerves, each cycle per second so that the muscle mass maintains tension development to an approximately uniform degree as long as energy is flowing through the muscle, even though the individual muscle fibers *do not* maintain their shortened state throughout the entire time course of several seconds or more that the stimulus is applied. If the same intensity is used, but with a surging rather than continuous stimulus, intermittent

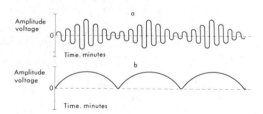

Figure 3-2. (a) AC, sine waveform, surging modulation. Note the regular fluctuation in amplitude over and above the regular rise and fall of voltage within a cycle, as well as the regular reversal of direction of electron flow once each cycle.
(b) DC, surging modulation. There is a gradual rise and fall in amplitude but no reversal of direction of electron flow.

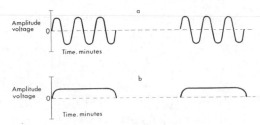

Figure 3-3 (a) AC, interrupted modulation. When current is flowing, it is at a uniform amplitude. There are regular intervals of current flow and no flow. As is *always* the case with AC, there is reversal of direction of electron flow once each cycle.

(b) DC, interrupted modulation. When current is flowing, it is at a uniform amplitude. There are regular intervals of current flow and no flow. As is usually the case with DC, there is no reversal of direction of electron flow. Apparatus with automatically reversing polarity is available, but such sophisticated apparatus is not in common clinical use.

muscle contraction and relaxation will occur. There will be a *gradual* rise and fall in tension development occurring several times *per minute*. If all parameters are the same except that an interrupted modulation is used, there will again be intermittent tetanic contraction and relaxation. This time, the rise and fall in muscle tension will be much more abrupt.

As the frequency of stimulus is decreased from 50 Hz and approaches ½ Hz, fewer and fewer motor nerves will be stimulated by each energy peak. More and more of the nerve fibers will accommodate to the more gradual rise and fall in the applied voltage. Consequently, the muscle response will be less tetanic and more like a twitch.

When a stimulating current is applied in similar fashion to a denervated muscle, the energy must flow *in one direction* for a longer period of time (milliseconds) before membrane depolarization can occur, with subsequent contractile response. In a denervated muscle, the motor nerve is no longer functioning and the muscle membrane has a larger capacitance than its axon membrane. Hence, current must flow for a longer period of time, in one direction, before denervated muscle will contract.

When stimulating current of adequate duration is applied to a denervated muscle at a uniform rate, there will be only a single, brief twitch response, regardless of whether the current flows at that rate for milliseconds or for seconds. The twitch response results whenever either AC or DC having stimulus frequency of ½ to 20 Hz is applied. If intensity is raised from zero to peak too slowly, accommodation will occur and no contraction will take place. If these same frequencies are used, but with a surging modulation, there will be a single muscle mass contraction with each surge. If an interrupted modulation is used, but all other factors are the same, the contractile response will be stronger. The more abrupt the change in intensity, the greater the number of muscle fibers that will respond at the same instant.

There can be widely varying degrees of deficit in motor nerve supply to a muscle mass. Trauma or disease anywhere in the peripheral nervous system commonly will result in loss of ability to conduct impulses by some, but not by all, of the motor nerve fibers supplying that muscle mass. The greater the number of malfunctioning axons, the lower the stimulus frequency necessary to elicit a contractile response. When nearly all axons are unable to conduct, the stimulus frequency must be 20 Hz or less (AC or DC) in order to have current flow in one direction long enough to bring about adequate depolarization. If a muscle mass is completely denervated, sometimes DC with a low interrupted modulation rate is the only feasible means of causing muscle membrane depolarization. A DC interruption rate of five times *per minute* can give rise to a current flow in one direction with nearly uniform intensity for over *one second* each time the current is flowing. If the rest period between interruptions is long enough, there is ample time for recovery of membrane potential to its resting level.

Variable *frequency* controls can be used to reduce the risk of injury (chemical burn of the skin) or discomfort to the patient. Such problems are less when AC is applied, at any frequency, as compared to DC at any frequency. The chances of abnormal chemical buildup in the skin are negligible with AC. Electron and then ion flow reverse in direction each half cycle with AC. The net effect is no residual acidic or alkaline buildup under either electrode. Such buildup is inevitable with application of

DC because there is no periodic reversal of direction of electron or ion flow.

Even though present-day stimulating apparatus permits use of DC at almost any frequency that is used with AC, high frequency DC is usually less comfortable to persons whose sensory nervous system is intact. Although ion flow with 60 Hz DC is clearly intermittent, it is still ion flow in one direction only, rather than ion flow with periodically reversing direction, as is the case for AC. When DC is applied to the skin, free oxygen and acid are formed at the anode and free hydrogen at the cathode. This results in cauterization of tissues closest to the electrodes if the concentration becomes high enough.[37] Visible hyperemia is an anticipated reaction, even when current density is insufficient to cause skin damage. Hyperemia is rare when the stimulating current is AC.

The preceding two paragraphs apply to the widely used low volt-milliampere (lv-mA) nerve and muscle stimulating current devices. They do *not* apply to the high voltage-microampere (hv-μA) devices which started to come into clinical use in the 1970s and which will probably come into widespread use in the 1980s because they usually are significantly more comfortable for the patient.

High voltage stimulators deliver to the patient paired subthreshold pulses (DC only) of extremely short duration (microseconds). When DC flows for less than 150 microseconds at a time and has a paired pulse frequency of less than 150 pulses per second, there is no significant irritation of the skin and no visible hyperemia.

SAFETY STANDARDS FOR CLINICAL ELECTRICAL STIMULATING APPARATUS

It is obvious that any device that is applied to a patient should at least do no harm. Federal regulatory agencies establish, revise, and enforce safety standards, after consultation with physicians, bioengineers, biophysicists, and manufacturers of equipment. Two federal agencies that have major responsibility over equipment that physical therapists use are the Bureau of Radiological

Health, with its Acoustic and Electromagnetic Divisions, and the Federal Communications Commission.

Ultimately, it is the physical therapist's responsibility to see to it that the devices used cannot harm the patient. This is especially important in applying electrical energy directly to the patient's skin. This occurs when nerve and muscle stimulating apparatus is used, as well as in the diathermies, where high frequency electrical and magnetic energy is directed toward the patient, and in ultrasonic energy, wherein electrical energy is converted into acoustic energy, which is then transmitted directly through the skin and into the patient. In the latter case, both electrical and acoustic energy are sometimes transmitted simultaneously.

It is simple to perceive macroshock, which can occur from defective equipment. It is more difficult to be aware when microshock occurs.* Both can be fatal. Patients with cardiac lesions, especially those who are wearing pacemakers, are particularly susceptible to microshock. Current leakage is most apt to occur when there is improper grounding of the apparatus. This can be due to poor quality control on the part of the manufacturer, to deterioration of electrical or electronic circuitry after extensive use, or to a defect in the institution's provision for grounding through line outlets.

Microshock testing of all apparatus from which there is any possibility of uncontrolled low or high frequency electrical energy reaching the patient should be done at least annually by persons trained in these technics. Adequate maintenance of all stimulating current, diathermy, and ultrasonic apparatus more than justifies the costs when the alternative is improper treatment or possible physiological or psychological harm to the patient.

EQUIPMENT CONTROLS

With the exception of battery-powered units, all nerve and muscle stimulating current apparatus (NMSC) is designed to modify standard house (wall outlet) current. The standard current is 110 v, 60 cycle, sine wave alternating current. Current

---

* The American Association for the Advancement of Medical Instrumentation defines microshock as current leakage of less than one milliampere. Macroshock is current leakage greater than one ma. (AMI: *Seven Steps to Electrical Safety*, 1970).

delivered to the patient may be AC or DC, or a simultaneous combination through two or more circuits. The NMSC units in most common use deliver to the patient relative low voltage, moderate amperage electrical energy. The voltage range to the patient may be from 0 to 50 v (AC) or to 100 v (DC). The amperage range may be from 0 to 100 millamperes. The waveform may be sine, square, faradic, pulse, or exponential. Modulation may be continuous, surging, or interrupted. In modern equipment, all modification is electronic rather than mechanical. As of the 1980s there is steadily increasing use of high voltage galvanic stimulators. These units deliver to the patient DC only, with precisely controlled voltage up to 500 v, with correspondingly low amperage, rarely exceeding 0.5 mA peak value. The general principles involved in such modification of line current are outlined in Chapter 8.

The more kinds of modification available with any single piece of apparatus, the better the chances of being able to achieve the desired contractile response with maximum patient comfort. It also follows that the more modifications available, the greater the cost of the unit. Very few NMSC generators will have all of the above modification capabilities available. The most elaborate models are intended for teaching or research rather than clinical use.

Many stimulators will have one or more electrical meters which measure the amperage, voltage, or wattage delivered to the patient with an acceptable degree of precision. Such meters can be used by the therapist to provide an objective record of energy needed to produce the desired response through a series of treatments. This kind of record can indicate improvement or deterioration of a patient's condition.

Regardless of size or cost of the apparatus, all stimulators will have provision for the following.

1. on-off control
2. intensity control
3. waveform and/or modulation selection
4. polarity control (DC only)

The intensity control should be at zero (no energy in the patient circuit) when electrodes are being applied to the patient or whenever any change is to be made in the parameters of the energy to be delivered to the patient. Also, any change in intensity should be made slowly, over a period of several seconds, rather than going up or down as rapidly as possible. The Law of DuBois Reymond is operative whenever the patient circuit is complete. If change in intensity is too rapid, so many muscle fibers will contract simultaneously that the contraction will be unnecessarily painful.

CURRENT TYPE

Some stimulators will deliver to the patient only AC, others only DC. Most units in clinical use can deliver either current type to the patient. Patients with peripheral nervous system involvement may respond to low frequency AC (20 to 60 Hz) or may need DC (0 to 20 Hz), depending upon the stage of degeneration or regeneration of peripheral axons. Patients whose primary problem is some form of organic occlusive peripheral vascular disease usually will respond to AC, although if their circulatory inadequacy is accompanied by long-standing diabetes mellitus, low frequency AC, or DC, may be needed. The patient with chronic diabetes may have a peripheral neuropathy. The individual whose loss of voluntary control over joint motion is related to psychosomatic rather than neurological deficit should always respond to AC. If the loss of voluntary control over joint motion is due to a central nervous system defect but the peripheral motor axons are intact, an AC stimulus should be effective. If there is concomitant peripheral nerve deficit, low frequency AC (less than 60 Hz) may be needed.

Most of the lv-mA stimulators presently in clinical use can deliver AC at a frequency of 20 Hz or less. These low frequencies will usually cause direct depolarization of the muscle fiber membrane and thus elicit a contractile response in denervated muscle. Only in patients where the great majority of motor nerve supply to a muscle mass is nonfunctional is DC required. The key to muscle or nerve response to an externally applied current is whether the current flows long enough in one direction, *or* whether the voltage is high enough to cause depolarization of the membrane being stimulated. The less excitable the membrane, the greater its capacitance and the longer the stimulus must flow in one direction (up to 10 ms) *or* the higher the voltage (up to 500 v). High voltage stimulators deliver pulses of not more than 75 μsec duration. Even with a normal subject, a response may require at least 75 and more commonly well over 100 v. Normal axons are *always* much more easily depolarized than are denervated muscle fibers.

When lv-mA stimulators are used, more than 90 percent of all patients who have an intact cutaneous sensory nervous system will feel more comfortable with AC at any frequency as compared to DC at any frequency. Presumably, this is due to negligible alteration of acidity or alkalinity on the skin when AC is used.

If current flows in one direction for more than a few seconds, an unnecessary and painful chemical irritation of the skin is likely to occur. This does not occur with AC at any frequency because of the automatic reversal of direction of current flow each cycle. This can and does occur whenever DC is applied to the skin and occurs to the greatest degree when the modulation is continuous (zero frequency). The preceding can be easily demonstrated. Apply two pad electrodes (5 × 5 cm or a little larger are convenient) to any area of the body. The electrodes may be close together or far apart. Attach each electrode to a lead cord. Attach the lead cord to the machine circuit. The patient circuit is now complete. Use AC of 60 Hz or higher, with continuous modulation. Turn up intensity to the subject's tolerance. A muscle contraction is not necessary. Let the current flow for at least two minutes, with a flow for five minutes being better. Adjust the intensity to the subject's comfort if necessary. Observe and record the percent of available power used, or voltage and amperage if such meters are available. When five minutes are up, turn the intensity down to zero. Remove the electrodes, and inspect the skin. There will be little or no hyperemia. Replace the electrodes at the same or adjacent areas. Switch the current type to DC, continuous modulation. Turn up the intensity to the same level as with AC. If the subject will tolerate this intensity, let the DC flow for the same time interval as with AC. Adjust intensity to the subject's comfort as needed. Turn the intensity to zero, remove the electrodes, and inspect the skin. There will be a strong hyperemia under one or both electrodes. This may not appear for a minute or two after electrode removal if treatment time was less than two minutes. Very likely, the hyperemia will become steadily stronger during the next five to ten minutes and will remain plainly visible for several hours.

The hyperemia is due to the local release of histamine or a histaminelike compound by cutaneous cells in response to a significant change in their environment. If voltage, amperage, and wattage were identical for AC and DC treatment, then the experimental variable has to be duration of current flow *in one direction*. With a five-minute treatment with DC, electrons and then ions have been flowing in one direction infinitely longer as compared to electron and ion flow induced by AC.

If the DC had been pulsed at the same rate as AC, the DC-induced hyperemia would be less intense than if the DC had an infinite wavelength, but it would still be visibly greater than that seen with AC at any pulse rate. Thus, whenever DC is used, regardless of modulation or other parameters, there is a greater chemical irritation of the skin. The same events take place with AC, but during each AC cycle there is a regular reversal of electron and ion flow so that there is insufficient time for a significant irritation of the skin. Hence, occurrence of pain or numbness is extremely rare when AC is used but common when DC is applied.

Another way to demonstrate the fundamental difference between lv-mA AC and DC is to fill any transparent container (200 ml is a convenient volume) with tap water. Place the bare metal terminals from two lead cords in the water, keeping them separate. Plug the other lead cord terminals into appropriate terminals of any NMSC generator that can deliver either AC or DC. Start with intensity at zero. Turn up intensity to any desired level, and observe the terminals in the water. When DC is transmitted by the lead cords, bubbles will appear at both terminals, always in greater quantity at the negative pole. Turn intensity down, reverse polarity of the leads, and note the rapid shift in quantity of bubbles at each terminal. The bubble formation is due to the partial dissociation of water into H^+ and O^- ions. Since approximately twice as many hydrogen ions are formed as compared to oxygen ions, and since ($+$) ions are attracted to the

(−) pole, more bubbles appear at the (−) pole. This reaction does not take place to any significant extent when AC is delivered to the lead cords. Since the DC-induced chemical reaction is *not necessary* for the formation of action potentials in nerve or muscle, usually AC of some frequency can be used as an adequate and more comfortable stimulus to cause muscle contraction. This is true regardless of the cause of denervation, and there is far less risk of skin damage.

Occasionally, a patient's skin chemistry will be such that DC is tolerated better than AC. Once in a great while, the degeneration-regeneration process will be such that DC of continuous modulation and uniform amplitude will be needed to elicit a contractile response. In most cases, however, the desired response can be achieved with some variety of AC.

WAVEFORMS

The therapist may have need of the sine, pulse, square, faradic, or exponential waveform to obtain the desired contractile response. Figure 3-4 shows a schematic representation of these waveforms. The sine wave has a gradual buildup and a gradual decline of intensity two times each cycle, with reversal of direction of electron flow once each cycle. The pulse wave has an abrupt increase and decrease in amplitude, along with reversal of direction of electron flow. The square wave has an abrupt increase in intensity, followed by a plateau, followed by a much larger change in intensity simultaneous with reversal of direction of electron flow.

With one exception, if DC is converted into similar waveforms, there is no reversal of direction of electron flow. The exception is DC with automatically reversing polarity, which physiologically becomes identical to AC.

The true faradic waveform is obsolete. Equipment with waveform selection that is labeled faradic (derived from standard wall outlet current) is actually producing a pulse wave. The amplitude of the first segment of the true faradic wave is small in proportion to the amplitude of the second segment. If the peak of the second segment is clinically tolerable, the peak of the first segment is not of sufficient amplitude to cause depolarization.

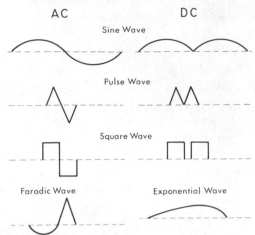

Figure 3-4. (a) *Sine Wave.* (1) AC — Note the gradual rise and fall of amplitude twice in each cycle, with reversal of direction of electron
flow once each cycle. (2) DC — Note the gradual rise and fall of
amplitude once each cycle, with no reversal of direction of
electron flow.
(b) *Pulse Wave.* (1) AC — Note the rapid rise and fall of amplitude
twice in each cycle, with reversal of direction of electron flow
once each cycle. (2) DC — note the rapid rise and fall of
amplitude once each cycle. Unless the apparatus has automatically reversing polarity, there is no reversal of direction of
electron flow.
(c) *Square Wave.* (1) AC — Note the abrupt rise and fall of amplitude twice each cycle. There is a plateau wherein the intensity
is uniform twice each cycle. There is reversal of direction of
electron flow once each cycle. (2) DC — Note the abrupt rise
and fall of amplitude, with a plateau occurring once each cycle.
There is no reversal of direction of electron flow.
(d) *Faradic Wave.* This waveform *always* has reversal of direction of
electron flow once each cycle and hence is always AC. However, the net effect is that of a rapid DC pulse because of the
significant difference in amplitude of the two segments of the
waveform. Whether this waveform stimulates nerve or muscle
depends on its frequency. If the frequency is 60 Hz or higher,
only nerve will be stimulated. If the frequency is lower, nerve
or muscle will be stimulated.
(e) *Exponential Wave.* (Also called the triangular or sawtooth
wave.) This waveform was developed in the 1940s specifically
for stimulation of denervated skeletal muscle. Note its slow
amplitude rise time and rapid amplitude decline. This wave-

Frequently, what the manufacturer labels "Faradic" will be of higher frequency (100 to 250 Hz) than that which is labeled "Sine" or "Pulse" (50 to 100 Hz). The faradic waveform derived from a house current source is physiologically the same as the pulse waveform. The most effective way to determine what waveform and frequency is actually being delivered to the patient is to display the patient circuit output on an oscilloscope. It is recommended that the derived data be permanently attached to each device.

The exponential waveform features a slowly rising amplitude, followed by an abrupt decline. It is sometimes referred to as a sawtooth or triangular rather than exponential waveform. In theory at least, this waveform permits stimulation of denervated muscle that lies deep to normally innervated muscle without painful massive contraction of the superficial muscle. The muscle with a functioning motor nerve supply tends to accommodate to the slowly rising ion flow, and hence depolarization is less apt to occur.

It is obvious that as frequency is increased, with any of the above waveforms, all will tend to appear more and more like the pulse waveform. In part for this reason, fewer and fewer manufacturers are providing any choice in waveform. When the waveform is limited to one, it usually approximates the ideal pulse form.

The waveforms as drawn (Fig. 3-4) are theoretical or ideal. They are rarely generated exactly as shown. Only oscilloscopic display will reveal what is actually delivered to the patient circuit. Periodic recheck of the display is a useful means of determining whether the generator is undergoing electronic deterioration, in which case repair or replacement may be indicated.

The house current modification of sine wave into other waveforms, other frequencies, and other current types requires a number of steps. Filtering of electron flow through various

---

form is not commonly available on apparatus used in this country. It is always DC. Selective stimulation of denervated muscle without stimulation of intervening normally innervated muscle is possible with this waveform as well as with other waveforms of slowly rising amplitude.

circuit components is perhaps the most important for patient comfort, expecially for the rectification of AC into DC. The better the filtering, the less discomfort. The better the filtering, the greater the cost. Chapter 8 discusses in detail house current modification for nerve and muscle current stimulators as well as for all other equipment that physical therapists use.

CURRENT MODULATION

Most modern stimulators offer a choice of continuous, surge, or interrupted modulation for AC or DC or both. The term *continuous modulation* can be difficult to grasp. In terms of NMSC, continuous modulation means that the amplitude is uniform and nonvarying for a prolonged period of time, i.e. seconds to minutes. Yet continuous modulation DC (Fig. 3-5a) is obviously physically different from continuous modulation AC (Fig. 3-5b). From the viewpoint of neurophysiology, if the stimulus repeats itself more than fifty to sixty times per second, with equal peak amplitude for each cycle, enough motor nerves, and the muscles they supply, will be stimulated by each cycle to give rise to a sustained contraction. Note that if the stimulus repeats itself less than about fifty times per second, an incomplete alternate contraction and relaxation of the muscle mass will occur. This response is sometimes called an intermittent tetanic contraction in order to distinguish it from the twitch response which is invariably produced by true continuous modulation DC, irrespective of whether the muscle is innervated or denervated.

When DC is pulsed rather than being truly continuous (Fig. 3-5c) at a rate of less than fifty times per second, it too will produce an intermittent contraction and relaxation, i.e. an intermittent tetanic response. This will hold true for any DC waveform. DC pulsed at a rate of greater than about fifty times per second will cause a true tetanic response. Because of concomitant skin chemical changes, it is usually less comfortable and usually requires a higher voltage to produce a equivalent response.

Placement of a voltmeter and a milliamperemeter in the patient circuit will confirm this fact. Stimulate a muscle on one side of the body, obtain a palpable response, and note both the volt

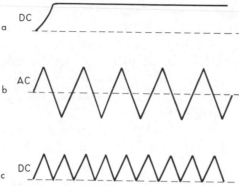

Figure 3-5. (a) DC continuous modulation. For any given intensity, the rate of electron flow is uniform. There is no reversal of direction of electron flow. The stimulated muscle responds only with a twitch and only upon rise or fall of amplitude (make or break of circuit).

(b) AC continuous modulation. For any given intensity, there is constant variation in rate of electron flow. There is reversal of direction of electron flow once each cycle. If the frequency is high enough, the stimulated muscle mass maintains a level of tension development that is clinically designated as a tetanic response. If the frequency is lower than about 50 Hz, there will be intermittent muscle mass contraction and relaxation.

(c) DC, *pulse wave*, continuous modulation. If the pulses occur at 50 Hz or higher, the muscle mass response is designated as tetanic because of a maintained level of tension development within the stimulated mass. If the pulse rate is lower, there will be intermittent mass contraction and relaxation because there is significant fluctuation in amplitude.

and ma readings *at the time of stimulation,* using either AC or DC. Replace the electrodes in the contralateral position and repeat, using the other current type, and obtain an equivalent palpable response. Again, record the meter readings at the time of stimulation. In normal subjects, the voltage will always be higher when DC is used (5 to 10 v). The ma reading may be higher, the same, or very slightly less when DC is used. Since watts equals volts times amperes, the milliwattage will always be higher when DC is used.

It should now be clear that the key to understanding variation in contractile response to continuous modulation is knowing what is the frequency of stimulation (per second) as well as what is the modulation, as much or more than being aware of the current type (AC or DC).

Contractile responses to other available modulations are easier to understand. The term *surging modulation* means there are alternate periods of current flow and no flow, with a gradual buildup and decline in intensity (*see* Figs. 3-2a and 3-2b). Most stimulators will permit a choice of surges through a range of about five to sixty times *per minute*. Oscilloscopic monitoring of the various surge rates will show that the control systems for variation in surge rates tend to be rather imprecise.

Some stimulators also permit variation in ratio of surge to the rest period between surges, irrespective of surge rate. This can be useful when the lesion is such that the stimulated muscle is slow to relax after the stimulus has ceased. In this case, the rest interval needs to be long. Also, if the patient has a chronic arterial insufficiency, the surge rate may need to be low and the rest interval long so that the impaired arterial flow can adequately meet the demand for increased blood supply as the muscle is regularly contracting and relaxing.

The term *interrupted modulation* means periodic current flow and cessation of current flow. The difference between interrupted and surging modulation is that with interrupted modulation, the shift from energy flow to no flow is abrupt rather than gradual. The net effect is that when a muscle is stimulated with an interrupted modulation, more fibers contract simultaneously because stimulus adequate to cause depolarization occurs in a shorter period of time. This obviously can be less comfortable, but it may be needed when skin impedance is high or many muscle fibers are denervated.

Perhaps the most important modulation of house current (110 v, 60 cycle AC) is that of frequency. Most stimulators that give the operator a choice will do so for AC only. If the unit will deliver only DC, variation in frequency rate is often not available. In sophisticated apparatus, one may select either AC or DC through a wide range of frequencies ($\frac{1}{2}$ to 3000 Hz) as well as DC with automatically reversing polarity. Where variation in frequency rate is permitted, it may be for only a few fixed frequencies, or stepless, or for many fixed frequencies. An AC frequency range of 20 to 1000 Hz with four or five choices within that range is probably adequate for the department that used NMSC on only one or two patients a day. For the teaching hospital with an active neurological service, a wider choice of frequencies can be justified. The greater the capability of choice of both AC and DC frequencies, the greater the likelihood of being able to obtain the desired contractile response with minimum discomfort to the patient.

THE PATIENT CIRCUIT

The patient circuit consists of lead cords that connect the stimulator to the electrodes, the electrodes themselves, and the patient. The circuit must have a minimum of two lead cords and two electrodes to be complete. When AC is delivered to the patient, each electrode is carrying energy to the patient for one half of the cycle and returning energy to the apparatus for the other half at precisely opposite times. Hence, each electrode is both stimulating and dispersive during each complete cycle.

When DC is delivered to the patient, the situation is different: One electrode is always active (stimulating) and the other is always inactive (dispersive). Usually, it is advisable to have the active electrode be of negative and the inactive electrode be of positive polarity because the negative pole electrode is almost always more stimulating than the positive pole. This is in part due to the fact that chemical changes on the skin exposed to the negative pole tend to be irritating whereas changes at the positive pole tend to be sedative. Also, the charge separation between the inside and outside of excitable membranes is normally (+) on the outside and (−) on the inside. If the stimulating electrode is (−), the requisite depolarization is readily achieved. If the stimulating electrode is (+), hyperpolarization will occur and a greater intensity is needed to produce equivalent response. This point can be simply confirmed.

Use any apparatus that delivers DC of continuous modulation and has a built-in voltmeter and an ammeter. Select any muscle mass to be stimulated and do so, noting the voltage and milliamperage needed to produce a palpable response. Reverse polarity, and stimulate the contralateral muscle, keeping all other factors equal. In the normal individual, it will invariably require at least 10 volts more when the stimulating electrode is (+) than when it is (−) because the excitable membrane is being hyperpolarized rather than depolarized.

Connecting the Patient to the Stimulator

It is advisable to check that the components of the patient circuit are in good order before attaching them to the patient. After making sure that the lead cord terminals are tightly connected to their lead cords, plug the appropriate cord terminal into one of the apparatus terminals. Do this for each of two lead cords. Then place the distal lead cord terminals together and turn up the intensity part way. The ma meter should give a reading. If not, either the lead cord terminals are not fitting tightly in the machine terminal sockets, one of the lead cords itself has a short circuit (broken wire underneath its insulation), or the connecting terminal between lead cord and electrode is loose. If the ma meter does read when the intensity is above zero, turn the intensity down and attach a tap water soaked electrode to each of the two lead cords. Hold them firmly together. Turn up the intensity control, and again the ma meter should rise above zero, indicating that the metallic part of the patient circuit is ready for use. If the meter does not read after connecting the electrodes, either the electrodes have not been adequately soaked or an electrode plate is corroded or broken and should be discarded. If the electrode was completely dry prior to use, it may need to be soaked for at least one half hour in warm water before it will conduct safely and effectively. If the electrode was in use within the last twenty-four hours, soaking it for five to ten minutes will usually be adequate.

If the NMSC apparatus does not have an ammeter, the procedure outlined above can be followed with substitution of moistened fingers when checking the lead cords themselves; for electrodes plus lead cords, place the electrodes firmly on any skin surface. In both cases, as intensity is turned up slowly, the subject should perceive a gentle tingling. If such a sensation is not achieved when the intensity control reads 50 percent of available power, something is defective in the patient circuit.

If the apparatus has both a voltmeter and an ammeter, the voltmeter will indicate whether the instrument circuit *(not patient circuit)* is in good condition. One does not need to have the patient circuit attached for this test. Being sure that the on-off control is set at zero and that the apparatus is plugged in, proceed to turn up the intensity. The voltmeter should rise above its zero reading. If it does not, the chances are that the line cord (not lead cord) is defective, a machine circuit fuse has blown, or the line current supply has been interrupted. If the line current is on, as indicated by the wall panel fuse or circuit breaker, trouble-shooting of a possibly defective machine circuit may be done by the institution's electrician. All NMSC apparatus will have a machine circuit fuse. Most often this fuse is readily accessible, but in some units, one or more chassis panels must be removed to locate the fuse. Spare fuses of appropriate type and size should be kept on hand, as this is the most common component failure. Fuses are designed to be safety valves and to be the weakest link in any electrical circuit. The most common cause of fuse failure is a brief surge in line current. Line current circuit fuses (or circuit breakers) commonly have a rated capacity of 20 to 30 amperes. Machine circuit fuse capacity is usually 2 to 5 amperes. Patient circuit fuses, which are integral parts of many NMSC units, will have a capacity of $\frac{1}{16}$ to $\frac{1}{4}$ ampere. Thus, a small, uncontrolled current surge will cause only the patient circuit to fail. A much larger surge is needed to interrupt the line current supply.

One word of caution: Before attempting to check any fuse, always unplug the apparatus from the line current supply. Many times a defect in a fuse is not visible. Fuses are cheap. If after replacing a suspect fuse the apparatus still does not work, the chances are good that the fuse was functioning and that the problem is in another circuit component. If the replacement fuse blows on attempt to test the apparatus, the problem is more serious and professional servicing is needed.

HIGH VOLTAGE STIMULATORS

During the 1970s high voltage-low amperage nerve and muscle stimulating apparatus came out of the laboratory and into slowly increasing clinical use. Its major advantage over the low voltage-moderate amperage equipment that was widely available in earlier decades is a dramatic increase in patient comfort, regardless of type or degree of nervous system deficit.

This new generation of stimulators can deliver up to 500 volts and up to 1.2 milliamperes at peak intensity (600 milliwatts). These are peak values deliverable to the active electrode. Because pulse rise time is very fast, the average voltage and amperage for each pulse is substantially less, approximately 170 volts and 0.5 ma at maximum intensity. Very few patients require maximum intensity to elicit the desired stimulation of axons and/or skeletal muscle. The voltage and amperage transmitted through the patient is lower still and is variable within the tissues through which energy is flowing. These stimulus parameters are in marked contrast to the low volt stimulators. The latter have the capability of delivering to the active electrode not more than 100 volts at not more than 80 ma (8000 milliwatts).

Further, with the high voltage stimulators, individual pulse duration is measured in microseconds and rarely exceeds 100 μsec. Low voltage stimulators rarely have a pulse duration shorter than 2,500 μsec. The duration is commonly much longer. It follows that with extremely short pulse duration, the rise time must be very fast. In the most sophisticated of the high voltage stimulators, the pulse rise time is on the order of 100 nanoseconds. In the best of the low volt units, rise time is 100 to 1000 microseconds.

Lastly, the high voltage units use paired subliminal amplitude pulses, a refinement previously available only in laboratory research stimulators for stimulation of isolated muscle nerve preparations, where patient sensation of stimulus is no factor. The paired pulses, through temporal summation, add up to a stimulus causing greater partial depolarization of excitable membranes, either of axons or muscle fibers directly if there is a somatic motor nerve deficit. The more advanced high voltage stimulators also have the capability of varying the interval between each pulse of a pair, through a range of 1 to 100 μsec. The majority of the high voltage units have only a fixed interval of about 70 μsec between each pulse of a pair. Both the variation in distance (time) between the individual pulses of a pair and the variation in distance (time) between pairs of pulses make it possible to elicit a contractile response in normally innervated skeletal muscle as well as in muscle with widely varying degrees of motor nerve deficit. The variation in time between pulse pairs is equivalent to the stimulus frequency control available on most low volt stimulators.

When applied to normal human subjects in areas where there is average skin impedance and subcutaneous fat, the high voltage stimulators will require an intensity of 75 to 250 v to elicit an easily palpable contractile response. Subjects with above-average impedance or who have an above-average thickness of subcutaneous fat in the area to be stimulated will require, and tolerate well, higher voltages. Patients with a peripheral motor nerve deficit and/or high impedance and/or an exceptionally thick fat layer may require close to 500 peak volts to produce a useful contractile response. Even at these intensities and with these problems, the high voltage stimuli will be well tolerated.

It is particularly in the problem patients that the two operator controlled pulse-time variations become particularly advantageous in insuring both comfort and generation of a functionally useful contractile response. The only exception to patient comfort that has been noted to date is that when the muscle to be stimulated is small and underlying bone is close to the skin, i.e. stimulation of a denervated frontalis muscle, the stimulus may be slightly noxious. Even here, patient comfort is greatly improved over what it would be were a low voltage apparatus used.

A simple way to convince yourself of the significant difference in patient comfort with use of high voltage stimulation is to locate the motor point of the gluteus maximus on a normal volunteer. This can be done even on a subject who is 5 feet tall and weighs 200 pounds. Then try the same stimulation on the contralateral area with any low volt stimulator. The chances of obtaining a useful contractile response at an intensity that a patient with normal cutaneous sensation will tolerate are negligible.

The reason(s) for the difference in patient comfort are not clearly established. A useful working hypothesis is that the greater driving force (higher voltage) leads to less cutaneous nerve stimulation. Perhaps because of the higher voltage, plus the faster rise time of the individual pulse, more of the energy leaving the active electrode penetrates through the skin and subcutaneous fat and is thus available for causing depolarization of deeper-lying sensory and motor axons. It might also be, but it has not been demonstrated, that the high impedance tissues, i.e. skin and fat, do not enter into resonance with the electromagnetic field established by this highly pulsatile stimulus whereas the low impedance excitable membranes do enter into resonance with the high voltage field. The magnetic field-resonance effect induced by high voltage stimulators is negligible. It is known, as established by the Law of DuBois Reymond, that a pulse with a rise time of nano- or picoseconds will be more stimulating than a pulse with a rise time of micro- or milliseconds, at any given intensity.

Possibly of equal importance is the fact that the high voltage stimulators are constant voltage, rather than constant current, devices. This means there is less hazard of generation of an electromagnetic field within tissues of high electrolyte content. The less the induced magnetic field, the less the likelihood of eddy current formation and consequently the less chance for inducing pinpoint pathologic tissue temperature rise.

All high voltage stimulators deliver to the patient only DC, whereas low voltage stimulators commonly deliver either AC or DC or a combination of the two current types. It is important to remember that because of its extreme pulsatile characteristics, the DC from the high voltage units does not and cannot cause significant irritation of the skin (i.e., hyperemia) or cutaneous receptors. This is because the energy flow is always pulsed, never true continuous modulation, and the pulses are of such short duration (nano- to microseconds) that no chemical alteration of the skin can accrue. Indeed, the energy delivered to the patient is so unlike low voltage DC that it is impossible to use high voltage stimulators to treat a patient by iontophoretic techniques.

ELECTRODES

Down through the years, many electrodes have been designed. Those in widespread use have some sort of connector for attachment to the lead cord on one side and the surface to be in contact with the patient on the other. The connection for the lead cord should always be tight for efficient conduction of electricity from cord to electrode. Hence, a spring-loaded snap fit or a spring clip is commonly used. The connector is permanently attached to a slightly flexible metal plate or screen mesh. On the terminal connecting side, the plate or screen is covered by an insulating material, usually a synthetic rubber or an insulating plastic. Loosely attached to the other side of the plate or screen is a layer of orthopedic felt or layers of asbestos paper to a thickness of about 1 cm. This in turn is covered with a loosely woven fabric, commonly cotton, which is sewn to the insulating cover. The fabric is porous and will admit any liquid into the felt or asbestos paper. Tap water is ordinarily used in the clinic as the electrical conducting link between the metal plate and the patient. When this kind of electrode is dry, the electrical circuit cannot be completed. If the felt is not thoroughly soaked, current may be concentrated in a small area, since current always follows the path of least resistance. The purpose of the electrode is to spread or diffuse the current delivered by the lead cord. For patient comfort, the current should be diffused uniformly throughout the electrode. Soaking the electrode in warm (37° to 40°C) water will always add to patient comfort.

Since the same electrode will be used on many patients (unless the patient is known to have a communicable disease that could be transferred by the electrode), most therapists prefer to insert a disposable cover between the electrode patient surface and the skin. Any soft, absorbent paper toweling is the most readily available and cheapest disposable cover. It should be cut to fit the patient surface of the electrode rather than left with a wide margin. Roller bandage gauze or a thin layer of cotton can also be used. The disposable cover must also be thoroughly wet, or there can be conduction problems.

The above described electrodes are available in many sizes, ranging from about 5 × 5 cm to about 20 × 25 cm. The smaller the electrode, the greater the stimulus for any given intensity. When selecting one large and one small electrode, the smaller will be the active electrode and the larger will be the inactive or dispersive electrode.

Some therapists prefer using bare metal electrodes with a

layer of electrode paste or jelly placed between the electrode and skin. Lead cords are then attached with alligator clips to a turned-up corner of the metal plate.

Electrodes need to be securely fixed to the skin to assure uniformity of contact. Body weight, of either trunk or extremity, is frequently used to insure good uniform contact. Elastic bandages or sandbags are also adequate.

When stimulating a single muscle, a different type of electrode may be useful. The contact surface is much smaller, ranging from 1 to 3 cm in diameter. This is always the active electrode, and it is commonly referred to as the tap-key stimulator or diagnostic handle. It is always held in place by the therapist's hand and so can be readily moved from one muscle to another within a treatment period. The usual design includes a flat spring attached to an insulated handle the size of a pencil, adjusted so that when no pressure is applied to the spring, the circuit is open and no current can flow. Thumb or finger pressure will close the contact and complete the circuit. Some tap-key electrodes are designed so that they may be used as above, or if the lead cord is attached at a different terminal, the circuit is made upon contact of the patient surface with skin and the circuit is broken when the electrode is lifted away. When the electrode offers this choice, one needs to be aware of which terminal is attached to the lead cord. In both cases, the patient surface contact consists of a small metal disc covered with ½ to 1 cm of felt and then the usual thin layer of fabric. The therapist should add a disposable cover for use with each patient. A small piece of roller bandage gauze is adequate and easily held in place with a rubber band. The tap-key electrode does not require prolonged soaking in water. Five minutes is adequate, but because the volume of felt is small, it needs to be rewet every few minutes during a treatment session.

Electrodes for the high voltage stimulators are more nearly standardized in size and composition as compared to those used in low voltage stimulators. The dispersive electrode is usually large — approximately 20×25 (500 cm^2). This limits the areas where the dispersive electrode can be applied. The stimulating electrode is much smaller and can range from 1 to 65 cm^2 in total area, depending upon whether group or individual muscle stimulation is desired. From one to four stimulating electrodes can be used simultaneously.

MONOPOLAR VERSUS BIPOLAR STIMULATION

The term *monopolar stimulation* indicates that only one electrode is placed on or near a muscle mass that is to be stimulated. The other electrode is remote from that area and should be placed on the skin overlying any muscle that is not an antagonist to the muscle to be stimulated. When electrodes are far apart, a relatively small amount of energy reaches the intervening motor nerves. The smaller the amount of current per unit volume of tissue, the more comfortable the patient will be, and, as long as the desired contractile response is obtained, this approach constitutes the most effective treatment. The monopolar technic can be used in individual muscle stimulation (IMS) problems if degeneration is not severe, but frequently IMS problems will require a bipolar technic.

On occasion, bipolar technics are also necessary in CNS and vascular problems. Once in a while, one of the effects of a CNS lesion will be to cause impairment of peripheral motor nerve's ability to propagate impulses. An example would be a lesion in the spinal cord resulting in continuing edema formation in the cord. Pressure from the edema in the ventral horn area of the cord could give rise to dysfunction of the motor neurons in the edematous area. A major cause of organic occlusive peripheral vascular impairment is diabetes mellitus of long-standing duration. This can lead to a peripheral neuropathy which can affect both sensory and motor peripheral axons.

In the bipolar technic, one electrode is placed at each end of a muscle or muscle group. When the current is flowing, the concentration of energy is much higher per unit volume of tissue than is the case when only one electrode overlies the muscle. Consequently, for a given intensity of stimulus, more energy is reaching the muscle that needs to be stimulated. The bipolar technic may be necessary when skin impedance is unusually high, when massive edema is present in the area to be stimulated, and/or when a majority of the nerve supply to a muscle has been physiologically or anatomically interrupted. Any of these complicating factors may occur in any of the categories of disease that have been discussed, except that of impaired motor nerve conduction, which does not often occur unless there has been a PNS lesion.

The bipolar technic can create a problem of overflow of energy into normally innervated synergistic or antagonistic muscles. The problem is usually solvable by careful replacement of electrodes, by lowering of skin impedance, or by alteration of stimulus parameters. The same adjustments can be used if this problem arises with monopolar stimulation.

TECHNIQUES FOR REDUCING SKIN IMPEDANCE

Patients with central (CNS) or peripheral (PNS) neurological deficits, as well as those with peripheral circulatory or emotional disturbances, are apt to have a significantly higher skin resistance than normal individuals. Washing the area to be stimulated with soap or detergent and then rinsing thoroughly with water is usually adequate to remove skin debris and any excess oil. The washing will very likely cause sufficient hydration of the skin to adequately lower the impedance. If that does not permit the desired response with reasonable comfort, a five- to ten-minute application of a hot pack or an infrared lamp should be helpful. This will increase skin hydration and electrolyte content. When neither of these methods are successful, soaking the electrodes in tea or in a fresh "Sine-Solution"* before use will be highly effective in lowering skin resistance. The tannic acid in tea and the lactic acid in the "Sine-Solution" are very effective at dissolving the waxy coating that may accumulate on the epidermis. However, tea will permanently stain the electrode and may transiently darken the skin. Occasionally, the patient will develop a dermatitis after exposure to the "Sine-Solution." This irritation will disappear within a few days after exposure to lactic acid ceases. The use of continuous modulation DC (−) pole is

---

* "Sine-Solution" consists of 2½ oz. lactic acid in 95% ethanol to make one quart. Enough distilled water is then added to dilute to one gallon. This solution was developed by Frank H. Krusen, M.D., at the Mayo Clinic in 1956. It is not stable and must be made up fresh at least once a month.

also effective in dissolving the outermost dead portion of the epidermis but is apt to be painful when used for the necessary three- to five-minute period, even though intensity is kept low enough so that there is no significant motor nerve depolarization.

GROUP VERSUS INDIVIDUAL MUSCLE STIMULATION

Positioning of the inactive or dispersive electrode will vary according to the type and severity of the disorder being treated, as well as in accordance with complicating factors such as scars, cuts, or other skin lesions, and cardiac status. Two general technics of stimulation are in use, namely group muscle stimulation (GMS) and individual muscle stimulation (IMS).

Group Muscle Stimulation

Stimulation of groups of muscles will be most often used with patients with disorders other than peripheral nerve lesions (PNS). In GMS, two or more pad electrodes are used. Choice of size is dependent on the area of application. If the electrodes are of equal size and AC is delivered to the patient, each electrode will be equally stimulating. If the electrodes are of different size, the smallest will be more stimulating. If DC (but not AC — at ½ to 20 Hz) is used, the ($-$) electrode will be more stimulating unless the ($-$) electrode is significantly larger than the ($+$) electrode.

Since in all lesions other than those involving the motor division of the PNS the axons supplying the muscles are functioning normally, a vast number of muscle fibers within several muscle masses can be adequately stimulated simultaneously with a relatively small concentration of current. Thus, for a CNS lesion, it is possible to apply one electrode to the skin over the posterior midshaft of the humerus and the other to the skin of the middorsal forearm and stimulate the elbow, wrist, and finger extensor muscles simultaneously. In the case of generalized arteriosclerosis, one electrode can be applied to each posterior calf and adequately stimulate ankle plantar flexor muscles bilaterally.

If the patient has any known cardiac pathology, bilateral upper extremity stimulation should be avoided. A small amount of the applied current inevitably will pass through the cardiac muscle or its motor nerve supply. This can be hazardous in any cardiac condition, especially if the patient uses a cardiac pacemaker.

There also may be a slight risk of causing irritation of the coughing reflex with bilateral upper extremity stimulation. The chances of this occurring, in this author's experience, is somewhat greater if DC is used. The reasons for this difference between AC and DC are not known. For the same reason, it is better to avoid placing one electrode on the anterior and the other on the posterior thorax. Risk from positioning one electrode on the anterior and the other on the posterior abdomen is negligible, except in the case of major unstable cardiac disease.

A useful contractile response would not occur if the dispersive electrode were to be placed on the antagonist of the muscle to be stimulated. Thus, if elbow extension is desired, one electrode should be placed over the extensor muscles and the other on almost any group except the elbow flexors. The dispersive electrode would be much more effective and comfortable on the posterior thorax, lumbar area, or dorsal forearm.

CHRONIC CENTRAL NERVOUS SYSTEM LESIONS

Lesions within the telencephalon, diencephalon, mesencephalon, or spinal cord may give rise to loss of voluntary control over some of the patient's skeletal muscles. In the acute stage of the lesion, the most common clinical picture is a reduction of normal resting muscle tension plus inability to increase tension on attempt to cause joint motion. Clinically, this picture of loss of control is called flaccidity. The flaccidity may persist for days to weeks (moderate lesion) to months (severe lesion). The flaccidity may continue indefinitely. As time goes on, frequently the flaccidity will disappear, being replaced by an abnormal increase in skeletal muscle tension, especially on attempt at motion or in response to external stimuli. Clinically, such an abnormal increase in tension is usually designated as spasticity.

In addition to causing loss of volitional control over skeletal muscle, if the lesion is within the cranial vault it may cause disruption of awareness of body image. The patient may not even be aware that the paralyzed segments are a part of his body, as well as having either an increased or decreased awareness of pain or other normal sensory input. The patient's ability to comprehend written and/or spoken language or his ability to express himself verbally or in writing may be altered.

If the lesion is within the spinal cord, usually the sensation normally present in the trunk or extremities is diminished or absent distal to the level of the lesion. Thus, the sensations of pain, touch, heat or cold, and proprioception are lost. Most commonly, this loss is permanent. More rarely, sensation may be heightened after onset of lesion, especially the sensation of pain.

The pattern of loss of volitional control over skeletal muscle and of altered sensation will vary with the individual patient. Even though a hundred patients may be labeled as hemiplegic (or paraplegic) on the basis of their gross motor deficits, the individual pattern of motor and/or sensory disruption is likely to be demonstrably different. The pattern of deficit within an individual patient will vary in accordance with location and severity of the lesion.

If the lesion is congenital rather than with onset later in life, any and all problems with sensory and/or motor deficits may be compounded because the child has never known normal sensation and has never had a chance to feel what it is like to move his joints in the normal sequence. There is increasing speculation, at least in that category of congenital lesions clinically labeled as the cerebral palsies, that sensory nervous system input, such as proprioception, is misinterpreted rather than not being transmitted supraspinally.[8] The misinterpretation could add to the abnormal motor response to external stimuli.

Nerve and muscle stimulating currents can be used to help the patient gain or regain sensory awareness and to gain or regain volitional control over skeletal muscle, although the NMSC cannot be regarded as a solution to the problem since they will not alter the CNS pathology.

It has been this author's experience that a majority of patients with CNS deficits as described will tolerate application of NMSC better than will patients with PNS lesions or those with no known neurological lesion as a basis for loss of voluntary control over their skeletal muscles. There are at least two reasons for this impression. Patients with CNS lesions will usually require far less intensity of stimulus to their affected muscles as compared to their unaffected muscles in achieving equivalent response, regardless of whether the affected muscle is flaccid or spastic. Presumably, this is because the affected motor neurons have been largely released from normal CNS inhibition and they tend to be hyperactive in response to any stimulus. Also, since their peripheral motor nerves are intact, there is only rarely need to use either DC or AC of less than 60 Hz. For reasons detailed earlier in this chapter, AC at a frequency of 1,000 Hz or better is usually more comfortable than either AC or DC of lower frequencies and is entirely adequate to obtain muscle contraction. The major exception is where there is massive chronic edema between the skin and muscle to be stimulated. When this occurs, it will usually be in the distal extremity. Modification of standard stimulation technics to insure adequate localization of stimulus through edema is discussed in the technic section of this chapter.

In both flaccid and spastic states, there may be circulatory impairment in the involved extremities, even in the absence of vascular disease. The impairment is in large part related to the loss of intermittent skeletal muscle contraction. Such contraction is normally a major factor in the return of venous blood to the heart. Daily use of NMSC to cause regular intermittent muscle contraction can be helpful in maintaining more nearly normal circulation in the extremities, especially in the presence of flaccidity and while the patient is confined to bed. The benefit of such treatment can be objectively monitored by regular digital skin temperature recording.

Many patients who have suffered upper motor neuron lesions resulting in paralysis will undergo an eventual shift from flaccidity towards spasticity. A factor in this shift may be the resorption of the cranial and/or spinal cord edema that accompanies the acute phase of many CNS lesions. When large numbers of neuron cell bodies and their processes are subjected to an abnormal increase in intra- and extracellular pressure, the affected nerves can no longer function. As the excess fluid is gradually resorbed, the nerve may return to erratic or to normal function, depending upon the degree of residual damage. When upper motor neurons are not functioning, the clinical picture is flaccidity. If large numbers of these neurons suffer residual damage and/or chronic impairment of function but have regained some capability to function, the clinical picture may be that of spasticity.

Many CNS lesions are vascular in origin. Some common vascular lesions are a plug of a blood vessel because of a thrombus or an embolus or a hemorrhage out of a vessel at a weak point in the vessel wall at a time when the blood pressure is transiently high. Any of these lesions will cause edema, which may take weeks to months to be resorbed. If the pressure on the neuron cell body or its processes is great, metabolism may be impaired and the cell dies. If the volume of edema is not too great, cells in the periphery of the edematous area may gradually return to some level of function. Neurons so affected tend to become hyperirritable. The clinical result, when areas affecting motor divisions of the CNS are involved, is inappropriate reaction to a given stimulus. This phenomenon is often described clinically as release from normal CNS inhibition. There is often an inappropriate skeletal muscle response to voluntary attempts at change in muscle tension. Vascular lesions within the cranial vault commonly affect the motor areas of the brain and give rise to that collection of symptoms clinically labeled as hemiplegia. Frequently, on one side, the facial muscles will be paralyzed. On the other, some of the muscles of the trunk, arm, and leg will suffer equal or greater loss of voluntary control.

In addition to the problem of circulatory stagnation, loss of ability to move joints at will can rapidly lead to muscle shortening, which can become permanent and lead to contracture formation. This can evolve into soft tissue and eventually bony ankylosis, in extreme cases. Rapidity of onset and the severity of these common sequelae to the loss of voluntary control over joint motion can be minimized by regular use of passive motion and regular use of NMSC to cause intermittent muscle contraction and relaxation. Appropriate application of NMSC can be useful when one muscle group, i.e. knee flexors, becomes hyperactive in response to any stimulus while its antagonist (knee extensors) has lost its ability to respond to normal stimulus. Such imbalance in response can lead to contracture formation. Careful application of NMSC to the antagonistic muscle group (knee extensors) can do much to prevent contracture formation and/or ankylosis.[3-11]

Stimulus parameters and other details are critical for successful application of NMSC to patients with either acquired or congenital lesions within the CNS. Many therapists are reluctant to take the time required for effective utilization of these procedures. In the author's opinion, it is usually time well spent with properly selected patients.

GROUP MUSCLE STIMULATION FOR THE PATIENT WITH HEMIPLEGIA

In the acute and subacute phases of cerebral vascular insults, even though the patient may be conscious, he frequently is not aware that the involved arm and leg are part of his body. This lack of awareness may be retained for weeks to months after his vital signs are stable. If the patient is not aware that these limbs are a part of his body, it is difficult to encourage him to try to use them. Appropriate use of nerve and muscle stimulating currents can be useful in helping the patient regain this awareness. Such treatment is best started as soon as the vital signs are stable and should be discontinued as soon as the patient exhibits ability to assist the stimulating current in tension development on command.

It must be recognized that if the patient is not verbally encouraged to work along with the intermittently stimulating current and perceive that the current is causing contraction which the patient could not voluntarily induce, he will often develop the attitude that the current alone will restore control of joint motion. After the therapist is satisfied that the patient is aware that the intermittent current flow is causing alternate muscle contraction and relaxation, he should ask the patient to try to help perform the movement when the current comes on. Palpation by the therapist will tell whether there is an increase in tension development with the patient's attempts at assistance. If not, the NMSC should be used passively a few more days, and then another attempt should be made for patient assistance. As soon as the patient can assist in tension development, the intensity of the electrical stimulus should be decreased. Once the patient can assist the use of NMSC for that muscle group, treatment with NMSC in that area can usually be discontinued within a week or two. If the patient cannot comprehend instruction, then the NMSC utilization must be entirely passive. However, within any time period, NMSC will be capable of causing a greater number of intermittent contractions and relaxations than any therapeutic exercise technic, with the net result of better maintenance of muscle elasticity, with minimal energy expenditure on the part of the therapist.[12-14]

When attempting to stimulate *extensors* in the presence of either spastic or flaccid flexors, the patient with a stroke commonly will have a flexion reaction first, especially when stimulus is at low intensity. If the surge or interrupted current modulation is at a sufficiently low rate, the flexion reaction will be followed by contraction of the extensor group. As *intensity* is increased, the flexion reaction will diminish and the extensor response will increase. A modulation rate of five to fifteen surges per minute will usually be effective in management of this problem. Although there has been much speculation as to why attempts at extension often lead to flexion, with and without application of NMSC, the reasons for this reaction in the stroke patient are not known. Perhaps it is because nerves supplying flexor musculature respond faster, or the flexor muscles themselves have the capacity for faster response to equal stimulus, or because the ratio of flexor nerves (gamma as well as alpha) to flexor muscles is different from that of extensor nerves to extensor muscles. Although not entirely comparable because of difference in type of stimulus, Bishop's discussions of vibratory stimulation amply point up the complexity of the neurophysiology involved in stimulus through the skin.[38]

The first response to NMSC applied to extensors or abductors is likely to be flexion or adduction, respectively, in the patient with a CNS lesion. However, if the modulation rate is low and the intensity is high enough, the unwanted response will be overridden by the slower-appearing desired response. The dual response usually disappears within a few treatments, leaving only the desired response.

Increase in intensity must be slow when using NMSC on patients with spasticity. Otherwise, a massive, whole-body flex-or-adductor response is likely to occur with the first few surges of current, regardless of location of electrodes.

Consider a chronic severely involved hemiplegic patient, one who has deltoid atrophy leading to subluxation, loss of both active and passive range in shoulder flexion and abduction, spasticity in elbow flexors with elbow flexion contracture, marked forearm pronation, wrist and finger flexor contracture with spasticity, and wrist ulnar deviation. The hand and fingers are edematous. How can NMSC be best utilized? The starting point should be with the proximal muscle groups. Something must be done to minimize the shoulder muscle atrophy and pain or the patient will not make any attempt to use his shoulder.

Until such time as the patient regains capability of voluntary deltoid contraction, an effective physical therapy approach is application of one small pad electrode to the posterior and another to the anterior deltoid, followed by stimulation with a high frequency (1000 Hz or higher) slowly surging AC for five to ten minutes several times daily. This can be done safely with the patient supine or semireclining. This treatment will cause far more intermittent muscle contraction and relaxation of the entire deltoid than any amount or type of therapeutic exercise that can be given manually in an equal time span. The therapist should not forget to instruct the patient, as soon as he can comprehend such instruction, to attempt to try to aid contraction when he feels the current come on; stimulus intensity should be decreased as soon as he can voluntarily increase contraction on command. As soon as active motion toward shoulder flexion and abduction is possible, the electrical stimulation can be discontinued. The therapist should not expect significant return of deltoid bulk. This will rarely occur. Return of a functional degree of strength is considerably more important as well as more common.

Similar treatment may be applied to the elbow and wrist extensors, with either a monopolar or bipolar technic, depending upon how responsive the extensors are to electrical stimulus. Usually, this can be done during the same treatment period in which the deltoid is stimulated, but not simultaneously. When the monopolar technic can be used, one electrode should be positioned over the midposterior humerus, the other on the middorsal forearm.

If this sort of treatment accomplishes nothing else, it minimizes the circulatory stasis that is so common in long-standing flaccidity or spasticity. The reduction of circulatory stasis will be due to the induced intermittent contraction and relaxation of paralyzed skeletal muscle.

The wrist and fingers are commonly more severely involved than the more proximal musculature, so that with initial treatment, the bipolar technic is often mandatory. One electrode should be placed on the proximal dorsal forearm and the other on the distal dorsal forearm. This can be conveniently done with the patient supine or sitting. When sitting, it is easier to have the forearm supported in pronation with the elbow and wrist in comfortable flexion, and frequently it is easier for the patient to see as well as feel what is happening when the current flows. If overflow to antagonists is a problem that has not responded to variation in current parameters or to previously discussed methods for reduction of skin impedance, then smaller electrodes can be used. Sometimes it is necessary to use two tap-key electrodes, connected for automatic rather than manual make and break of the patient circuit. The tap-key electrodes are held in place by hand rather than with bandages. Use of two tap-key electrodes is especially valuable when grossly visible edema is present. The smaller the electrode, the greater the concentration of current immediately deep to the electrode. The high electrolyte content and volume of gross edema tends to diffuse or dilute the circuit.

Similar procedures can be used throughout the lower extremities. Such treatment can be very effective in helping the patient regain awareness of sensation generated by intermittent contraction in hip and knee extensors. Again, as soon as the patient can comprehend instruction to attempt to assist contraction, he should be asked to do so. As soon as he can significantly increase tension on command, the electrical stimulus intensity can be decreased and then discontinued.

Since ankle dorsiflexor muscles are small and weak in comparison with plantar flexor bulk and strength, bipolar stimulation is almost mandatory. As soon as the patient can walk with any degree of safety, if ankle dorsiflexion during the swing phase of his step is a problem, a battery-powered patient foot switch device can be used.[5, 6] There appears to be reasonable carryover after training with such devices. Evidence is accumulating that male patients benefit more than female from use of such devices.[39, 40] Reasons for this are not known at this time.

It cannot be stressed too strongly that use of NMSC in hemiplegic lesions will not restore function to normal. The same can be said for any other procedure the physical therapist may use. However, when used as outlined above, it can be very useful in increasing rate of return to whatever level of function the residual deficit will permit. Active patient cooperation in assisting intermittent muscle contraction and relaxation is essential. Without it, it is all too easy for the patient to sit back and believe the magic black box is going to "cure" him.

SPINAL CORD LESIONS

Similar technics can be used for the para- and quadriplegic patient. In traumatic lesions resulting in such paralyses, there is usually less expectation of partial return of function as compared with the hemiplegic patient. Benefits will be largely in minimizing circulatory inadequacy, slowing onset of contractures, and possibly in decreasing rate of onset of osteoporosis. Once the patient is able to stand or walk, by whatever means, the intermittent spasticity usually produced by these activities will probably do as much to minimize the common sequelae as would regular use of NMSC. However, if the patient must be confined to bed because of intercurrent disease or other malfunction, regular use of NMSC is indicated, as outlined for the hemiplegic patient, until the cord lesion patient can be mobile again. The setback in rehabilitation progress will be minimized by such treatment. Treatment can be easily done in the patient's room.

In the late 1970s reports began to appear giving strong clinical evidence of the usefulness of electrical stimulation for the management of pain and spasticity in multiple sclerosis[9, 10] and knee flexor spasticity in paraplegia.[11] For the patient with multiple sclerosis, as is the case with the hemiplegic, the effects are cumulative. Daily stimulation frequently will induce marked reduction in spasticity — lasting from treatment to treatment — within a month. The stimulation can then either be discontinued or continued once or twice a week as the individual patient symptoms present themselves. The principal merit of stimulation in such patients is reduction of severity of contracture formation.

Depending upon the individual patient problem, either a bipolar or monopolar technic may be indicated. The involved extremities may be treated separately or simultaneously. Weekly or monthly passive range of motion testing will provide objective evidence of reduction of spasticity.

If the paraplegic individual is flaccid distal to the lesion, simultaneous stimulation of the quadriceps and gluteus maximus bilaterally can be very effective in assisting the patient in rising from sitting to standing.

For the great majority of patients who are either flaccid or spastic due to a CNS lesion, high frequency AC (100 Hz or higher) with a slow surging modulation (five to ten surges per minute) will elicit a functionally useful contractile response. Risk of skin damage is then negligible, and no special stimulating equipment is needed. Standard treatment time is ten to twenty minutes.

CHRONIC PERIPHERAL NERVOUS SYSTEM LESIONS

Peripheral nervous system (PNS) lesions may involve sensory, motor, or autonomic nerves or any combination of these three functional types of nerves. The patient most likely to be seen by the physical therapist will be the one who has some motor deficit. This may be a result of trauma or a disease process within the anterior (ventral) horn area of the spinal cord or anywhere peripherally, including malfunction of the myoneural junction. The chronic stage of any peripheral motor deficit invariably results in muscle flaccidity because of loss of ability of the motor nerve to conduct the stimulus needed to generate the muscle action potential.

Peripheral nerves, unlike those within the central nervous system, do have a capacity for regeneration. Where the sheath of Schwann remains intact, the prognosis for regeneration is good, but by no means does regeneration always occur, and it will never occur if the cell body (the anterior horn cell) has been killed by the lesion. If the sheath of Schwann has been damaged, the likelihood of regeneration is much less, but chances of regeneration are improved with appropriate surgical repair.

The usual sequelae of skeletal muscle flaccidity, namely circulatory stasis, edema, muscle shortening, contracture formation, fibrous ankylosis, and bony ankylosis, can and do occur. This is especially likely if most of the nerve supply to a major muscle mass controlling a joint motion is lost while the motor nerve supply to its principal antagonist remains intact and functional.

The physical therapy procedures available, including the use of NMSC, do nothing to alter the nerve lesion per se, but it is hoped that adequate use of NMSC will help to maintain denervated muscle elasticity — the capability to contract and relax. Intermittent muscle contraction and relaxation will help to minimize circulatory stasis, thus maintaining better nutrition and more adequate removal of waste products while waiting to see how much, if any, regeneration is going to take place. If regeneration is to occur, it will be no faster than at the rate of one millimeter per day. If an axon has been anatomically severed at the level of the midshaft of the humerus and was supplying an intrinsic muscle of the hand, for an average size adult this would mean that the distal axon must grow more than 450 mm. Functional regeneration over distances such as this do occur, with subsequent return to useful function of the denervated muscle,[41] but it may take two to three years. If all other factors are equal, the shorter the distance between site of start of degeneration and the point of the myoneural junction, the better the chances for regeneration.

In considering a muscle mass, i.e. biceps brachii, which is denervated, if enough of its motor nerve axons do not regenerate, eventually the denervated muscle fibers will atrophy. These muscle fibers may be infiltrated by noncontractile components such as fibrous connective tissue. Such deterioration of the muscle fibers usually does not take place until eighteen months to two years after denervation. When such deterioration has taken place, there can be no contractile response to any kind of stimulus. Use of NMSC will not prevent this process from occurring but can delay the rate at which it occurs.

The person who has suffered a peripheral motor nerve lesion but whose peripheral sensory nervous system has not been impaired will as a general rule have more acute sensation of any externally supplied electrical stimulus than either the individual whose entire nervous system is intact or the patient who has suffered both sensory and motor nerve malfunction. The classical example is the patient with anterior poliomyelitis, which is a disease process that involves anterior horn (motor nerve cell bodies) but not the dorsal ganglia (sensory nerve cell bodies) or dorsal horn cell bodies. Fortunately, this formerly common epidemic disease is rarely seen in this country now, subsequent to wide utilization of appropriate vaccines. For patients with an intact sensory nervous system but with a nonfunctioning or partially functioning motor nervous system, it is difficult to provide adequate electrical stimulation to cause denervated muscle contraction using intensities that the patient can tolerate.

Stimulation of denervated muscle requires a longer duration current flow in one direction to generate a muscle action potential.[14, 41] One of the skin's reactions to this longer duration flow appears to be accumulation of abnormal and painfully irritating substances on or within the skin. The differences in skin reaction to DC as compared to AC are discussed in this chapter's section on current type.

Depending upon the number of axons involved, a PNS lesion may affect some or all muscle fibers within a muscle mass, or some fibers in each of several muscles. If more than one muscle is affected, it is more likely than not that they will be affected in varying degrees. For these reasons, in PNS lesions, individual muscle stimulation is indicated far more often than is group muscle stimulation. The standard procedure in IMS is to use one large (5 × 5 cm or bigger) dispersive pad electrode plus a tap-key electrode for stimulation of only one muscle or segment of that muscle. When the monopolar technic will produce the desired contractile response, there is less chance of an overflow problem than if the bipolar technic must be used. If the bipolar procedure is necessary, it is usually, but not always, more effective when the stimulating electrode can be distal to the dispersive electrode. If AC can produce the desired response, even if its frequency must be lower than 20 Hz, there is less risk of skin damage than when DC must be used.

When DC must be used, Erb's Polar Formula should be kept in mind. This formula states that in the normal individual, a cathode closing contraction (CCC) will be more stimulating than an anode closing contraction (ACC). Next in order of stimulus strength will be an anode opening contraction (AOC), and finally, a cathode opening contraction (COC) may produce the desired muscle contraction.[41] In the individual with a PNS lesion, anodal stimulation may give a response at a much lower intensity. With rare exception, contraction on opening the circuit requires far more intensity (five to ten times as much) so that neither COC or AOC will cause muscle contraction with a clinically tolerable intensity. An ACC will be more effective than a CCC only when degeneration of the axon has resulted in reversal of charge separation such that the outside of the membrane has an excess of negatively charged ions relative to the ionic charge on the inside of the membrane.

Care must be taken to avoid fatigue when using IMS technics. A muscle with deficit in its nerve supply will tire far more easily than a muscle with a normal nerve supply. The net result may be that for a few stimuli there may be a good contractile response, but then the response weakens, even though the intensity is gradually increased. As intensity rises, nearby synergistic or antagonistic muscle may start to contract. If stimulation is continued to a fatiguing muscle, there is some evidence that nerve regeneration may be delayed or arrested.[41-43] Clinical literature on poliomyelitis in the 1940s and early 1950s stressed that any kind of stimulus evoking a contractile response and repeated too often could cause a recovering axon to fail permanently. Laboratory experiments on denervated rat muscle[44] indicate that the hazard of regeneration retardation is minimized if the dener-

vated muscle is stimulated with short bouts (five to ten contractile responses) of stimulation four or five times each day rather
than providing twenty to one hundred stimuli within a single
twenty-minute period. In the presence of a PNS lesion, if stimulation is to be beneficial, treatment should be given *at least* once
a day until signs of fatigue appear.[41] It is better to give the
stimulation twice a day if possible. The need for short but frequent sessions of electrical stimulation is critical and may explain
the poor results obtained when stimulation is given only two or
three times per week.

Motor Points

When IMS is indicated, the therapist must be able to locate one
or more motor points over the muscle to be stimulated. A motor
point may be defined as that area on the skin which overlies a
point where many single terminal nerve branches connect to the
muscle fibers they supply. Most skeletal muscles are ovoid in
mass, and the greater number of muscle fibers are at the center
rather than at either end of the mass. Hence, the primary motor
point will be on the skin overlying the greatest bulk of that
muscle. Since some muscles are deep to others, it is fortunate
that all muscles have secondary motor points. Thus, it is easy to
find motor points of muscles like the biceps brachii or the gastrocnemius, since they are superficial, but much harder to find
motor points for the brachialis or soleus, which lie deep. A motor
point can be identified because far less intensity is required to
elicit an equivalent response at that point than anywhere else on
the skin over that muscle mass. This is because a greater number
of axons supplying a single muscle mass are collected in a small
volume of tissue. Appendix A at the end of this chapter gives the
location and result of stimulation of motor points throughout
the body. Location of these points will become very easy for the
therapist who works with patients with PNS lesions on a regular
basis.

In general, motor point stimulation is more comfortable in
muscles that are remote from bone. Stimulation of shoulder or
hip musculature is not as disagreeable as stimulation of intrinsic
hand or foot muscles, or, most of all, the facial muscles. At least

part of the reason for this difference is that when muscle lies close to bone, an appreciable amount of energy reaches the sensory receptors in the underlying periosteum as well as the cutaneous receptors. The more the sensory stimulation, the greater the discomfort.

Obesity and Hirsute Skin

The more obese or hirsute the subject (insofar as location of electrodes is concerned), the more uncomfortable is any electrical stimulation. The more obese the individual, the thicker the subcutaneous fat layer. Hydrated skin is a good conductor of electricity, since there are many openings on the surface — hair follicles, sweat glands, etc. — all of which have a high electrolyte content and thus easily transmit electrical energy through the skin. Subcutaneous fat is a poor conductor. It has a low water content as well as a poor blood and lymph supply, and hence a low electrolyte content. Since NMSC penetrate fatty layers largely via the blood vessel and lymph channels, the thicker the fat layer, the more trouble the electrical energy has in reaching the motor axons. Therefore, the more subcutaneous fat overlying the muscle to be stimulated, the higher the intensity needed. The normal overlying fat layer is a major reason why it can be difficult to find motor points of muscles such as the gluteus maximus or gluteus medius.

Hair follicles transmit NMSC readily because of their high electrolyte content. If the hair is dense and stiff, however, it is difficult to insure uniform contact of the patient surface of the electrode with the skin. This can lead to concentration of the current in an irregular manner and cause the stimulation to be more painful than it need be. If feasible, the easiest solution is to place the electrodes in areas where hair is sparse. If this is not possible, shaving the area may be necessary. An electric shaver is preferable, since even the slightest nick or cut in the skin will lower the skin resistance dramatically, leading to undesirable irregular current concentration.

Scar Tissue

It is not wise to place electrodes on either old or new scar tissue. Old scars (in Caucasians, more pale than surrounding skin) have a poor blood supply. They have no openings into subcutaneous tissue and a very high resistance to current flow, since electrolyte concentration is low. All of the above is equally true for old acne scars. On the other hand, new scar tissue and active acne or other eruptive skin lesions usually have an excellent blood supply. In the case of new scars, exposure to significant quantities of NMSC, especially DC, can arrest completion of wound repair. In all cases where there has been eruptive skin damage, current concentration is apt to be irregular and consequently more painful than it would be if it were feasible to apply electrodes elsewhere.

There are also skin lesions wherein, even though the skin may appear completely normal in the area where one wishes to place an electrode, the skin impedance will remain continuously high.[45] The patient with psoriasis is a prime example.

CHRONIC ORGANIC OCCLUSIVE PERIPHERAL VASCULAR DISEASES

As more and more of the population is living well beyond retirement age, more and more people are faced with the pain and other handicaps that are a direct result of increasingly impaired circulation. While the various chronic organic occlusive peripheral vascular diseases are usually systemic rather than local in effect, the fact that blood has a longer way to go to return from the lower extremities to the heart than from elsewhere in the body means that circulatory insufficiency is apt to be more of a problem in the legs than in the arms, even though the effects of equivalent impairment in cerebral or coronary vessels may be more life threatening. The major reason why the chronic vascular diseases are more severe in the lower extremities is the stronger effect of gravity on the return of blood to the heart. More work must be done both by venous valves and skeletal muscle. The weight of the much longer column of blood on the valves frequently leads to a need for additional intermittent skeletal muscle contraction and relaxation, especially by the calf musculature. If there is arterial insufficiency due to intimal deposition and consequent decrease in lumen size, there is apt to be an instinctive decrease in ambulation. The net result is often a marked venous stasis. Clinically, valvular venous incompetency is frequently seen as a factor in varicose veins.

In all of the organic occlusive vascular diseases, there is a gradual deposition of minerals (chiefly calcium salts) or lipid complexes on the inside lining of the walls of arterial vessels. There may or may not be significant mural irritation and thrombus formation. As the deposits accumulate over the years, the lumen of the arterial vessels gradually decreases in diameter. This increases resistance to blood flow. At first, the vasoregulatory system compensates for this increased resistance by raising the blood pressure, thus insuring adequate circulation. In time, this may lead to other problems such as cardiac enlargement or vascular aneurysm formation. All of these and many more vascular changes make treatment more complex as the pathology progresses. This is especially true since the early and potentially reversible changes are relatively pain free. By the time the pain is persistent and severe enough for the subject to seek medical attention, the impairment is often quite severe and largely irreversible. Two very useful books detailing these problems are the volumes by Shepard[46] and Abramson.[47]

When the patient cannot or will not engage in enough ambulatory activity to make enough intermittent use of calf musculature to keep the circulatory insufficiency within tolerable limits, regular use of NMSC can be a useful adjunct in overall management of the patient. A major reason why NMSC can be useful in chronic circulatory impairment is that intermittent skeletal muscle contraction with the patient prone puts less demand on circulation than does ambulation but more demand than if the patient is confined at rest in a bed or wheelchair. It is generally accepted that when a patient with a chronic occlusive peripheral vascular disease must be confined, the rate of increase in circulatory stasis goes up sharply. As the degree of diminution of blood flow goes up, the risk of thrombus formation increases. Wakim[31] and Martella[32] were among the first to demonstrate that regular use of NMSC can be helpful in combatting this kind of circulatory inadequacy.

Just as is the case when using NMSC in the presence of central or peripheral nervous system deficits, here again the physical agent does not resolve the cause of the disorder, but it can help to delay or arrest further damage. If one can delay or arrest the progression of circulatory impairment so that amputation does not become necessary, the time and effort involved in the procedure is certainly worthwhile. There are other physical therapy procedures that can and should be used concurrently with treatment by NMSC, but they are not within the scope of this book.

In most cases of chronic arteriosclerosis or atherosclerotic peripheral vascular disease, the simplest use of NMSC is to position the patient prone (or supine with the lower extremities elevated 10 to 20 degrees with pillows) and apply one electrode to each posterior midcalf. Surging AC of 60 Hz or higher frequency will produce adequate intermittent tetanic contraction and relaxation of the ankle plantar flexors. Ideally, the treatment would be given twice daily, for twenty to thirty minutes each time. The modulation rate would be adjusted so that there would be five or ten contractions per minute. Digital skin temperature measurement before and after treatment and/or weekly checking of distance that can be walked before onset of intermittent claudication will provide an objective record of effectiveness of treatment.

If the patient has chronic diabetes mellitus, with a resultant peripheral neuropathy, a bipolar technic may be necessary. In this case, each calf should have two electrodes applied, one proximal and the other distal. If the neuropathy is far advanced, it may be necessary to use an interrupted modulation DC, but the skin should be carefully inspected before and after each treatment because of the greater risk of skin damage with DC as well as the fact that the neuropathy may involve sensory as well as motor nerves. If there is a marked difference in severity of involvement in the two extremities, it may be necessary to treat them separately because of the difference in current intensity and other electrical parameters necessary to elicit the desired response. However, if the intermittent contraction and relaxation is approximately equal in the two extremities, they can be treated simultaneously. Many models of NMSC have provision for simultaneous use of two or more circuits.

If this type of treatment is effective for a given patient, it will produce a transient rise in toe skin temperature on the order of 5° to 10°C as well as an increase in pain-free walking distance of better than 10 percent within three weeks of daily use. If such results have not occurred within a three- to four-week period, there is little reason to continue this type of treatment.

PSYCHOSOMATIC DISORDERS

Patients who suffer from apparent skeletal muscle weakness or from other loss of volitional control despite apparently intact nervous and circulatory systems may benefit from NMSC. The procedure may help the neurologist or psychiatrist decide whether there is neurological damage or whether the apparent paralysis is the result of extreme emotional conflict. If the loss of voluntary control is entirely related to a nonneurological crisis, the quantity of energy required to induce a contractile response is likely to be significantly greater as compared to that needed for response in the patient's contralateral uninvolved muscles. There are at least two reasons for this. The skin impedance is usually much higher in the apparently paralyzed area, and the circulation, both cutaneous and deep, is apt to be diminished, as compared to the contralateral muscles. Earlier in this chapter, the hyperirritability of motor nerves in patients with central nervous system lesions was pointed out. This rarely occurs in patients whose nervous system is intact. In the patient where emotional conflict has led to loss of control over skeletal muscle, the skin is frequently very dry, and significant vasospasm is likely to be present in the paralyzed area. Hence, the quantity of energy necessary to elicit a contractile response is likely to be higher than it is for uninvolved areas. If the paralysis is actually the result of a peripheral motor nerve deficit, involved muscles would not respond to current flow of short duration in one direction, i.e. 60 Hz or higher AC, but would respond to low frequency AC or to DC. The patient whose apparent paralysis is related to an emotional crisis will always respond to 60 Hz or higher AC. Hence, it is easy to rule out nervous system lesions as the cause of the paralysis.

At the conscious level, the patient may be firmly convinced that he cannot voluntarily move the affected joint(s). It is frequently helpful to the patient's attempts when he can see and feel the controlling muscle contract.

There is another category of patient who may quite sincerely believe that he can no longer move an apparently paralyzed body segment — the individual who was injured while at work and who stands to be awarded greater compensation for the injury the more severe the permanent damage appears to be. Again, appropriate use of NMSC can go far to demonstrate to all concerned whether the lesion is as damaging as it may appear to be.

TRANSCUTANEOUS ELECTRICAL NERVE AND MUSCLE STIMULATING CURRENTS (TENS)

The 1970s heralded a marked increase in use of electrical stimulation as part of the management of patients with chronic pain. This technique has probably been in use on an empirical basis for close to a century and certainly has been taught as a part of physical agents since the 1930s. Development of practical battery-powered sources of NMSC in the late 1960s and 1970s has made the various techniques clinically feasible on a large scale. During the 1970s use of TENS by therapists became so widespread that the journal *Physical Therapy* saw fit to devote an entire issue (Vol. 58 #12, 1978) to a series of papers dealing with rationale and techniques by a group of authors with extensive clinical experience. These papers provide the interested reader with over 400 references to research, both basic and clinical.

Chronic pain is standardly defined as that which persists for at least three and more commonly six months after onset and which has not responded in a lasting fashion to appropriate medication and/or surgery. The most common site of such pain is the low back area, but it may occur in any area of the body. There may be a palpable low grade skeletal muscle spasm associated with the pain. The referring physician will have ruled out pain due to a thalamic or cauda equina lesion.

The key to management of chronic pain by clinical electrical stimulation is to flood the large-diameter cutaneous axons with a high volume of stimuli at a uniform rate for up to thirty minutes at a time. Palpable skeletal muscle contraction is neither necessary nor desirable. The patient should not feel any increase in muscle tension during treatment; only a gentle tingling sensation, which is likely to diminish or disappear several times during a twenty-minute treatment. When this occurs, intensity should be increased until the tingling is perceived again, provided the patient does not also feel an increase in muscle tension. Therefore, the current modulation should be continuous rather than surge or interrupted. Current type can be either AC or DC, or a combination of the two.

For a majority of patients with chronic pain, relief can be achieved equally well with the clinically standard low volt-milliampere house current powered apparatus, the newer high voltage microampere house current devices, specially designed low volt-milliampere high frequency generators or battery-powered units of several different designs. The battery-powered units are light in weight, can be attached to a waistband, and permit patient self-stimulation whenever s/he feels the need for same. On the other hand, the battery-powered units have definite limitations as to frequency range and intensity levels available. For various reasons the battery-powered units are in more common use. However, it has been this author's experience over more than thirty years that when battery-powered devices do not give adequate pain relief, the house current powered stimulators are more effective, for reasons to be discussed later.

Almost all the patients for whom TENS is indicated have an intact sensory nervous system. Therefore, either AC or DC at 60 cps or higher will stimulate the sensory axons. Small capacitance axons can respond to each of 1000 stimuli per second. Large capacitance axons *cannot* respond to each of 1000 stimuli per second but can respond to lower frequencies, i.e. 50 to 250 Hz. Denervated muscles require a stimulus frequency of 20 cps or less because their capacitance is three or four or more times greater than that of any axon. When a stimulating frequency is too high for the normal axon to respond to each stimulus, it will fire each time that it can respond. Hence, to achieve a maximum number of nerve action potentials per unit time, the ideal stimulus frequency should be 1000 cps or higher. It is not practical for a portable battery-powered TENS unit to have a frequency higher than about 500 Hz. Most such units will have a maximum frequency of about 250 cps and a low frequency of about 50 Hz. This frequency range *is* adequate for relief of most chronic pain. The authors have in preparation (1981) a manuscript discussing a series of twenty-five patients with chronic pain who did not achieve lasting pain relief when treated with TENS at frequencies less than 250 Hz but who did perceive functional relief when TENS was delivered with house current powered apparatus at a frequency of 1000 cps.

In the latter 1970s it was established that a major reason for pain relief by TENS is that most of the cutaneous axons of small capacitance produce their own endogenous opiates. These opiates are the neurotransmitter across axonal synapses. This has been demonstrated by a measurable increase in opiate levels in the dorsal horn areas, where these axons are known to terminate, when the axons are stimulated with TENS. (*See* Figs. 1-2, 1-3, and 1-4 for a useful schema.)

On the other hand, sensory axons of large capacitance apparently do not produce or cause secretion of endogenous opiates within the spinal card. Sensory physiologists agree that typical pain stimuli are conveyed to the cord by axons of large capacitance. The interested reader should consult Bishop's articles on pain physiology for detailed documentation and interpretation.[48]

Apparently the gate control theory developed by Melzack and Wall (*see* Chapter 1), coupled with newer knowledge about endorphins and enkelphalins, can do much to explain pain relief from conductive heat and cold as well as pain relief from TENS. It now seems clear that heat, cold, and electrical stimulation all cause a clinically useful increase in endogenous opiate release in both the substantia gelatinosa and the marginal zone of the dorsal horn.[48] Whether there is a similar effect upon exposure of the large diameter cutaneous axons to the diathermies or to ultrasound has not yet been reported.

Techniques in Tens

In general, the painful area should be bracketed by two or more electrodes. If the painful area is small (500 cm^2 or less) and sharply localized, a one circuit-two electrode setup will usually be adequate. For larger and more diffuse areas of pain, four electrodes and two circuits may be needed, with various combinations of current type (AC and/or DC) and current parameters. In all cases the current modulation should be continuous rather than surged or interrupted. The apparatus to be used should have the capability of delivering different frequencies at least through a range of 50 to 250 Hz. Choice of frequency, current type, current parameters, and electrode placement will vary with the individual patient. As the therapist accrues clinical experience and utilizes apparatus that offer a reasonable variety of choice of variation of current parameters, the amount of time needed to determine that combination of parameters which gives the individual patient effective pain relief usually should not be longer than one, or at the most two treatment periods.

When two circuits are indicated, they may be parallel (one on the right and the other on the left side) or diagonal (one electrode upper right, the other lower left) from the same circuit, with the electrodes from the second circuit being placed in the opposite fashion. Very occasionally when two circuits are used they are placed horizontally (one electrode on the right, the other on the left side). If two circuits are set up in this fashion for simultaneous use, the second circuit would be distal or proximal to the first, but still horizontal.

When two circuits are used, they may emanate from the same or separate NMSC devices, may be of the same or different frequencies, and may be of the same or different current types (AC and/or DC). Most experienced therapists will utilize the simpler setups on any given patient first. If that treatment does not produce substantial pain relief lasting one to two hours after treatment, within three treatments, it is time to consider the more complex setups.

Indication of pain relief is inevitably a complex physiological and psychological mix (*See* chapter 1). A clinically useful indicator of whether the TENS treatment is producing some benefit is stimulation of sensation by a rapidly moving fingernail before and after treatment. The fingernail should be run over the skin with uniform pressure and rate in the area of electrode placement as well as between electrodes. If the treatment is effective, the patient will perceive diminished sensation in the treated area for up to one half hour after the first treatment. The perceived degree of diminished sensation is expected to increase with each treatment and last longer after each treatment.

Perhaps the most logical approach to use for TENS is to repeat stimulation for twenty to thirty minutes b.i.d. or t.i.d. for three days to a week, then gradually taper the number of treatments as indicated by individual response. During this time the ideal current parameters for that patient will have been established. If the patient perceives good pain relief but of short duration (one to two hours), it is then time to consider use of a battery-powered unit. These are available with either one or two channels (two or four electrodes). All will have intensity and pulse frequency controls. Many will also have an individual pulse duration (width) control. Output waveform will vary with different manufacturers. The battery-powered units are equipped with rechargeable batteries of various designs. If not abused and if used only for several hours out of each twenty-four, and if recharged every night, life expectancy of the battery pack should be at least three months, and more commonly far longer.

Choice of electrodes for TENS are a debatable issue. As of the early 1980s it appears that the standard fabric-covered orthopedic felt electrodes soaked in tap water present the least problem with skin irritation.[49] On the other hand, they cannot be kept in place for more than several hours without rewetting, which may cause incorrect positioning or placement.

The second most widely used electrode is some form of carbon-impregnated rubber. These electrodes require use of an electrical conducting jelly between skin and electrode, but they can be left in place for twenty-four hours or more and still be functional. Some patients are allergic to long-term use of readily available electrode gels and may develop a contact dermatitis. This skin irritation will usually disappear within three days of avoidance of the gel. If not, almost all will respond favorably to a topically applied hydrocortisone ointment used once or twice. Only rarely does TENS have to be discontinued because of skin irritation.

There are several other more esoteric and more expensive

types of electrodes that have been developed to combat electrode placement slippage while ambulatory and/or to prevent skin irritation.[49] They appear to be less efficient as electrical conductors as compared to felt or carbonized rubber, but they do give rise to less skin irritation.

Some patients require capability for use of TENS for more than eight hours per day to keep their pain at a tolerable level. Obviously, these patients must use battery-powered units and be thoroughly instructed as to electrode placement and skin care. It is the author's opinion that if a patient requires steady increase in intensity and/or hours of use per day appreciably beyond eight hours, the treatment is losing its initial benefit and alternate methods of management of chronic pain need to be considered.

ION TRANSFER

Ion transfer is a technique that utilizes NMSC with DC continuous modulation only. This technique *cannot* be done with the battery-powered TENS stimulator or with high voltage stimulators. In both cases the DC output is always pulsed rather than truly continuous. Ion transfer *can* be done with the standard house current powered low volt-milliampere current source if it is designed to deliver continuous modulation DC to the patient.

The objective of the treatment is to drive topically applied medication into the epidermis and dermis for slow release (hours to days), or in the case of selected medication, into systemic circulation. A reliable source of iontophoretic techniques as used in clinical practice in the 1970s is that written by Kahn.[50]

Ion transfer has also been variously called iontophoresis, electro-osmosis, electrophoresis, and dielectrolysis. Use of this technic has been largely abandoned in this country because of major hazards, controversy of efficacy, and improved management of many of the lesions for which it was previously prescribed.[37, 41]

The medication to be introduced is topically applied. It may be in liquid or ointment form. No advantage is gained through medication strength greater than 1% or 2%.[37, 51, 52] In the late 1920s, it was demonstrated that inorganic ions rarely penetrate deep to the epidermis. This is in large part due to the difference in rate of mobility of ions upon exposure to DC. The H^+ ion is the lightest in weight and hence moves the fastest, about twice as fast as $(OH)^-$ and approximately five times faster than K^+, Cl^- and Cu^{++}.[37] Since hydrogen, in one form or another, is normally occurring and in plentiful supply in the human body, excitation into H^+ utilizes much of the DC that passes through the epidermis, leaving relatively little energy to mobilize the heavier atoms. When compounds such as KI, NaCl, $ZnCl_2$, or Cu_2SO_4 are used, their major effect is to liquify (I^-, Cl^-) or to dehydrate (Zn^{++}, Cu^{++}) the skin.

Organic compounds react differently when ionized by DC and do penetrate rapidly into systemic circulation.[51, 52] However, careful preparation of the medication, with particular attention to pH, is essential. Then, primary penetration through intact skin and to a depth of 1 cm is possible.[51, 52]

For both inorganic and organic compounds, the manner in which the specific compound ionizes must be known, as well as whether the effective ingredient will be repelled from the positive or the negative pole. If a medication can be ionized by DC, one or more of the component atoms will be dissociated from the others. Some will become deficient in electrons (H^+, K^+, Zn^{++}, Ca^{++}) and thus are driven into the skin from the positive pole. Other ions will acquire an excess of electrons [Cl^-, I^-, $(SO_4)^{--}$] and hence are driven in from the negative pole. When the component atoms are dissociated by exposure to DC, the primary reaction is the formation of chemical active atoms; second, there will be chemical recombination of these atoms with electrolytes within the living tissue through which they are being driven (and with the electrode metal); third, there will be a reaction of the living tissue to the newly formed chemicals.[37] All of the above reactions will almost always be rapidly attenuated as soon as the driving force is removed.

Electrodes to be used for ion transfer should be separated from those used to cause a contractile response. Some of the inorganic compounds used, i.e. NaCl, will be corrosive to the conducting metal plate. Other compounds will tend to dissolve the felt and/or fabric that normally intervenes between the skin and the metal. Furthermore, it is difficult to rinse out traces of medication from pad electrodes. Thus, if later used for muscle stimulation, an ion transfer treatment may be inadvertently done simultaneously. For these reasons, when medication is in liquid form, many therapists use bare metal electrodes, with care being taken to avoid direct contact with the skin or mucosal surface undergoing treatment.

If the electrodes are of equal size, current density will be equal under each. If they are of different sizes, current density will always be greater under the smaller electrode. If one wishes to treat a large area, or one of irregular contour, i.e. distal forearm, wrist, and hand, an immersion technic is convenient. The contralateral body segment can function as the dispersive area. With an immersion technic, the active and the dispersive electrode should *not* be placed in the same bath. More than 99 percent of the current would then flow through the conducting medication and bypass penetration into the body, thus serving no useful purpose.[15] With the immersion technic, care should also be taken to avoid direct electrode-skin contact.

When treatment is by ion transfer, a major hazard is burn of the exposed tissue. This is due to the use of continuous modulation DC, not the medication. Normal skin will not tolerate an intensity higher than 1 ma/cm^2 of skin surface exposed to this form of DC.[37, 41] If the current is applied to scar tissue or to an area where the skin is abraded or lacerated, the risk of damage is great, since impedance is dramatically lower in such areas. Because of the numbing effect of continuous modulation DC (flooding of the cutaneous receptors), neither the therapist nor the patient may be aware of skin damage until the electrodes are removed.

For all of these reasons, it is recommended that the current density used never exceed 1 ma/cm^2 and that the initial treatment duration not exceed ten minutes. The standard treatment is ten to twenty minutes. Hyperemia is to be expected as skin reaction (capillary dilation) to DC, both poles, irrespective of the medication used.[41]

At this time, at least insofar as complex organic compounds are concerned, when introduction of medication by topical application is indicated, the technic of phonophoresis would appear simpler as compared to iontophoresis.[53-55] This technic is discussed in Chapter 7.

CONTRAINDICATIONS TO USE OF NERVE AND MUSCLE STIMULATING CURRENTS

There are three major contraindications to the use of stimulating currents. The most important is the patient with significant unstable cardiac pathology, especially if the lesion requires use of a pacemaker. Most of the externally applied energy will flow from electrode to electrode in the patient circuit, but inevitably some of the energy will reach the cardiac motor nerve supply, the cardiac muscle, and/or the pacemaker leads. This can interfere with normal function of the pacemaker and hence cause cardiac arrest. Even if the patient is not wearing a pacemaker, if he has an uncontrolled arrhythmia, the stimulus could cause further irregularity in heartbeat. Obviously, the risks would be greater if one or both electrodes were applied anywhere on the thorax, or one on each upper extremity, but it is recommended that nerve and muscle stimulating currents not be used anywhere on the body if there is significant cardiac pathology. Patient selection is the responsibility of the referring physician.

It is also important to realize that if there is clinical evidence of phlebothrombosis or thrombophlebitis, stimulating currents should not be applied adjacent to or distal to the area of mural irritation. There is a definite risk of the induced skeletal muscle intermittent contraction and relaxation causing a fragment of a thrombus to be converted into an embolus. Phlebothrombosis and thrombophlebitis are far more common in the lower extremities than elsewhere in the body.

Lastly, electrodes should not be applied in an area of abnormal skin. The skin impedance may be abnormally high (psoriasis) or low (abrasion or laceration). If impedance is high, high intensity must be used, increasing the risk of skin damage, especially with DC. If impedance is low, this will raise current concentration in a small volume of tissue and can lead to burn, especially with DC.

ELECTROPHYSIOLOGICAL TESTING AND BIOFEEDBACK

DEAN P. CURRIER

Introduction

A neurological examination many encompass many measurements that aid the physician in making a diagnosis. Two such measurements involving electrophysiological procedures are nerve conduction tests (NC) and electromyography (EMG). Nerve conduction tests measure the response of muscle and nerve to externally applied electrical stimuli, while electromyography is the study of the electrical activity produced by muscle as observed from insertion of electrodes in them. These two procedures, together with other tests and measurements, provide valuable information about the status of the motor unit and of the large (alpha) sensory nerve fibers.

The peripheral nervous system (PNS) is the communicative link of neurons outside the central nervous system (CNS). The neuron is the integrator, conductor, and transmitter of pooled information.[56] It consists of cell body (soma), an axon, and dendrites. Of major concern to electromyographic and nerve conduction testing are (1) the somatic afferent neurons connecting the skin to the central nervous system, (2) the somatic efferent neurons linking the CNS to skeletal muscle, (3) the neuromuscular junctions, and (4) the skeletal muscle fibers. Sensory nerve conduction (SNC) procedures examine the functional integrity of afferent neurons (sensory fibers), while motor conduction (MNC) and needle examination procedures assess the functional integrity of motor units. The motor unit consists of the muscle fibers and the neuromuscular junctions in addition to the efferent neuron that supplies them. The recorded electrical activity from muscle and, in the case of sensory conduction, from the nerve branch enables the electromyographer to assess locations of neuron lesions of the peripheral nerves. These locations include the anterior horn cell, spinal nerve roots, plexus, nerve branch, neuromuscular junction, and muscle.

In this division of the chapter on Nerve and Muscle Stimulating Currents we will discuss three procedures of electrophysiological testing and the therapeutic approach of biofeedback. Motor and sensory nerve conduction and the needle examination comprise the procedures used in electrophysiological testing. Techniques of muscle relaxation and reeducation, and thermal control are presented in the discussion of biofeedback.

Fundamentals of Muscle/Nerve Electrophysiology

The cell is the basic source of the electrical activity of muscle and nerve. The cell consists of a semipermeable membrane that separates ions concentrations; the concentration gradient (Na^+ and Cl^- on the outside, K^+ and Cl^- on the inside) forms opposite electrical charges that act as a force. This force serves as potential energy (potential difference) for work. The potential is measured in millivolts; at rest, the voltage gradient or difference is -70 to -90 mv polarity inside the cell relative to the outside. Ions move freely inside the solution of the cell and carry the electrical charge. The potential difference is called the *resting membrane potential.*

If the resting membrane is appropriately stimulated (volitionally, electrically, mechanically, chemically, or thermally), its equilibrium is upset by an *action potential.* In nerve an impulse results, and in muscle a contraction occurs as a result of the action potential. A number of sequential events occur in the resting membrane for the development and propagation of an action potential.

When a stimulus of sufficient strength is produced, its intensity causes the resting potential of the cell to rise from -90 mv to a critical point (-50 to -55 mv) called *threshold.* Threshold intensity is sufficient to upset the equilibrium (voltage gradient) of the resting cell to bring about a rapid reversal of the concentration gradient. A large number of Na+ ions from outside the cell rush in, while a large number of K+ from inside the cell move out momentarily to cause a polarity reversal (transmembrane potential). That is, the Na+ gradient now inside the cell is sufficient to cause the intracellular environment to become positive with respect to its outside. The change in polarity is known as *depolarization.* After the depolarization peaks, the membrane undergoes a recovery period called repolarization (all events last only for several milliseconds), but local circuit currents of threshold intensity flow to another point along the muscle or nerve to depolarize adjacent areas which are in equilibrium.

The events are repeated along the muscle or nerve to cause development and propagation of action potentials along the tissue. These *compound action potentials* constitute the electrical activity of excitable tissue (muscle and nerve), which can be recorded and displayed for convenience of interpretation. If the action potential is produced by an electrical stimulus, the recorded event is a compound action potential that is the summated responses of the individual muscle fibers. In practice, the compound action potential is referred to as a motor unit potential when taken from muscle and a nerve action potential when measured from nerve. Motor unit potentials produced by voluntary effort are referred to as volitional motor unit potentials or simply MUPs, while those produced by electrical stimulation are often referred to as evoked motor unit potentials.

Instrumentation

The measurement of the electrical activity of muscle and nerve requires an electronic system to detect and transfer signals (electrodes) to conditioning components (preamplifiers and amplifiers) for amplifying and modifying them for display (graphic recorders and oscilloscopes). The electrical activity is produced and recorded when muscle and nerve cells are in depolarizing or repolarizing states; otherwise *electrical silence* is observed when excitable cells are in equilibrium (polarized state).[57] In electromyographic or needle examinations and in EMG biofeedback, the above general components are used because action potentials are produced by volitional effort. In nerve conduction tests an electrical stimulator (generator) is used in addition to the above general components to evoke compound action potentials. Nerve and muscle electrodes stimulating generators and electromyographic instrumentation are discussed in Chapter 8.

Electromyographic and biofeedback (BFB) units include an audio amplifier and loudspeaker in addition to visual display components. The harmonic content of the inputted electrical signals is converted into audible sound vibrations by the loudspeaker after being processed and amplified by the amplifier. Audio monitoring systems transmit most signals of the EMG sound spectrum, which are helpful to the examiner for clarifying various potentials and to both the therapist and patient in biofeedback for sensory input of the levels of activity. The audio system used must reproduce sounds accurately (fidelity). The frequency range of the amplifier needs to be 2 to 10,000 Hz for EMG. In both EMG examinations and EMG biofeedback training, the frequency of the sound (pitch) must be clear so that changes in the recorded potentials can be distinguished easily. The electrical activity produced by normal and abnormal motor units can be distinguished by both visual and auditory means

Although the electromyographic unit used for nerve conduction and needle examinations can be used for EMG BFB, it is usually too costly for BFB use, not always available when BFB training is needed, and limited to EMG measurement. Less costly modules with broader capabilities (temperature, skin conductance, heart rate, and blood pressure) are available for BFB. Since only EMG and temperature BFB are considered in this chapter, the instrument differences are discussed.

In EMG BFB the electrodes and amplifiers are similar to that used in electrophysiological testing. Display components differ, depending on the needs of the therapist. In place of the oscilloscope, a ammeter or voltmeter and various lights might have more clinical application in BFB. The meter provides quantitative data of the recorded signals instantaneously, averaged over different periods of time, or both. The advantage of the quantified signals is the digital display. In BFB the shape, frequency, duration, and amplitudes of individual motor unit potentials are of little value. The total voltage (duration, amplitude, and frequency) is the indicator needed to assess a muscle. Lights that change intensities or color are easier for some patients to follow or to monitor electrophysiological signals than a meter or oscilloscope. The audiomonitor can be the same for both testing and BFB functions, but often BFB training regimens can be enhanced if a variety of auditory signals are available to the patient.

Automated printouts of the recorded data are available in BFB instrumentation that add to the convenience of record keeping and monitoring patient progress.

Different instruments are needed to measure temperature data. Electronic thermometers are very useful in BFB training to monitor skin temperature changes. A thermometer that uses a moving coil meter is adequate in BFB training, since temperature changes occur relatively slowly. An electronic thermometer having an accuracy of $\pm 0.5°C$ is desirable for detecting skin temperatures varying over small ranges. A chart recorder interfaced with the electronic thermometer is necessary if progression of the thermal changes is required or continuous monitoring by the therapist is impossible. Variously sized and shaped thermistor probes are commercially available that can be used for monitoring skin, intramuscular, and oral temperatures.

Skin temperature is a function of body surface circulation and environmental temperatures. The ambient room temperature in which BFB training occurs should be controlled within reasonable limits. Room temperature for summer should range between 24° and 27°C and for winter between 18° and 21°C.

The thermistor probe, a semiconductor element, is a sensing device in which the resistance decreases curvilinearly 4 to 6 percent per degree C rise.[2] The circuitry of the thermometer compensates for the nonlinear resistance response to temperature change, so that the operator merely has to read the value indicated on the meter. Electronic thermometers can be adapted to produce changes in sound corresponding to the fluctuations in temperature.

Motor Nerve Conduction (MNC)

The purpose of motor nerve conduction testing is to provide objective information on the involvement or noninvolvement of the motor unit in patients suspected of peripheral nerve problems. Motor nerve conduction, along with sensory nerve conduction and needle examination of muscles, serves as one test of a battery to aid physicians in making a diagnosis or in collecting evidence for assessing the functional integrity of the motor component of a mixed peripheral nerve. Collectively, these examinations can clarify existing or suspected problems such as malingering, hysteria, upper motor neuron lesions, normal conditions, myelopathies, neuropathies, and myopathies. As a separate test, motor nerve conduction can assist in determining hysteria, malingering, and neuropathies. It is in the latter grouping that motor nerve conduction (MNC) characteristics are abnormal (prolonged latencies, slowing of velocity, and decreased amplitude of the MUP).

Preparation of Patient and Electrodes

After the patient is psychologically prepared for the examination, he is placed supine or in a semireclining position to obtain optimum relaxation, comfort, and convenience of procedure. The muscle is selected that anatomically adds convenience to the procedure. For example, the following muscles and their respective nerve supply are commonly selected for MNC testing: abductor pollicis brevis — median; abductor digiti minimi manus — ulnar; extensor pollicis brevis — radial; extensor digitorum brevis — peroneal; vastus medialis — femoral; and abductor hallucis or abductor digiti minimi pedis — posterior tibial. The motor point (point on the skin where nerve enters the muscle, which is usually at the center of the muscle's belly and is the most "electrical point") is located. The skin is cleansed with acetone or alcohol over the areas where the recording electrodes are to be placed (motor point and tendon) to reduce skin imped ance. The bare metal recording electrodes are moistened with electrode jelly; the recording electrodes are then secured in position with tape or rubber straps.

The active (negative) recording electrode is located over the motor point and the indifferent (positive) electrode over the tendon 3.5 to 5.0 cm distal to the active one. Figure 3-6 shows variations of recording electrode positions and their relative effects on MUP amplitude or areas of muscle contributing to the MUP. Davis has shown some possible differences of electrode positioning over normal muscle by using vectors (Fig. 3-6A, B, E, F).[58] The closer the surface recording electrodes are placed over muscle, the larger the amplitude of the MUPs, but the area of muscle contributing to the MUP is less than if the electrodes are widely separated (Fig. 3-6A, B). Figure 3-6F shows the effect of reducing the MUP amplitude when changing the electrodes placed in series to the fibers (unipennate muscle) to a position in which they are parallel to the direction of the muscle fibers. Figure 3-6G is hypothetical but shows that electrode positioning may affect amplitude of the recorded MUP from a bipennate muscle. Figure 3-6H shows that the amplitude of the recorded MUP is affected by recording over certain sections of a multipennate-shaped muscle like the deltoid.[59]

The ground electrode (*see* Chapter 9) is likewise prepared and secured in the appropriate position. Preferred locations for the ground electrode are on the skin between the stimulating and recording electrodes and over bone, tendon, and muscle in order of preference.

The stimulating electrodes (bipolar technique) are moistened with electrode jelly also. Both electrodes are placed (held manually) along the nerve branch, with the cathode (negative) always placed distally. Note that this is opposite to positioning of the recording electrodes. The cathode electrode must be placed over the exact course of the nerve and at a point where the nerve

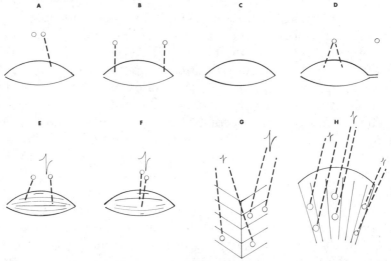

Figure 3-6. Possible influences of electrode positions on recorded motor unit activity.

is closest to the skin surface. Accurate placement of both the stimulating and recording electrodes is essential. In the case of the stimulating electrodes, accurate placement ensures evoking all available alpha motoneurons of the desired nerve and reduces volume conduction. Since the body is a volume of electrolytes, electrical potentials and voltages easily spread (conduct) throughout the surrounding area when stimuli are induced. This spread or conduction of electrical signals in the body is called *volume conduction.* Excessive volume conduction caused by imprecise electrode placement results in recording MUPs generated by adjacent muscles as well as by the selected muscle, and produces excessively large induced stimulus artifact. Volume conduction of this nature is a source of error. The distances at which the stimulating electrodes are located from the recording electrodes can be standardized somewhat (relative to patient's limb length) to increase reliability and accuracy of measurement (Table 3-I).

Procedure

In motor nerve conduction testing, the evoked motor unit potential is recorded and studied to assess the functional integrity of the motor unit. The nerve innervating the selected muscle is stimulated electrically while the motor unit potential is recorded. This, of course, is an oversimplification of the procedure.

Once the recording electrodes are located, the stimulating electrodes are placed on the skin over the nerve branch at a distance previously identified and marked with a felt-tip pen (Table 3-I). The stimulating electrodes are usually manufactured so that their polarity is easily identified (black = negative and red = positive) and can be held manually during the procedure. The stimulating intensity is increased moderately rapidly until a maximum MUP is produced, and then the intensity is increased an additional 15 to 25 percent. A supramaximum stimulus assures the examiner that all large axons supplying the muscle are elicited (stimulated and responsive). A brief single pulse (1 pps) of short duration (0.1 to 0.5 msec) is customarily used.

TABLE 3-I

NORMAL NERVE CONDUCTION AND MEASUREMENT VALUES

Nerve and Procedure	Distal Latency (msec)	Velocity (msec)	Amplitude (sensory = μv, motor = mv)	Distal Distance (stim-to-record = cm)
Femoral				
motor	<4.0	≥56	≥3	9.0-16.0
Median				
motor	<4.5	≥48	≥3	5.5-7.0
sensory	<3.8		≥15	11.0-13.0
Peroneal				
motor	<6.7	≥40	≥2	6.0-8.0
Posterior Tibial				
motor	<7.2	≥40	≥2	14.0-19.0
Radial				
motor	<3.0	≥50	≥4	11.8-13.0
sensory	<3.0		≥15	
Sural				
sensory	<4.8	≥40	≥5	14.0
Ulnar				
motor	<3.6	≥48	≥5	6.0-7.5
sensory	<3.1		≥5	9.0-11.0

Although the selection of pulse durations is arbitrary, short durations cause less skin irritability and patient discomfort than longer durations. Occasionally pulse duration of 1 msec or longer is used when the voltage stimulus is maximum and skin impedance is reduced but no muscle response is recorded. Principles of the strength duration curves must be observed (*see* Chapter 8). The response is then recorded. Be sure that the sweep speed of the oscilloscope is appropriately adjusted to accommodate the responses (2 or 5 msec/division) and the amplifier gain is set at 1 to 5 μv/division. The nerve is again stimulated but at a point more proximally than the first site (the recording electrodes remain in place at initial location). The stimulation and recording procedures are repeated over the second site. The muscle response is again recorded. Precautions must be taken to assure accuracy of locating the electrodes over nerve and to prevent excessively large stimulus artifact by properly locating the ground electrode.

Measurements

The accuracy and dependability of the recorded values depend on techniques of recording and measuring. The *latency* of the recorded response is measured from the beginning of the electronically induced stimulus artifact to the initial deflection (negative or positive) of the electronic baseline (electron beam) of the oscilloscope (Fig. 3-7A, L_1). Both latencies produced by stimulating the distal and proximal sites of the particular nerve are measured. Latencies are measured in milliseconds. (Note: The horizontal lines on the grid [between the vertical lines] of the oscilloscope are used to measure time, msec/division. The vertical lines [between the horizontal lines] denote magnitude in μv/division and are used for measuring amplitudes of compound action potentials.)

The *length of nerve* examined is measured between the two sites of cathode stimulation (from center to center of negative electrodes) and between the distal site of stimulation and the center of the active recording electrode. The distance is measured in

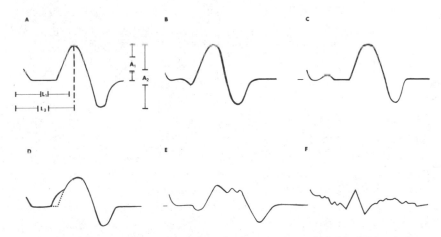

Figure 3-7. Waveforms of normal evoked action potentials and variations caused by disorders. A. Measurement of action potentials. B. Triphasic MUP. C. Nerve AP preceding MUP. D. MUP from atrophied muscle. E. Multiphasic MUP. F. Nerve AP (see text for details; drawings not to scale).

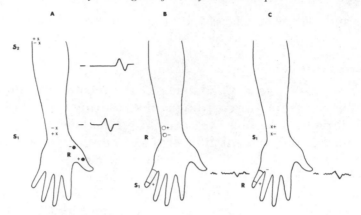

Figure 3-8. Techniques to record — (A) motor unit potentials from the median nerve, and sensory nerve potentials from the ulnar nerve using (B) orthodromic and (C) antidromic methods.

millimeters by the use of a tape measure. If the distance between stimulation sites is divided by the difference of the distal latency subtracted from the proximal latency, motor nerve conduction *velocity* is calculated. $V = \frac{d}{l_2 - l_1}$ where d is distance (mm) between distal and proximal stimulation sites (Fig. 3-8, $S_2 - S_1 = d$), l_2 is latency from proximal stimulation site to negative recording electrode (msec), and l_1 is latency from distal site to negative recording electrode placed over the selected muscle. The following is an example of a median nerve MNC test:

$$V = \frac{220 \text{ mm}}{7.5 - 3.5 \text{ msec}} = \frac{220 \text{ mm}}{4 \text{ m sec}} = 55.0 \text{ meters/sec}$$

Motor conduction velocity values are presented with one decimal place accuracy; the procedure does not warrant more accuracy. Marking the locations of the stimulating cathode with a felt-tip pen will facilitate measurements.

The *amplitude* (size) of the evoked motor unit potential is measured from the baseline to the negative peak of the motor unit potential (Fig. 3-7, A_1). (Note that in electrophysiological measurements negative phases are above the baseline of the oscilloscope, while positive phases are below the baseline.) This measurement can be done either by placing the baseline on a horizontal line of the oscilloscope grid and comparing the height with the calibration signal while stimulation is occurring, or by photographing the signal and comparing it to the calibration signal at a later time. The amplitude is reported in millivolts. Values of the upper range of normal latency and lower range of normal amplitude and velocity are shown in Table 3-I.

Factors Affecting Measurement

Several factors are important for accurate and repeatable measurements of conduction testing.

WAVEFORM AND AMPLITUDE. If the active recording electrode is placed on the skin over the motor point of the muscle in MNC, the propagated electrical signal will reach the motor point of the muscle and the active recording electrode simultaneously. The recorded evoked MUP will then be a biphasic wave with an initial negative phase and maximum amplitude (Fig. 3-7A). The location of the active recording electrode should be changed if the MUP begins with a positive (deflection) phase of its waveform, which indicates that the active recording electrode is not located over the motor point of the selected muscle (Fig. 3-7B). The initial positive deflection indicates that muscle fibers are being depolarized prior to the detection of the compound action potential rather than at the motor point. Also, the waveform recorded from the proximal stimulation site must appear similar to that of the distal site. Exact appearance assures that the same population of muscle fibers was sampled. Any movement of the recording electrodes might negate the exact-appearing waveforms.

Because of the cable properties of nerve and distances involved, the waveform recorded from the proximal stimulation site may be somewhat smaller in amplitude, but 1.5 mv is the maximum allowable difference in normal recordings. For example, the MUP amplitude recorded when stimulating the median nerve at the supraclavicular notch should not be more than 1.5 mv smaller than that recorded when stimulating at the wrist. An abnormal amplitude reduction may also be attributed to the stimulating electrodes not being close to the nerve branch. The size of the MUP represents the number of motor units being elicited by the induced electrical stimuli and is a value to be assessed (Table 3-I).

Other evoked MUP waveforms are also noteworthy. Figure 3-7C shows a normal evoked MUP preceded by a small nerve action potential (NAP). Ignore the NAP when measuring latency in the MNC test. An evoked MUP containing muscle fibers of both the selected muscle, which is atrophied (dashed lines), and an adjacent muscle, which is healthy and has a lower threshold (initial negative deflection) is shown in Figure 3-7. The amplitude of the MUP recorded from atrophied muscle is often reduced. Use of a needle recording electrode rather than a surface electrode will usually avert this situation.

The multiphasic waveform seen in Figure 3-7E shows temporal defects and long duration. Its amplitude may also be decreased from the expected value of healthy muscle. An evoked sensory nerve action potential is shown in Figure 3-7F. Note that the baseline is not straight like that shown for MUPs. The amplifier gain must be greatly increased when recording sensory nerve action potentials, and this increase permits excessive electrical noise. The increased amplifier gain is essential to record the small-sized sensory nerve action potentials that range from 1 to 50 microvolts amplitude.

Intensity of the electrical stimulation effects MUP amplitude. A maximum MUP amplitude is not assured unless a supramaximum stimulus is used. Other effects that reduce the MUP amplitude might be electrode sizes, placement separation, and active recording electrodes placed outside of the motor end plate region.

LATENCY AND VELOCITY. Both the cathode and anode of the stimulating electrodes excite nerve. Muscle and nerve are more sensitive to the physical properties of negative polarity and respond more vigorously to it than to anodal or positive electrode effects. Also, modern electricity theory has current flowing from the negative to positive electrode, which will provide the shortest latency when the negative stimulating electrode immediately opposes the negative recording electrodes (Fig. 3-8). If the polarity of stimulating electrodes is reversed at one site by error, the latency will be prolonged as much as 0.2 to 0.3 msec. In the previous example, if the proximal stimulating electrodes were reversed to produce a latency of 7.8 msec rather than 7.5 msec, the velocity would become 51.2 msec over the same nerve segment of 220 mm. Although these values from polarity reversal are within normal limits, the velocity is nevertheless decreased, and if a patient had borderline values, the examiner's interpretation may be equivocal or wrong.

The position of the limb can influence the latency. Usually a fully extended or flexed joint places nerve on a stretch, depending, of course, on the nerve. Motor conduction measurements have shown that the stretched position may increase conduction velocity. The differences are small, however; limb positions must be standardized if reliable measurements are to be recorded.[59]

DISTANCE. The use of a tape measure placed on the skin overlying the nerve branch is satisfactory for following the anatomical course of the nerve. Measurements taken over joints, particularly the shoulder, can be inaccurate and unreliable unless the joint positions are standardized. The examiner must mark the stimulating and recording sites carefully to assure proper measurement.

TEMPERATURE, LENGTH, AND SIZE. Nerve conduction latency decreases with cold (0.3 msec with each 1°C decrease)[60] and increases with heat (about 0.05 msec with each 1°C increase).[61, 62] The former is of concern if the subject's limbs are cold. Cold limbs are heated to rule out environmental effects from pathological injury factors. Pathological effects of nerve conduction remain in spite of heating a limb by physical means. Conduction is increased upon application of infrared, ultrasound, exercise, and diathermy.[61-63]

Higher conduction velocities occur in the proximal segments than in the distal segments of nerves. This may be accounted for by increased temperatures and by the fact that the size of the nerve branch is generally larger in proximal segments than in distal segments of an extremity.[64] Conduction is slower in the lower extremities than in the upper extremities.

Age

The effect of age on nerve conduction values must be considered when the patient's age is at the extreme ranges. Studies have revealed mean velocities (m/sec) of the ulnar nerve effected by various ages: premature newborn = 20.7; full-term newborn = 27.9; 1 to 3 months = 36.5; 4 to 8 months = 46.0; 9 to 12 months = 50; 2 to 3 years = 52; 20 to 30 years = 58.4; 30 to 40 years = 57.4; 40 to 50 years = 56.8; and over 50 years = 51.3.[65, 66]

Special Motor Conduction Procedure

Motor and sensory nerve conduction are normal in disorders of the neuromuscular junction, myasthenia gravis, and botulism. Evoked MUP amplitudes are usually normal in size with single stimuli, but with repetitive stimuli to the nerve innervating the examined muscle, their size decreases. This decrease in amplitude is accounted for by defects of acetylcholine release and neuromuscular transmission.

Disorders of the neuromuscular junction often show a progressive decrement or an early, but brief, decline in the MUP amplitude following exercise and repetitive stimuli. A brief explanation of the procedure is offered using an electromyograph that has permanent recording capabilities (paper at 2 cm/sec or time-delay photography).

A conventional MNC test is performed on the ulnar nerve of the patient. Without removing the recording electrodes from the abductor digiti minimi manus muscle, the hand to be examined by the special procedure is taped so that the thumb and fingers cannot be abducted or moved. In addition to the taping, the hand and wrist should be clamped between two wooden boards to assure stability and to prevent any movement at the wrist and in the fingers. Movement will mimic the myasthenic defect and result in misinterpretation.

A stimulus rate of 2 pps is selected, with the stimulating electrodes placed on the skin over the ulnar nerve at the wrist. The nerve is stimulated by short trains of stimuli for a total of three stimuli at each step at this rate. The first set of stimuli is applied followed by 15 seconds of rest. The patient is then asked to spread his fingers maximally for 15 seconds (isometric contraction). The next set of stimuli is applied immediately after the exercise and at 15 and 30 seconds after exercise. Stimuli are continued in sets at 30-second intervals until 4 minutes and thereafter at 1-minute intervals until a total of 6 minutes has elapsed following the exercise. Following exercise a total of 12 sets of stimuli (12 × 3 at 2 pps) are applied in step one.

Because considerable variation in response to repetitive stimulation exists among patients having myasthenia gravis, the stimulus repetition rates are increased to 5, 20, and 50 pps. At each step of these varied rates a total of 10 stimuli are applied, and then the rate is increased. Thus, the total procedure involves rates of 2 pps at intervals over 6 minutes and then 10 stimuli each at rates of 5, 20, and 50 pps. The recorded MUPs will show an early drop in amplitude followed by an increase that levels off and remains constant but decreased in size for myasthenia gravis as compared with healthy muscle.

Sensory Nerve Conduction (SNC)

Measurements of sensory nerve conduction differ from those of motor conduction because compound action potentials are recorded from a cutaneous or mixed nerve rather than from muscle. The procedures of measurement differ also. Sensory nerve conduction measurements are more difficult than those of motor nerve conduction because the recorded responses of nerve are smaller than muscle, and because of anatomical factors. Sensory nerve action potentials, however, can be recorded in either direction from the point of stimulus, whereas motor unit potentials are always recorded distally over muscle. SNC tests are often more sensitive to early and mild neuropathies than motor conduction studies.

Preparation of the patient for sensory nerve conduction tests is similar to that for motor nerve conduction tests; that is, skin cleansing and positioning. Patient cooperation is very important to prevent movement during the test procedure.

The noise level of the amplifier may mask the small nerve potentials unless good grounding, patient relaxation, and good technique are used. Good technique includes cleansing of the skin to reduce resistance to the transfer of the signals at the skin-electrode interface, and optimum positioning of all electrodes.

Procedure

Although sensory nerve conduction can be performed on most large afferent fibers, some sensory nerves require special technique or equipment because of their testing difficulty. The median, ulnar, radial, and sural nerves can easily be tested for their sensory conduction without special equipment. Two approaches to testing sensory nerves are available — orthodromic and antidromic methods. The orthodromic method records ascending compound nerve action potentials, while descending compound nerve action potentials are recorded by the antidromic method.

The orthodromic method is performed by stimulating the sensory nerve branch distally and recording the nerve action potential proximally. For example, the ulnar nerve can be stimulated by placing electrodes circumferentially over the skin of the little finger (cathode over proximal phalanx and anode over distal phalanx). The orthodromic method provides stimulation of the digital nerves of the little finger. The recording electrodes are positioned on the skin over the mixed nerve proximal to the wrist. The active electrode is located 2 to 4.5 cm distal to the indifferent recording electrode (Fig. 3-8B). The ground can be positioned on the dorsum of the hand or over the thenar eminence of the thumb. Fortunately, sensory nerve fibers have a lower threshold than motor fibers, and therefore less stimulus intensity is required for evoking compound action potentials. Because of the small size of the potentials, the gain on the amplifier is usually set at 5 or 10 μv/division, while the sweep speed of the oscilloscope is set at 1 or 2 msec/division. The rate of the stimulus is one per second with a pulse duration of 0.1 to 0.5 msec.

Since nerve depolarizes in both directions when electrically stimulated, the antidromic method can be used in sensory nerve conduction testing. The electrode locations are identical to those used in the orthodromic method. The difference between the two approaches is that in the antidromic method the stimulating and recording electrodes change relative to their location (Fig. 3-8C). The stimulating electrodes are positioned proximally (cathode is now distal relative to anode), while the recording electrodes are placed distally. For example, the sural nerve can be stimulated over the skin surface of the mediolateral gastrocnemius 14 to 21 cm proximal to the lateral malleolus using the bipolar stimulating approach with the cathode positioned distally. The evoked nerve action potentials can be recorded by placing the active electrode (negative) over the nerve branch located 1 to 2 cm posteriodistally to the lateral malleolus. The nerve branch can often be palpated at this location near the lateral malleolus. The indifferent electrode can be positioned about 2 to 4.5 cm distally to the active electrode, while the ground plate can be positioned on the skin over the fibula just proximal to the lateral malleolus. The amplitude of the compound NAP recorded by the antidromic method is larger than that evoked in the orthodromic method because anatomically digital nerves are nearer to the skin surface than are mixed or large sensory nerves[67] (Figure 3-8C).

As mentioned, the sensory nerve action potential is quite small (microvolts compared with mv for MNC) and a high amplifier gain (5 to 10 μv/division) is used. Repetitive stimulation, averaging, and storage oscilloscopes are often used in sensory nerve conduction testing. Repetitive stimulation (5 to 25 pulses at 1 pps) can often improve the action potential's image on the grid. The baseline may move during the stimulation, so its position changes horizontally on the grid; however, the compound NAP will remain uniform in waveform at the same point in time on the baseline. Repetitive stimulation then provides a summating effect that can be photographed using the time exposure technique. The baseline will appear all over the photograph, while the superimposed AP will appear in a fixed point on the photograph. The storage oscilloscope provides the opportunity of clarifying the NAP by temporarily storing the repetitive responses for visual inspection and measurement. That is, each time the nerve is stimulated, the NAP is displayed on the grid at a different location in a predetermined pattern (raster) so that each response can be examined for clarity.

Buchthal et al. have offered some tips that help to reduce the stimulus artifact seen in SNC when using high amplifier gain. The stimulus artifact is reduced by grounding with a relatively large ground placed between stimulating and recording electrodes, by not placing electrodes over blood vessels, by separating fingers with cotton to avoid skin contact, and by keeping skin between all electrodes dry.[67]

Measurements

The method of measuring the *latency* and the compound *NAP amplitude* differs from that described for the technique of motor nerve conduction testings. Again the difference in techniques can be attributed to the small NAPs.

The latency of the recorded response is measured from the beginning of the electronically induced stimulus artifact to the center of the negative peak of the nerve action potential (Fig. 3-7A, L_2). Often the initial deflection of the NAP from the baseline is indistinguishable from the baseline, and error can result from the required interpretation. Thus, the negative peak is easy to define and measure. The second latency may be determined by stimulating another location along the nerve branch like that described for the MNC method. Since SNC is more difficult and the compound action potential is smaller than that of MNC, velocities are not usually calculated. By deleting the velocity values for SNC, only the terminal or distal latencies are necessary. The *distance* from cathode stimulating electrode to active recording electrode is measured and recorded so that measurements can be duplicated in serial testing. Latencies should be identical for orthodromic and antidromic methods.

The amplitude of the evoked compound nerve action potential is recorded in microvolts (μv). Amplitude is determined by measuring the distance between the negative peak and the larger of the positive peaks or phases of the NAP (Fig. 3-7A, A_2). The NAP is often a triphasic wave having one large negative peak and two positive peaks (Fig. 3-7F). If the NAP is diphasic, the peak-to-peak distance is recorded. The measured distance between peaks is compared with the calibration of the amplifier for that particular recording to calculate the amplitude. For example, if the recorded peak-to-peak distance of the NAP's amplitude measured 2 cm, or 2 divisions on the grid with an amplifier calibration setting of 10 μv/division, the size of the

NAP is 20μv (2 × 10 μv/division). Normal values of SNC traits are shown in Table 3-I.

The Needle Examination

Following the motor and sensory nerve conduction testing of the patient, the needle examination is performed. The needle examination consists of inserting a needle electrode into a selected muscle, exploring various areas of the muscle, and interpreting the electrical responses observed on the oscilloscope of the electromyograph. The electrical responses of healthy muscle differ from those found in muscle associated with myelopathies, neuropathies, and myopathies.

The electrical activity occurring during a needle examination is described by its waveform, amplitude, duration, frequency, and sound. Electrical activity is recorded and studied by the examiner upon insertion of the active needle electrode; at rest; and during weak, moderate and strong voluntary contractions. Electrical activity occurs concurrently with voluntary contraction of muscle.

The waveform of a compound action potential is described according to its number of phases. Phases are the number of peaks of the motor unit that cross the baseline (isoelectric line) of the oscilloscope. A diphasic potential would have one large negative peak, cross the baseline to form a positive peak, and then return to the baseline. The triphasic waveform is a potential beginning and ending with a positive phase with a negative phase between the two positive phases. MUPs may have jagged peaks, peaks that may approach but not cross the baseline; these peaks are not phases.

In the needle examination the amplitude is assessed from peak-to-peak. The peaks are the largest appearing negatively and positively. If the baseline of the oscilloscope is positioned along the central horizontal line of the grid, the number of lines containing the waveform are counted and compared with the calibration (amplifier gain). For example, if a MUP occupies the space between six horizontal lines and the gain is set at 100 μv/division, the amplitude of the particular MUP is 600 μv (6 lines × 100 μv/division).

The duration is time that occurs between the initial deflection from the baseline until the form of the MUP returns to the baseline. The vertical lines are used to make this assessment. For example, if the sweep speed of the oscilloscope is set at 10 msec/division and the MUP occupies the space between the two lines, the duration is 10 msec.

Assessing the frequency of MUPs is more difficult and subjective than assessing its other traits. If the sweep speed is set at 10 msec/division and the grid contains 10 divisions, the sweep traverses the grid every 100 msec or 0.1 second. The examiner, for example, observes that the same MUP occurs twice during the sweep of the baseline. Since the 100 msec sweep is 0.1 second, it occurs 10 times per second and the MUP is repeated twice during each sweep; the frequency is then 20 per second (2 MUPs per 100 msec × 10 sweeps/sec).

Sounds of the electrical activity are usually characteristic of the potentials appearing on the oscilloscope but may be described differently by different examiners. Some examiners can identify electrical activity by its sound and never look at the oscilloscope, while others may not listen to the sounds. The combination of audiovisual input is often the preferred approach to identifying various electrical signals.

Preparation of Patient and Electrodes

As for nerve conduction testing, the patient should be supine or lying in a semireclining position. Although pillows and sandbags may add to patient comfort, they may not be needed during the needle examination because it requires less time and the patient participates more than in nerve conduction testing. Psychological preparation of the patient is also very important in this phase of the examination because complete cooperation is essential. The patient must be informed about the procedure and assured that every effort will be made to minimize discomfort of the needle insertions. Usually an explanation of the procedure and its importance along with adequate positioning will be sufficient to obtain the patient's cooperation and relaxation.

The ground electrode should be placed on skin overlying bone or tendons on the limb or area of the body where the muscle or muscles to be examined are located at the same site. The specific muscle to be examined is selected. The skin overlying this muscle is thoroughly cleansed with alcohol or a solution that is recommended by the local medical review committee. If a surface electrode is to be used as a reference, it is prepared with electrode jelly and then secured firmly in place over the selected muscle. The sterilized needle serving as the active or exploring electrode is ready for insertion. Caution should be exercised at all times during the examination to avoid its contamination by touching clothing or uncleansed skin of the patient. If the needle becomes contaminated by such accidents, it is replaced immediately by a sterilized needle electrode before proceeding with the examination.

Procedure

The muscle undergoing examination should be completely relaxed. A rapid plunging motion of the needle electrode held at a right angle to the skin surface will minimize patient discomfort. Needles with smaller diameters (25 to 27 gauge) usually cause less discomfort than those with large diameters (19 to 20 gauge). Once the needle electrode has been inserted into the muscle, the oscilloscope grid should be observed. In a healthy muscle that is relaxed, the baseline of the oscilloscope should remain horizontal and only slight hissing sounds should be heard on the audiomonitor. This condition of a relaxed healthy muscle as seen on the oscilloscope is called *electrical silence*. If the needle is moved slightly, electrical discharges from cell membranes can be observed.

Without moving the needle electrode, the next step is to ask the patient to contract the selected muscle weakly, moderately, and finally with a strong contraction. The gain of the amplifier may have to be increased from 100 to 200 or 500 μv/division during maximum muscle contraction in order to observe the peaks of the MUPs. The electrical responses obtained on the oscilloscope grid are observed and noted at each phase of this procedural step. This complete step is repeated by advancing the needle (still at the right-angled position) to two additional depths.

Whenever the position of the needle electrode is to be moved for exploration of another depth or area of muscle, the examiner should withdraw the needle slightly within the muscle (not enough to remove from the skin) and then advance it quickly to a new depth or area. This procedure is repeated step by step many times while examining a single muscle. The examiner should think of a selected muscle as being the dial of a clock. After exploring three depths of the muscle at the initial right-angled position (center of clock dial), the areas of muscle underneath the imaginary three, six, nine, and twelve o'clock positions of the clock are also explored, each at three depths. Each muscle in most cases should be explored at 15 total locations (5 positions of clock dial × 3 depths). Incomplete exploration may often lead to erroneous muscle assessments.

Most skeletal muscles can be examined with needle electrodes, some more easily than others. Muscles representing different dermatomes and innervated by different peripheral nerve fibers of the posterior primary ramus are also explored. Selection of the exploring needle electrode is optional, but the examiner must remember that traits of motor unit activity vary with the type of electrode used.[68] The same exploring and reference electrodes can be used throughout the entire needle examination on the same patient if not contaminated.

Electrical Activity of Healthy Muscle

On insertion of the active needle electrode, cell membranes or fibers are depolarized or irritated, causing a brief burst of electrical activity, which is called *insertional activity*. This electrical activity lasts only for a fraction of a second, and its size (amplitude) is relatively small (40 to 300 μv). Its sound is difficult to describe but has been likened to a "burr" sound.[69] The electrical activity ceases when needle movement is stopped and will recur when the needle is moved.

Because the center of the muscle is usually a site for needle insertion, the tip of the electrode may enter the motor end-plate region, disrupting a small number of vesicles containing acetylcholine. If this occurs, distinctive electrical signals may occur spontaneously at rest — *end-plate potentials*. These potentials are characterized by having an initial negative deflection, short duration of 2 msec or less, small amplitude 10 to 100 μv, and a sound like that heard from a seashell. These potentials occur randomly and independently of nerve impulses and disappear if the needle is advanced slightly to a deeper location.

The *nerve potential* is another type of potential that may occur at rest after the needle electrode is inserted. The tip of the needle may come in contact with a small intramuscular nerve or "twig," which produces potentials having 2 to 3 phases of about 3 msec or less in duration, amplitudes ranging from 20 to 200 μv, regular frequencies (10 to 100/sec), and a continuous rushing sound. The patient perceives pain with the concomitant electrode position. The pain is completely relieved by advancing the needle slightly to a deeper location. The continuous rushing sound may be likened to "seashell" sounds similar to those of end-plate potentials. Nerve potentials occur spontaneously when the muscle is at rest because they are mechanically stimulated by the needle tip.

On weak voluntary contraction, motor unit potentials (MUPs) from single or several units may be recorded and observed. The potentials represent the electrical summation of the action potentials of all muscle fibers of one or more motor units. The characteristics (waveform, amplitude, duration, frequency, and sound) of the MUP are best studied during very weak voluntary contractions. During this condition the MUP may have two to four phases, a duration of 2 to 15 msec, an amplitude ranging from about 100 μv to 4 mv, occur 1 to 15 times per second, and sound like sharp, clear thumps. The amplitudes of MUPs will vary according to the size of the muscle fibers within units, their distribution within the muscle, and the particular muscle.[70, 71] The facial muscles produce small MUPs, while those of the intrinsic muscles of the hand and triceps are large.

Since the strength of muscular contraction determines the number of motor units activated, the *recruitment pattern* is recorded and studied during graduated contractions. Normally, recruitment of motor units increases with increased contraction force until with maximum voluntary effort individual motor unit characteristics cannot be recognized. When maximum effort causes the electrical activity to obliterate the grid, the situation is called *interference* or recruitment pattern. Individual MUPs fuse and summate (increased numbers and frequency of MUPs) to prevent study of the traits of individual units. The gradated recruitment pattern is studied and at maximum voluntary effort it is reported as "full" in healthy muscle.

Electrical Activity of Abnormal Muscle

Insertional activity in healthy muscle ceases when needle movement stops but is often prolonged when the muscle has been injured or diseased (e.g. myotonia). Although assessment of this activity is very subjective, it is often the only abnormality observed as a positive finding in abnormal muscle. This is especially true in some conditions where the muscle appears irritable (very slight prolonged insertional activity) and no other electrical findings are abnormal. Excitability of muscle decreases in muscular atrophy induced by peripheral nerve lesions and thus results in a reduction of insertional activity. However, in most conditions of abnormal muscle the activity is increased because the mechanical stimuli produced by the moving needle may evoke positive sharp waves and fibrillations that may occur when needle movement has ceased.

Electrical potentials occurring after needle movement has stopped constitute *spontaneous activity* in the muscle. Other than the normally occurring insertional activity, end-plate and nerve potentials, spontaneous activity is an abnormal finding in completely relaxed muscle. Positive sharp waves, fibrillations, fasciculations, and high frequency discharges comprise the abnormal spontaneous signals.

Positive sharp waves are characterized by their sharp initial positive deflection from the baseline. They are monophasic or often diphasic with the positive phase dominant. When diphasic, the initial positive phase appears to slowly decay into the shorter negative phase, while the total duration of the potential may last up to 100 msec, occasionally longer. The amplitude is quite variable and may range from 50 to 1,000 μv. They usually occur about 8 to 12/sec but may range from 2 to 100/sec and disappear abruptly. A dull thud may describe their sound.

Fibrillations can be recognized by their biphasic or triphasic form with the initial deflection occurring positively. They have short durations (2 or less msec), relatively small amplitudes (10 to 500 μv), slow rates of 2 to 20 per second, and high pitched sounds that are sharp, resembling wrinkling and crackling of cellophane.[69] These potentials can also be observed on weak voluntary contractions of muscle. Like positive sharp waves, fibrillations can be graded according to their occurrence. A graded scale might be as follows: 0 for absence, + for a single occurrence in a sampling, + + for a few fibrillations in a sampling, + + + for many fibrillations occurring in most samplings, and + + + + for numerous occurrence of fibrillations in all samplings. They can be observed most commonly in neuropathies and myopathies.

Fasciculations may resemble normal motor unit potentials but more often have multiphases (>4) and occur spontaneously. They are associated more commonly with myelopathies involving the anterior horn cells than with neuropathies involving axons. Fasciculations often have prolonged durations (>15 msec), amplitudes similar to normal, and appear arrhythmic at rates of 2 to 15 per second. They may make loud "thumping" sounds. When fasciculations appear on the oscilloscope, nonvolitional muscle twitching can be seen.

Electrical discharges may occur at high frequencies, vary in waveform, and appear as trains of potentials. This group of potentials that usually defy description are called *bizarre high frequency discharges* and are characterized mostly by their variable rates of occurrence. They may appear at frequencies as high as 150/sec and then suddenly slow to 10 to 20/sec. These bizarre electrical discharges can be seen in myelopathies, neuropathies, and myopathies. In the myotonias, these high frequency discharges sound like a "dive-bomber" and are distinctly characteristic of those muscle diseases. In neuropathies, their sound changes with their frequencies, but they do not sound as dramatic as the discharge of the myotonias.

Recruitment patterns of abnormal muscle vary from those of healthy muscle. Any change from the normal pattern is noted. In neuropathies the pattern may contain gaps or "holes" because of diseased motor units, while in myopathies the pattern may be full but the amplitude of the pattern is reduced in size.

Weak to moderate voluntary muscle contractions may reveal two different potentials. *Giant motor unit potentials* are signals that have exaggerated amplitudes, greater than 4 mv. They may also have prolonged durations (around 20 msec) and more than 4 phases. These are seen in diseases of the anterior horn cell where surviving units may hypertrophy to provide the large amplitudes. Other findings are usually associated with these potentials which help to clarify the location of disease. Motor unit potentials having more than 4 phases but differing from those pre-

Table 3-II

USUAL CHARACTERISTICS OF NORMAL AND ABNORMAL COMPOUND ACTION POTENTIALS

	Waveform*†	Number of Peaks	Duration (milliseconds)	Amplitude (microvolts)
Normal				
Motor unit potential		2 to 4	2 to 15	100 to 4,000
Nerve potential		2 to 3	$\lesssim 3$	20 to 300
End-plate potential		1	$\lesssim 2$	10 to 100
Abnormal				
Fibrillation		2 to 3	$\lesssim 2$	10 to 500
Positive sharp wave		2	$\lesssim 100$	50 to 1,000
Fasciculations		$\lesssim 2$	> 15	100 to 4,000
Polyphasic		> 4	2 to 30	50 to 4,000

*Figures not scale
†Negative phase is above baseline

viously described are called *polyphasic* or *complex potentials*. These potentials have durations lasting between 2 and 30 msec, amplitudes between 50 and 4,000 μv, rates of 2 to 30 per second, and sounds that are rough and rattling. Polyphasic potentials can appear in healthy muscle but are considered abnormal when appearing as more than about 10 to 15 percent of all observed signals in a muscle. The deltoid and extensor digitorum brevis muscles may exhibit a higher number of polyphasic potentials than other normal muscles because of the repeated trauma resulting from injections and shoe irritations, respectively. They can occur in increased numbers in myelopathies, neuropathies, and myopathies.

Table 3-II summarizes the characteristics of some normal and abnormal compound action potentials.

Clarifying Electrical Findings

The absence of or combination of positive findings from sensory and motor nerve conduction tests and the needle examination aids the examiner in clarifying the patient's problem. Findings can be grouped as myelopathies, neuropathies, myopathies, or other. The other grouping may include normal, upper motor neuron disease, or malingering and hysterical paralysis. The findings of the "other grouping" essentially are within normal limits (WNL), while those of the other groups need elaboration.

MYELOPATHIES. Spinal muscular atrophy (Werdnig-Hoffman and Kugelberg-Welander syndromes), amyotrophic lateral sclerosis (ALS), spinal tumors, and poliomyelitis are conditions affecting the anterior horn cells within the spinal cord. These conditions are some of the myelopathies. Sensory and motor nerve conduction values are generally normal. Occasionally conduction rates may be slightly reduced but most often are WNL. In severely involved patients, evoked motor unit potential amplitudes may be reduced. Increased insertion activity, positive sharp waves, fibrillations, decreased recruitment patterns, increased polyphasic potentials, bizarre high frequency discharges, giant motor unit potentials, and fasciculation potentials may all be found with the needle examination. Different diseases with the myelopathy grouping may have varied findings from each other, but as a group the distinguishing features of the needle examination are the giant motor unit potentials, fasciculations, and large number of polyphasic potentials.

NEUROPATHIES. In diseases and injuries involving the axons of motor units, changes of conduction traits are strong evidence of pathology. Although not all neuropathies produce positive nerve conduction findings, nerve conduction tests usually reveal normal characteristics in conditions of the other groups (myelopathies and myopathies).

Neuropathies may be caused by (1) exogenous intoxications (lead, arsenic, Dilantin®, thallium, and mercury); (2) degeneration due to lacerations and wounds; (3) segmental demyelination (diptheria and metachromatic leukodystrophy); (4) polyradiculitis (neuronitis, Guillain-Barré syndrome); (5) hereditary (Charcot-Marie-Tooth, Dejerine-Sottas, and Friedreich's ataxia); (6) pressure and ischemia (carpal and tarsal tunnel, and Volkmann's contracture); and (7) metabolic disorders (alcoholism, uremia, rheumatoid arthritis, and diabetes mellitus). Conditions in the various subgroupings of neuropathies can be clarified by variations in the sensory and motor nerve conduction results, and in the findings of the needle examination. Often the clarification is based on whether the motor conduction abnormalities are local or diffuse, or whether sensory conduction disturbances are normal, slowed, or absent. Information gathered from the electrophysiological testing coupled with history, physical data, and laboratory data of the patient assist the physician in making a definitive diagnosis. The general electrophysiological test findings of the various subgroupings are given brief elaboration.

Neuropathies are conditions affecting the myelin and axons of peripheral nerves to varying degrees. Some neuropathies seem to involve both myelin and axonplasmic components of neurons. The rate of conduction in motor and sensory nerves is often slowed and their evoked action potential amplitudes are reduced when the myelin is affected. In conditions with axonal defects, the conduction rates are within normal limits, while the evoked action potentials are decreased in amplitudes. Needle examination may reveal such electrical changes as increased insertional activity, positive sharp waves, fibrillations, polyphasic potentials, reduced recruitment patterns, and increased duration of MUPs. Electrophysiological abnormalities may be difficult to detect on needle examination in mild neuropathies, and no abnormality is revealed immediately after the development of a neuropathic lesion.

Numerous conditions could be listed under neuropathies, but only a few will be discussed, outlining briefly the clinical condition and EMG characteristics. Detailed information can be obtained in books on the subject (*see* Selected Readings).

Certain drugs (nitrofurantoin, diphenylhydantoin, and vincristine) and chemicals (lead and arsenic) are toxic to the peripheral nerves. Neuropathies resulting from these conditions involve mostly changes in the neuron and axon. Toxicity from *lead* commonly is caused by paints and nonethanolic alcohol and may produce slowing of motor and sensory conduction rates, reduced evoked action potentials, and abnormal findings on needle examination. The latter findings may be positive sharp waves and fibrillations in affected muscles. *Nitrofurantoin* (Furadantin®) toxicity may involve nerves of the upper and lower extremities and may cause slowing of motor conduction and decreased MUP amplitudes. *Diphenylhydantoin* (Dilantin®) may cause toxicity of motor and sensory nerves with a prolonged period of drug usage. The predominant motor involvement causes slowed conduction, fibrillations, and reduced recruitment patterns in EMG. *Vincristine* causes reduced MUP amplitudes, while motor conduction rates are usually within normal limits. Needle examination may reveal spontaneous activity such as fibrillations, and decreased recruitment of MUPs.

Charcot-Marie-Tooth disease is an autosomal dominant condition that can be detected in infants by nerve conduction testing, although symptoms may not manifest themselves for several years. Patients having this disease often display marked pes cavus, atrophy, and muscle weakness of the extremities. Motor nerve conduction is slowed. Amplitudes of evoked sensory nerve potentials may also be decreased, along with sensory conduction. On needle examination, fibrillation potentials are seen at rest, while reduced recruitment is found on effort. Another hereditary neuropathy found in some locations where inbreeding of families is high is *Friedreich's ataxia.* Both motor and sensory conduction may be slowed, along with decreased amplitudes of evoked sensory nerve potentials. Needle examination may reveal abnormal electrical activity of peripheral nerve involvement.

Pressure and entrapment neuropathies are identified electrophysiologically most frequently by motor sensory conduction tests. Often sensory nerve conduction abnormalities precede those of motor nerves and show slowing of conduction in the distal nerve branches. Sensory conduction findings may be positive without clinical evidence of impaired sensory perception. When motor nerve conduction traits are abnormal, distal latencies may be increased, along with decreased MUP amplitude and increased duration of the evoked potentials. Needle examination may be unrevealing in many cases, but in moderately severe cases, fibrillations may be found. Entrapment neuropathies may involve the median, ulnar, radial, peroneal, and femoral nerves at various locations along their course. The facial nerve can be included in this group of compression neuropathies.

The herniated disc may cause a root compression (radiculopathy) that results when the nucleus pulposus ruptures from its encasement, the annulus fibrosus. Usual intervertebral disc problems arise from the cervical and lumbrosacral areas with posterolateral protrusions, and occasionally midline rupture. Motor and sensory nerve conduction tests reveal values within normal limits, but this information is of value to establish the pattern of findings of the herniated disc. Needle examination must be done involving myotomes that represent and are supplied by spinal roots under suspicion. The paraspinal musculature must also be examined. Abnormal electrical activity that might be found includes increased insertional activity, positive sharp waves, fibrillations, polyphasic potentials, fasciculations, and sometimes bizarre high frequency discharges.

In addition to entrapment and pressure causing a neuropathy of a single peripheral nerve, neuropathies can result from trauma. Lesions of peripheral nerves may result from tears or stretches, lacerations, and gunshot wounds. The brachial plexus is often the site of such lesions, as well as the courses of the various peripheral nerves. Denervation and Wallerian degeneration often result in abnormal changes of motor and sensory conduction and EMG tests. These changes of peripheral nerve injuries are slowed motor and sensory conduction (latencies and velocities); reduced amplitudes of the evoked action potentials; absence of conduction traits; and such EMG findings as positive sharp waves, fibrillations, polyphasic potentials, bizarre high frequency discharges, increased insertional activity, and decreased recruitment patterns.

Alcoholic polyneuropathy is considered as a nutritional disorder that may result in motor and sensory disturbances in the extremities. If conduction abnormalities are found, sensory nerve conduction findings predominate. Conduction abnormalities may consist only of reduced amplitudes of sensory nerve potentials. Symptoms of burning feet and paresthesias may prevail, yet conduction is often not disturbed or is minimally disturbed. Needle examination of distally located muscles often reveal fibrillation and polyphasic potentials. The voluntary motor unit potentials may exceed 15 msec in duration.

In patients with *renal insufficiency,* both motor and sensory conduction is slowed. Often sensory nerve potentials cannot be elicited in the lower extremities. The amplitudes of the evoked potentials of motor and sensory nerves may be decreased, while EMG findings often show fibrillations. Uremic poisoning may involve both the axon and myelin of peripheral nerves.

Guillain-Barré syndrome is an infectious polyneuritis that strikes mostly adults, and its cause is uncertain. The course of involvement is spotty (segmental demyelination) along peripheral nerves, which may result in severe muscular weakness but normal nerve conduction tests. However, motor nerve conduction changes may occur in all stages of the syndrome and vary in abnormality. Findings on needle examination are often helpful and may reveal polyphasic potentials and some fibrillations. Abnormal EMG activity subsides with improved health of the patients.

These examples serve only to acquaint the reader with some neuropathies and the electrophysiological abnormalities that may follow the various stages of the condition. Books on neurology would serve the best interests of those who are not familiar with neuromuscular pathology.

In summary, the neuropathies can be clarified by abnormal conduction traits of both motor and sensory nerve, along with various EMG findings. Often the decreased recruitment pattern on needle examination accompanied by the slowing of nerve conduction typifies this grouping of conditions affecting peripheral nerves from an electrophysiological standpoint.

MYOPATHIES. Diseases of muscle, unlike the neuropathies, involve only the muscle fibers and the neuromuscular junction. Muscle diseases are fewer in number than conditions effecting the neuron. Myopathies include genetic, congenital, endocrine, metabolic, and infectious conditions.

Myopathies can be clarified electrophysiologically from myelopathies and neuropathies because of some specific differences. Motor and sensory nerve conduction test values are within normal limits in diseases of muscle. Findings on needle examination, therefore, are the distinguishing electrical factors in this group of conditions. Generally, the duration of motor unit potentials is shorter than those seen in healthy muscle and may decrease to values of 1 to 3 msec.[72] Because muscle fibers are involved (destroyed), the number and density of fibers that can be activated in the motor units is often greatly reduced. This situation of reduced numbers of muscle fibers then creates a loss of cross-sectional area of the motor unit territory, which in turn causes the amplitude of the voluntarily elicited MUPs to be smaller than that seen in healthy muscle on needle exploration. The recruitment pattern is full on maximum voluntary muscle contraction. The reduced fiber density is not uniform, however, throughout the affected muscle; therefore, a number of muscles and a number of areas within each muscle must be examined with the active needle electrode. Muscle diseases are often characterized by increased numbers of polyphasic potentials and increased insertional activity.

A group of genetically defined muscle diseases are the muscular dystrophies. They are classified genetically by their mode of inheritance. Severity of the disease ranges from the highly malignant Duchenne form to the benign Becker type. Levels of involvement are described as facioscapulohumeral, distal, limb-girdle, ocular, congenital, and pseudohypertrophic muscular dystrophies. Needle examination may reveal an excessive number of polyphasic potentials. When muscle fibers deteriorate, the surviving fibers do not discharge synchronously, so that many MUPs appear multiphasic. Polyphasic potentials are easily recognized by their complex waveform and distinguishing "rattling" sound. The duration of recorded action potentials is less than that seen in healthy muscle. Of course, not all motor units have muscle fiber destruction, and therefore, many normal motor unit potentials will be seen on the oscilloscope during needle exploration of muscles in patients with dystrophies. On maximum voluntary muscle contraction, the amplitudes of the recruited motor units should be slightly to markedly reduced in size but full in number. Spontaneously occurring potentials are not a common feature of the dystrophies.

Polymyositis is an acquired myopathy that presents inflammation of the muscle fibers, their supporting connective tissue, and overlying skin. Each of these features may occur separately, and therefore, polymyositis can be subgrouped according to structures involved. Muscular weakness is also present. Findings on needle examination are similar to those found in the various subgroup types of polymyositis. The usual findings of myopathies that are seen on needle examination are increased polyphasic potentials, full recruitment pattern with possible reduced amplitude, and decreased durations of many MUPs. Spontaneous electrical activity may be present in polymyositis, along with spotty abnormal findings among the muscle tissue explored.

The myotonias are another unique group of myopathies. Muscular atrophy and weakness are progressive. Distal musculature is often involved more than proximal from a functional point, but needle examination may reveal abnormal electrical activity in proximal as well as distal musculature. Some patients have difficulty relaxing muscles that have been stimulated volitionally, mechanically, or electrically. A distinguishing EMG feature is the high frequency discharges that suddenly decrease in rate and amplitude to produce a characteristic sound of a "dive-bomber" on the audiomonitor. These high frequency discharges may be encountered on movement of the active needle electrode or following voluntary muscle contraction.

Other types of myopathies involving metabolic (periodic paralysis and McArdle's syndrome) and endocrine (Addison's disease and Cushing's syndrome) disorders are seen less often than the dystrophies and myotonias and are not discussed here.

In summary, the distinguishing electrophysiological features of myopathies are normal motor and sensory nerve conduction traits and, on needle examination, increased polyphasic potentials, potentials having short durations, and the decreased amplitude of recruited MUPs on maximum voluntary effort. Other electrical activity such as fibrillations, positive sharp waves, and high frequency discharges may be found in some myopathies. The myotonias are unique among all conditions seen and heard on needle examination because of the "dive-bomber" sounds.

Forms for Electrophysiological Testing

Formats for recording findings during nerve conduction and needle examinations vary widely and are usually adapted to the convenience and needs of a particular facility. Certain basic data should be included for ease of reading, accuracy of interpretation, and convenience of recording. Forms require a means of identification, so the patient's name and record number are included. Demographic information may be provided in varied detail. Often demographic information is available from several sources, so great detail may be unwarranted or redundant on the form for electrophysiological testing. The patient's age may, however, be helpful, along with the date of examination and provisional diagnosis cited on the referral form.

Nerve conduction results can easily be recorded in outline in a predetermined format and area on the form. Useful information includes electrophysiological data. Two different forms are suggested for use in recording. Both forms contain basic data cited. One form should serve as a worksheet to the examiner and include some data not transferred to the permanent record form. Such data of value only to the examiner but not to other readers may include the amplifier gain, distances measured over nerve segments, temperature recordings if any, and any comments on needle examination not for the record. Both the worksheet and the permanent record forms should include (1) nerve stimulated, (2) muscle recorded from, (3) amplitude of MUP (mv) if motor and NAP (μv) if sensory, (4) conduction velocity if motor (m/sec), (5) and distal latency (msec) for nerve conduction tests. The sides of the body are included for all nerve conduction tests, and whenever amplitude, velocity, or latency values are recorded, the normal "cutoff" values should be given in parentheses for the reader's assistance. The name of muscle, insertional activity, spontaneous activity, and activity of voluntary motor unit potentials should be provided in outline format on both the worksheet and the permanent record forms. In addition, the worksheet may include a predetermined format for recording amplitude, frequency, durations, and recruitment patterns of the recorded electrical activity.

Space on each form should be provided for a narrative summary of the nerve conduction test results and for a narrative interpretation of the needle examination. The interpretation should include clarifying remarks about the compatability of the findings with a myelopathy, neuropathy, myopathy, normal response, or undetermined outcome. The examiner's name and signature should be affixed on both forms.

Biofeedback (BFB)

EMG biofeedback (BFB) is really an extension of the needle examination discussed earlier. Techniques of BFB differ somewhat from those of the needle examination, but both have reeducation in common. BFB branches out to involve training of several physiological traits such as temperature, skin conductance, blood pressure, gastrointestinal response, and brain wave control.

Whenever weakened muscles are examined with needle electrodes during an EMG examination, the patient is always encouraged to develop additional motor unit potentials. Patients often increase the electrical activity by activating dormant MUPs after observing the oscilloscope and hearing the sounds emitted from the MUPs. Thus, EMG biofeedback existed in the 1940s but was rarely used as treatment. Various time periods and individuals have been cited as starting biofeedback as a part of patient management. In 1960, Marinacci and Horande reported on the use of EMG for muscle reeducation.[73] Later, Basmajian used EMG to train and control single motor units.[74] Psychologists apparently coined the term "biofeedback" from the engineer's use of feedback and moved clinical research on the subject forward in the 1970s.[75] It should be remembered, however, that Jacobson was using similar techniques in his relaxation training prior to 1938.[76]

Biofeedback is a method or process of providing an individual with information about his/her current physiological status; that is, what is happening inside the body. Any explanation of the scientific basis of BFB must necessarily involve psychophysiological functions. Neural pathways involving sensory input (visual, auditory, tactile), cerebral influence, and motor output enter into the scientific explanation of BFB.

Therapeutically, BFB is used to achieve an improved status over some physiological trait by volitionally controlling or exerting influence on the malfunctioning trait, whether it be motor or autonomic activity.

The physiological basis of recording EMG for BFB training is similar to that discussed for the normal motor unit potential. The electrical activity produced by the contracted muscle or motor units is detected and measured.

The difference in BFB and the needle examination is the technique and a slight change in instrumentation. EMG BFB techniques usually use surface recording electrodes and display the signals quantitatively, while the needle examination displays the recorded electrical activity qualitatively. The basis for BFB using other than EMG signals differs only in instrumentation and the techniques of recording various bioelectrical potentials.

A simplistic concept of biofeedback can be reviewed as the monitoring of a maladjusted or faulty physiological trait (e.g. muscle contraction) by an appropriate instrumentation system so that the patient can make volitional modification of the trait. This instrumentation system detects the bioelectrical signals and displays them in a form that can be visualized or heard by the patient. In other words, knowledge of the operation of the muscle contraction can be gained by observing and listening to the instrument. The muscle contraction or lack of it is then perceived by means of sensory input. The sensory input goes to the central processor and cognitive areas of the central nervous system, where the input is translated and possibly adjusted. Processed input is then relayed from the cortex through the central nervous system back to the muscle. If the inputted information is properly processed, the output or the information fed back to the contracting muscle causes the muscle to adjust to the newly received command. Assuming that the central nervous system is capable of translating, processing, and conditioning input, then the muscle may respond by reducing its activity (relaxation) or increasing it (reeducation).

Biofeedback is incapable of establishing new anatomical pathways but is capable of freeing surviving tract fibers from psychological blocks by relearning. For example, a patient having had a cerebrovascular accident (stroke) may have forgotten how to dorsiflex his foot because of the inflammation, edema, and vascular destruction that may have taken place in the brain. If a few nerve fibers survived the trauma of the stroke and are intact between the brain and muscle, neural communication and control is possible again. BFB training can be of use in reeducating the patient on how to dorsiflex the ankle, but it cannot develop new pathways of communication if the corticospinal, spinocerebellar, and other pathways that connect the peripheral nerves to that particular muscle have been totally destroyed. Wolf has written a good discussion on the anatomical and physiological basis of BFB.[77]

In summary, the activity of a particular physiological trait is monitored by instrumentation, perceived by the patient as both visual and auditory sensory input, processed and conditioned by the central nervous system, and then fed back to the source in a modulated form for a change of function.

Uses of BFB

Biofeedback is a tool to aid the therapist and patient in the patient's therapeutic management. It has limitations like any modality and therefore is not a panacea for clinical use. BFB training has been used in treating cardiovascular problems such as control of heart rate to reduce levels of stress and anxiety, blood pressure reduction in cases of essential hypertension, and management of gastrointestinal disorders, involving the control against incontinence and esophageal spasms.[78] Two areas of BFB that can be used very successfully in physical therapy are EMG and temperature control techniques.

EMG biofeedback is used for increasing tension in neuromuscular reeducation or decreasing tension in muscular conditions requiring relaxation. Neuromuscular reeducation has been used in restoring muscular function in patients having peripheral nerve injuries, tendon repairs, muscle transfers, cerebrovascular accidents, and arthritis. BFB techniques are used for reducing muscular tension in patients with spasticity due to cerebral palsy, stroke, and head injuries, and with tension headaches and stress due to anxiety. Temperature BFB training is used to treat patients with migraine headaches and Raynaud's syndrome.

Method for Muscle Relaxation

Muscle relaxation through BFB training involves two types of conditions: spasticity and muscle spasm. Spasticity is a neuromuscular condition resulting from destruction of one or more of the afferent and efferent nerve tracts of the central nervous system, which in turn results in muscle weakness, dysfunction, and undesired resistance upon movement. Muscle tension, or spasm, is a condition in which the tone of muscle is increased by undesired stimuli from emotional stress, social pressure, or pain. These different types of conditions require different BFB approaches to achieve relaxation or inhibition of stimuli.

SPASTICITY. Spasticity is an abnormal neuromuscular condition that is associated with the chronic stage of lesions of the central nervous system (CNS). Lesions to the corticospinal tracts reduce the normal inhibitory effect of spinal motoneurons on afferent input.[79] Reduced inhibition of the presynaptic impact on afferent nerve fibers results in increased facilitation or overactivity of the gamma motoneurons supplying the muscle spindles of a particular muscle or muscles. The muscle spindles modulate stretch levels of muscles. Since the spindles contain intrafusal muscle fibers, the contraction of these intrafusal fibers serves to increase the sensitivity to stretch. The reduced inhibition of spinal motoneurons then results in a hyperactive state of gamma stimuli, which makes the muscle spindles very sensitive to stretch.

The velocity or rate of passive stretch influences the response of the muscular reaction. A very slow, passive stretch may not result in increased muscular resistance, but a quick stretch will increase resistance. The rate of movement overbiases the nuclear bag by increasing the muscular resistance proportionally to the velocity of stretch.

Spasticity is found predominantly in antigravity muscles.[80] It appears, then, as an overabundance of facilitatory activity in both motor and sensory tracts. It is the result of failure of the neural control system of the CNS.[81] The clinical result is loss of motor control and muscle function. Part of the dysfunction is also muscular weakness. Thus, spasticity prevents or reduces purposeful movement of the affected individual.

The goal of BFB in spasticity is to inhibit or reduce the excessive arousal (overactivity) that is present in muscles and to gain some degree of function in, for example, an extremity. The approach is to teach the patient to decrease the level of overactivity.

Electrodes are attached to the affected muscle after appropriate skin preparation. The initial measurement is a record of the electrical activity with the patient relaxed and the muscle is at "rest." If the resting activity is increased, the patient should be taught to reduce the MUP activity through relaxation. When resting activity of the muscle has been decreased to the therapist's satisfaction, s/he should proceed by passively stretching the muscle at graduated levels of speed. The patient is then taught to reduce the electrical activity of the stretched muscle, which in turn should decrease the resistance encountered to varying rates of stretch. The amplifier and audiomonitor of the BFB system should be set so as to establish targets for the patient to reach. In the case of spasticity, the amplifier gain is continuously reduced by resettings or change of target levels.

BFB seems to work well for training a single muscle and in some instances groups of muscles; however, it fails when complex movements or coordinated patterns are required of several muscles.[82] Individual muscles must be trained separately with BFB, and when satisfactory levels of achievement are reached, other methods of encouraging coordinated movements must be engaged.

DeBacher has suggested a training hierarchy for dealing with spastic muscles of patients. The first approach is to teach relaxation of the muscle at rest; that is, patients must first learn to control the level of muscular arousal when the limb is at rest or when the muscle is not engaged in purposeful movement. The next stage of training involves the patient's learning control of muscular activity during graduated passive and active stretch of the affected muscle(s). The final stage of training involves the relearning of elementary skills necessary for purposeful movement.[82]

Because muscles have neural connections to each other through interneurons, it may be necessary to monitor both agonist and antagonist muscles during the training of spastic muscle. In this manner, the patient knows when the desired action is taking place in the muscles relative to each other; one activates, the other inhibits. When the patient begins to accomplish the target of coordinated movements, BFB can be discontinued and resistance exercises substituted. Unless a major problem occurs in the training program, resistance exercise is minimized until coordinated movement is achieved. The patient is always encouraged to continue his program at home to supplement training with the therapist.

SPASM. Spasm is the discharge of motor unit potential resulting from increased arousal due to emotional or physiological states. Pain is often the contributing factor that causes increased and constant motor unit activity in a particular muscle. Spasm is not a result of neural lesion. The muscular tension produced by spasm can often be palpated but is more easily measured with biofeedback instrumentation. In cases of spasm, the patient may be unable to voluntarily relax the muscle or group of muscles in question. Spontaneous relaxation following a maximum or submaximum muscular contraction is often very slow. Relaxation may be achieved following sleep, special positioning, or treatment by thermal agents, ultrasound, or TENS.

Spasm seems to appear most frequently following strains, periarticular changes in arthritis, and emotional stress. These conditions cause muscle to remain hyperactive for sustained periods of time. Sustained muscular contractions cause increased patient discomfort, and after a period of time the muscle appears to physiologically adapt to the state of increased tension.[78]

The role of biofeedback is to obtain relaxation of the involved muscle. Muscles selected for BFB training often are the frontalis in tension headaches, the trapezius or neck muscles in tension caused by emotional states and cervical arthritis, and the erector spinae in cases of low back strain. The extensor muscles of the forearm may also be used, as well as other muscles, for monitoring muscular tension resulting from emotional states.

The BFB training procedure begins by preparing the patient psychologically and by positioning the patient in such a fashion (supine or sitting) as to encourage relaxation and to effect movement and observation by the therapist. An unaffected muscle may be measured before beginning the training of the affected muscle. This approach is taken to teach the patient about electrical silence when a muscle is at rest and about the recorded MUP activity at various levels of contraction (recruitment). Thus, the patient must understand what to expect in normal EMG training. A baseline measurement of the existing motor unit activity is taken, and target levels are set on the EMG biofeedback instrumentation.

BFB relaxation training of patients having muscle spasm is similar to that described in the treatment of spasticity. Target levels for the patient to achieve during training sessions are set and reset. The target values are documented in the patient's record for recall during serial sessions. Various imagery or phrases are used by the patient.[83] Imagery or phrases may be suggested by the therapist to support or reinforce the relaxation training. Deep breaths are also often helpful to the patient in achieving relaxation.

Muscle Reeducation

Many disorders of the neuromuscular system result in a hypotonic condition of muscle. Lesions of the central and peripheral nervous systems, muscle tendon transfers or repairs, hysterical paralysis, immobilization, and contractures may contribute to the decreased muscular activity. The role of BFB in these conditions is to teach the patient to regain control of muscle function. Whether muscle dysfunction is mild (paresis) or severe (paralysis), the patient must relearn the coordinated activity of nerve impulse transmission from the CNS to activate and control motor units. In the course of the existing disorder, the patient may have forgotten how to transmit nerve impulses to activate the muscle fibers that bring about contraction and joint movement. This is often the situation confronting the patient who has had a cardiovascular accident (CVA or stroke), in which the events of the disorder often result in a partial reversible physiological block of the nerve transmission in afferent and efferent tracts. This block of transmission may be due to the inflammatory and destructive process acting upon nerve cells.

The patient having a form of muscle hypotonus must undergo a relearning process. BFB training is successful only when some motor nerve fibers survive the destruction of the neuromuscular process. Patients with long-standing conditions in which muscle fiber fibrosis (replacement of contractile tissue with noncontractile fibrous or fatty tissue) has occurred have little chance of benefiting from BFB.

After psychological and physical preparation of the patient, the muscle is selected. Once selected, surface electrodes are properly applied. Since hypotonus may mean a scarcity of surviving motor units or limited CNS connection with normal motor units, surface electrode placement is critical. The possible influencing factors on electrode positioning is important in BFB, as explained earlier for nerve conduction tests. In BFB, the waveform of the recorded MUP is unimportant, but its voltage or size is important because this trait contributes to the value reached on the meter. In the case of a scarcity of recorded MUP activity, the therapist is advised to increase the distance separating the electrodes.[84] The risk of performing the latter is the increased chance of recording MUPs from an activated muscle lying beneath or near the particular muscle selected for training. The essential concern is to determine whether any motor unit activity can be recorded from the affected muscle. If this determination cannot be made satisfactorily with surface electrodes, then needle examination of the muscle must be made in the same manner as discussed previously. If needle exploration is performed and one or more MUPs are found, muscle reeducation takes place while the muscle is being explored.

Verbal encouragement by the therapist is very helpful, as well as the employment of internal imagery by the patient. Similar procedures are repeated during subsequent training sessions with the patient. The gains on the amplifier and audiomonitor are set so that targets are established for the patient's achievement. Once voluntary control is achieved, the patient is encouraged to repeat examples of contraction and relaxation. Target levels can be set on the BFB unit that challenge the patient's efforts to reach them. The patient must be able and willing to concentrate on the training procedures. In addition to verbal commands and patient imagery, electrical stimulation, tendon and muscle taps, brushing of the skin, reflex and PNF patterns, and passive movement or stretch of the limb may help facilitate motor unit activity. Whenever the patient can voluntarily contract the muscle to a poor grade, BFB may be discontinued on that particular muscle in favor of another that is weaker.

Temperature Biofeedback

Monitoring skin temperature of patients with migraine headaches and Raynaud's syndrome is a convenient and conservative way of managing the disorders. The tip of one or more fingers or the palmar surface of the hand is connected to an electronic thermometer by means of a thermistor probe. A baseline measurement is made and recorded after a few seconds. BFB training is then aimed at warming the hand.

The process of controlling temperature is usually considered a function of the autonomic nervous system. In BFB, the temperature of the skin is imputed to the thermometer, which the patient then visualizes. This information is then transmitted to the cerebral cortex to exert influence over the limbic system (emotional and mental responses) and hypothalamus. The processing and conditioning of the CNS results in a changed temperature of the hand.

Migraine headaches are apparently a result of vasodilation of branches of the external carotid artery. The continous state of dilation during periods of anxiety and emotional stress causes pain to the individual. The patient can be taught to increase his finger or hand temperature and by so doing can bring about constriction of the external carotid artery, which then results in decreased pain.[85]

After the therapist explains to the patient the rationale of BFB and the training procedures, the thermistor probe is attached to the middle finger or palmar surface of the dominant hand. The training sessions consist of imagery and phrases suggesting warmth. Having the patient close his/her eyes often helps relaxation. Green has suggested that the face of the electronic thermometer be turned away from the patient during the initial training session.[86] Personal experience indicates that having the patient face the thermometer is easier than having him/her not facing it. Several sessions may be necessary for the patient to achieve the established goals. Treatment can be dramatic when conducted during an episode of migraine headaches. Once the patient achieves relaxation and temperature control satisfactorily, measurements can be made before and after a session without the patient connected to the thermometer during the training. The ultimate goal of the BFB thermal training is for patient control of hand temperature during states of anxiety and emotional stress to prevent or reduce migraine headaches.

The BFB approach to patient with Raynaud's syndrome is similar to that for treatment of migraine headaches. The patient concentrates on warming his/her hands to diminish the discomfort of cold. Successful treatment is accomplished when the patient can reduce finger discomfort by internal control.

Training Imagery and Phrases

The patient is instructed to visualize and imagine the body responding to these phrases. They can be repeated by the therapist or imagined by the patient by means of autogenic training.[83]

RELAXATION EXAMPLES:

Imagine that you are a bird and are gliding with the air currents.
Imagine how it feels to lie in bed on Saturday mornings.
You are lying on an air mattress in a pool.
Your arms feel heavy and floppy.
Imagine tension running down and out of your arm.
Imagine that you are a rag doll.

WARMTH EXAMPLES:

You are wrapped in warm towels just taken from the dryer.
Imagine that you are jogging on a hot day.
Imagine rubbing your hands over a warm fire.
Think about lying on a hot beach.
Imagine cutting grass on a hot August day.
My body is relaxed, my hands are warm, they are getting warm-
    er.

BFB Training Program

Techniques and approaches of BFB used for neuromuscular disorders may vary, but some basic steps should be considered by therapists. This section outlines some of the basic steps.

EVALUATION AND ORIENTATION. Patient evaluation is essential on initial visit to determine whether BFB is needed and whether patient benefits are possible. Patients must be prepared for BFB evaluations through psychological and physical approaches. They must receive an explanation of the procedures, what to expect, and assurance that evaluation techniques are harmless. The explanations need not be as elaborate for the evaluation phase as for the treatment phase, but the patient's confidence and cooperation must be gained. The patient can be made comfortable by positioning and support with the use of pillows and sandbags. After this preparation, a normal muscle is tested and used to teach the patient what is being attempted. Affected muscles are evaluated, and measurements are taken and recorded.

If the patient is accepted for BFB training, roles of the therapist and patient should be discussed briefly, along with possible patient expectations. In addition to the therapist's customary responsibilities towards patients, s/he must constantly evaluate the patient to modify treatment when indicated, set target values and goals to be achieved, and select modes of training and their termination. The patient receiving BFB training must accept an increasing role in his/her treatment. The patient must be willing to learn, modify his/her life-style if it affects the outcome of the established goals, agree to cooperate fully with treatment procedures, and supply information.[78] Goals are established from this data and treatment is started.

TREATMENT. Baseline measurements are taken at the beginning of each session, and progress will be compared with these values. Target values are set for particular sessions. The therapist should get the patient started each session. Sometimes patients can be left alone during parts of the session, but periodic checks by the therapist are essential. The environment of the training area is very important and must be conducive to learning and concentration. Overstuffed chairs that can be adjusted are often useful in addition to a comfortable treatment table. The room should be free of extraneous noises and interruptions by others. The lighting should be soft and comforting. Because learning is most productive with short lengths of practice, sessions should last twenty to thirty minutes. Inpatients may benefit from two or more sessions per day, while outpatients should be seen two or three times per week until they can manage more on their own. Outpatients often benefit by using a BFB at home with several sessions daily.

Careful planning should be exercised when terminating treatment. The patient should undergo a trial period without use of the BFB instrumentation. Upon follow-up evaluation by the therapist, a successfully treated patient can be terminated. Of course, the number of treatment sessions depends on the results of the evaluation. If evaluations indicate little progress achieved with a few sessions, and that additional treatment is likely to fail also, BFB should be terminated. BFB treatment should be terminated when relaxation is achieved and when a poor grade of muscle tension is reached by reeducation procedures. Exceptions may be made when dealing with patients having spasticity. Spasticity is difficult to overcome and requires longer periods of training than many other conditions treated with BFB.

Training Theories and Approaches

Several clinical approaches to BFB have used learning theories. The theories and the BFB techniques differ. The physical therapist should have these approaches at his disposal whenever modification of treatment is indicated through evaluation.

OPERANT CONDITIONING. This approach rewards the patient for performance to achieve behavioral modification and learning. The recorded MUP activity is used as the reward, and when a particular level is reached by the patient, a new target level is set. The target levels of MUP activity are set according to whether the new performance should be easier or more difficult to achieve than the previously specified physiological goal. The reward of achieving a target level of MUP activity provides an opportunity for the patient to learn associations between stimuli encountered in the course of producing the given response and the rewarding outcome. The mechanism producing facilitative feedback is activated by increases and inhibited by decreases in anticipation of reward. Successful use of operant condition in BFB requires that the patient learn that altering a stimulus situation in one direction increases the chance of reward and changing it in the other direction decreases chances of reward. In EMG reeducation, the patient is instructed to increase his motor unit activity; the reward will be received whenever the target level of activity is reached.

Patients will differ in their rate of acquisition of perceptual motor skills. These rates may be related to differences in attentiveness to the procedure and verbal phrases or imagery used. The therapist can begin the training by setting target levels that can be easily achieved and then increasing the levels of difficulty. Verbal instruction can be altered with more or less encouragement or reinforcement. The effectiveness of the reward must be maintained in operant conditioning for continued success.

PROGRESSIVE RELAXATION. Jacobson was a pioneer in the work of relaxation. He maintained that stress was caused by demands of society, money, war, employment, and family responsibilities and that it resulted in heart attacks, ulcers, and high levels of tension manifested in personalities. His studies showed that stress and anxiety levels produced alterations in physiological traits such as irregular breathing, increased pulse rates and blood pressures, frequent frowning, and increased sensitivity to sudden noises.[87, 88]

His method of progressive relaxation advocated the avoidance of body positions that facilitate sensory input. He discouraged folding arms or crossing legs, which increases tactile stimulation, but encouraged supporting body parts while resting and closing the eyes when resting. He discouraged the use of verbal phrases to instruct patients in physical relaxation because he believed talk distracted mental awareness. He taught patient imagery that could be used in concentration of progressive relaxation procedures. Patients recognized tenseness by first strongly contracting muscles in different parts of the body. After the patient acquired a thorough understanding of Jacobson's method, he would practice relaxation by sitting or lying down in a quiet room. Muscles of the feet would be contracted, and then relaxation would follow with use of mental exercises. The procedure of contract-relax would then progress from the feet to the legs, trunk, arms, neck, and face. Patients were encouraged to learn to relax during active phases of their daily activities.[76, 78]

Autogenic Training

The autogenic method (self-generated physiological activity) was an outgrowth of therapeutic hypnosis. The patient practices relaxation by using self-suggested imagery. The self-suggested imagery usually involves abstract qualities, and the patient usually focuses his mental concentration on a single activity during the course of practice. Phrases such as "my hand is warm" and "my arm is floppy" are used for all parts of the body in relaxation training. By focusing attention on warming of the hand, the patient with migraine, for example, can elevate hand temperature while constricting the external carotid artery to effectively relieve headaches.

The procedure focuses on muscular tension and skin temperature with imagery of a single activity. The patient can begin with his eyes closed and concentration directed on the one activity. Imagery phases are repeated slowly by the patient. The physiological responses are monitored and target levels established according to the recorded values.

Conclusion

Nerve conduction tests and electromyography are performed together and use the same console equipment to clarify patient problems suspicioned as being myelopathies, neuropathies, or myopathies. They are electrophysiological test procedures.

In nerve conduction, the compound action potential is evoked to provide measurements of latency, amplitude, and velocity. The measurements are useful in studying various neuropathies because they become altered in these disorders. Measurements of nerve conduction traits are generally normal in myelopathies and myopathies. Various factors, such as nerve segmental distance, muscles selected, age, temperature, and axonal diameter, influence nerve conduction traits. The results of nerve conduction tests supplement the findings of electromyography.

The procedure for electromyography (EMG) uses the insertion of a needle in muscle to assess the functional integrity of motor units. Electrical activity of muscle is studied during needle insertion and when the muscle is at rest and at various graduated levels of contraction. Such motor unit traits as waveform, amplitude, duration, frequency, and sounds are studied during the needle examination.

Biofeedback (BFB) is a therapeutic agent using instrumentation to monitor various physiological traits and to feed this information to the patient by visual or auditory means. The patient, in turn, interprets the sensory input and modifies the physiological trait being monitored. BFB is a very useful tool to the therapist for achieving muscle relaxation and reeducation goals. Thermal BFB provides a convenient approach to treating patients with migraine headaches or Raynaud's syndrome.

This section constitutes an overview on the topics discussed. Readers seeking detailed information should consult the following books on electrophysiological testing and biofeedback.

Selected Readings

Aminoff, M. J. (Ed.): *Electrodiagnosis in Clinical Neurology.* New York, Churchill Livingstone, 1980, Chapters 6-9, 13.
Goodgold, J. et al.: *Electrodiagnosis of Neuromuscular Diseases,* 2nd ed. Baltimore, Williams & Wilkins, 1978.
Johnson, E. W. (Ed.): *Practical Electromyography.* Baltimore, Williams & Wilkins, 1980.
Lenman, J. A. R. et al.: *Clinical Electromyography,* 2nd ed. New York, Lippincott, 1976.
Mayo Clinic: *Clinical Examinations in Neurology.* Philadelphia, Saunders, 1976.
Smorto, M. P. et al.: *Electrodiagnosis: A Handbook for Neurologists.* New York, Harper & Row, 1977.

SUMMARY

Clinical use of nerve and muscle stimulating currents increased greatly during the 1970s. The biggest increases in demand have been for —

1. Relief of chronic pain (TENS)
2. More effective management of CNS lesions leading to spasticity
3. Biofeedback training

One must now be acutely aware of whether the generator delivers the classical low voltage milliamperage current (either AC or DC) or whether the generator delivers high voltage microampere stimuli (DC only). For the patient who is abnormally sensitive to electrical stimulation, the high voltage stimulators seem to be more comfortable in most cases.

Techniques, equipment, and rationale are discussed in detail. In the last several decades there have been two major developments in the classical stimulators — more and more models are supplying a wider continuous modulation frequency range. When this includes low frequency AC, the need for DC is diminished. The other major development in low volt stimulators has been the appearance of practical battery-powered stimulators, which have proven highly successful in management of chronic pain.

As of the 1980s, the practicing therapist should think about using electrical stimulation whenever the patient has lost (or never had) voluntary control over skeletal muscle, or whenever chronic pain is a significant handicap.

The major contraindication for use of electrical stimulation is in the presence of an unstable cardiac pathology, particularly if the patient wears a pacemaker. Electrical stimulation should also be avoided when there is clinical evidence of thrombophlebitis or phlebothrombosis underneath or proximal to desirable electrode placement.

APPENDIX A
EASILY LOCATED MOTOR POINTS—THEIR APPROXIMATE LOCATION AND RESPONSE TO STIMULUS

A. *Neck and Trunk*

Muscle	*Location*	*Action*
1. Sternocleidomastoid	Anterolateral neck, midway between the mastoid process and the sternal notch	Acting separately, the muscle laterally flexes the neck toward the shoulder on that side or, if the neck is fully rotated, flexes the neck toward the thorax
2. Upper Trapezius	Superior border of the shoulder, midway between the spinous and acromion processes	Elevation of the scapula with slight lateral rotation of the inferior angle
3. Middle Trapezius	On the posterior scapula, near the vertebral border and slightly inferior to the spine of the scapula	Adduction of the scapula toward the spinous processes
4. Lower Trapezius	3 to 5 cm lateral to spinous processes T9 or T10	Diagonal pull between spinous processes and acromion, resulting in medial rotation of the inferior angle and depression of the scapula

	Location	Action
5. Rhomboids	Between the spinous processes and the vertebral border of the scapula and inferior to the spine of the scapula	Diagonal pull of the inferior angle of the scapula up and toward the spinous processes
6. Latissimus Dorsi	Posterolateral aspect of the trunk, inferior to the scapula but usually on the thorax	Shoulder depression
7. Serratus Anterior	Lateral aspect of the thorax and on (*not* between) ribs 6 through 9	Scapular abduction
8. Pectoralis Major	Anteroateral thorax, 3 to 5 cm superior to the nipple	Humeral adduction

B. Upper Extremity (*cont'd.*)

Muscle	Location	Action
1. Anterior Deltoid	Anterior proximal third of the humerus, midway between the acromion process and the deltoid insertion	Flexion of the humerus
2. Middle Deltoid	Lateral proximal third of the humerus, midway between the acromion process and the deltoid insertion	Abduction of the humerus

Appendix A (cont'd.)

B. Upper Extremity

Muscle	Location	Action
3. Posterior Deltoid	Posterior proximal third of the humerus, midway between the acromion process and deltoid insertion	Extension of the humerus
4. Coracobrachialis	Medial proximal third of the humerus, best found when humerus is in 90° abduction and full external rotation. Caution — median and ulnar nerves are close and if stimulated will cause strong wrist and finger response	Adduction of the humerus
5. Biceps Brachii	Anterior middle third of the humerus	Flexion of the elbow
6. Brachialis	Lateral (usually) or medial distal third of the humerus	Flexion of the elbow
7. Triceps Brachii	Posterior middle third of the humerus	Extension of the elbow

8. Extensor Carpi Radialis Longus	Dorsal proximal third of the forearm, toward the thumb side	Dorsiflexion and radial deviation of the hand
9. Extensor Carpi Radialis Brevis	Dorsal forearm at the junction of upper and middle thirds, toward the thumb side	Dorsiflexion of the hand without radial deviation
10. Extensor Digitorum	Dorsal forearm distal third, toward the thumb side	Extension of the metacarpal phalangeal of the four lesser digits. Rarely will stimulation of the motor point cause all digits to respond
11. Extensor Carpi Ulnaris	Proximal dorsal third of the forearm, toward the ulnar side	Dorsiflexion of the hand with ulnar deviation
12. Extensor Indicis Proprius	Dorsal middle third of the forearm, midway between the radius and ulna	Extension of all joints of the index finger
13. Abductor Pollicis Longus	Dorsal distal third of the forearm, toward the thumb side	Abduction of the metacarpal phalangeal joint in the plane of the forearm along with extension of the distal phalanx
14. Extensor Pollicis Longus	Dorsal distal third of the forearm, toward the thumb side — usually more distal and more lateral than the abductor	Extension of the distal phalanx of the thumb

Appendix A (cont'd.)

B. Upper Extremity (cont'd.)

Muscle	Location	Action
15. Dorsal Interossei	Dorsal aspect of the hand, 2 to 3 cm proximal to the metacarpal phalangeal joints and between them	Abduction of the metacarpal phalangeal joints individually
16. Lumbricales	Usually found on dorsal aspect of the hand 1 to 2 cm proximal to the metacarpal phalangeal joints. If palmar fat pads or callus is not thick, it may be found on the volar hand at this level	Flexion of the metacarpal phalangeal joint plus extension of the distal phalanx
17. Volar Interossei	Dorsal hand between the motor point for dorsal interossei and lumbricales	Adduction of the metacarpal phalangeal joints individually
18. Brachioradialis	Proximal third anterior (volar) forearm, toward the thumb side	Elbow flexion plus forearm rotation toward neutral
19. Pronator Teres	Proximal third anteromedial forearm	Forearm pronation with slight elbow flexion
20. Flexor Carpi Radialis	Proximal third anterolateral forearm	Flexion and radial deviation of the hand

21. Flexor Carpi Ulnaris	Proximal third anteromedial forearm	Flexion and ulnar deviation of the hand
22. Flexor Digitorum Sublimis	Middle third anterior (volar) forearm midway between the radius and ulna	Flexion of the metacarpal phalangeal joints
23. Flexor Digitorum Profundus	Distal third anterior forearm, toward the little finger side	Flexion of the distal phalanges of the fingers
24. Flexor Pollicis Longus	Distal third anterior forearm, toward the thumb side	Flexion of the distal phalanx of the thumb
25. Abductor Pollicis Brevis	Proximal thenar eminence, close to the carpometacarpal joint	Radial (anterior) abduction of the carpometacarpal joint of thumb
26. Opponens Pollicis	Anterolateral thenar eminence, midway between the carpometacarpal and metacarpophalangeal joints	Rotation of the thumb so that the thumbnail rotates from lateral toward anterior
27. Flexor Pollicis Brevis	Medial thenar eminence	Flexion and adduction of the carpometacarpal joint of the thumb
28. Adductor Pollicis Brevis	Distal thenar eminence	Adduction and slight flexion of the carpometacarpal joint of the thumb
29. Flexor Digiti Minimi Manus	Anteromedial hypothenar eminence at the midpoint of the fifth metacarpal bone	Flexion of the metacarpophalangeal joint
30. Abductor Digiti Minimi Manus	Medial aspect of the hypothenar eminence either distal or proximal to the motor point of the flexor	Abduction of the metacarpophalangeal joint

C. Lower Extremity (cont'd.)

Muscle	Location	Action
1. Gluteus Medius	Lateral pelvis, 2 to 5 cm posterior to a line between the anterior superior iliac spine and the greater trochanter	Abduction of the femur
2. Gluteus Maximus	On the buttock within a circle of 2 cm radius surrounding the ischial tuberosity	Extension of the femur
3. Semimembranosus	Posteromedial thigh, midway between knee and hip joints	Knee flexion
4. Semitendinosus	Posterior distal third of the femur, slightly towards medial	Knee flexion
5. Biceps Femoris, Long Head	Posterior thigh at the junction of the upper and middle third	Knee flexion
6. Biceps Femoris, Short Head	Distal third of the posterolateral femur	Knee flexion
7. Rectus Femoris (Quadriceps)	Anterior thigh, midway between hip and knee	Knee extension
8. Vastus Medialis (Quadriceps)	Anterior femur, distal third, slightly medial	Knee extension

9. Vastus Lateralis (Quadriceps)	Anterolateral femur, distal third	Knee extension
10. Sartorius	Anterior proximal femur, on a line between the anterior superior iliac spine and the medial condyle of the tibia	Hip and knee flexion
11. Adductor Longus	Medial thigh at the junction of the proximal and middle third	Adduction of the femur
12. Gracilis	Medial middle third of the femur	Adduction of the femur
13. Adductor Magnus	Medial distal third of the femur	Adduction of the femur
14. Tibialis Anterior	Slightly lateral to the crest of the tibia, 5 to 10 cm inferior to the head of the fibula	Ankle dorsiflexion with inversion of the foot
15. Extensor Digitorum Longus	Lateral calf, 5 to 10 cm distal to the head of the fibula, on a line between the head of the fibula and the lateral malleolus	Extension of the distal phalanx of the lesser toes
16. Peroneus Longus	Lateral aspect of the calf, slightly posterior to a line from the head of the fibula to the lateral malleolus, 10 to 15 cm inferior to the head of the fibula	Ankle plantar flexion with eversion of the foot

Appendix A (cont'd.)

C. *Lower Extremity*

Muscle	Location	Action
17. Peroneus Brevis	Lateral aspect of the calf, 15 to 20 cm inferior to the head of the fibula	Eversion of the foot
18. Extensor Hallucis Longus	Distal third of the tibia, slightly lateral to the crest of the tibia	Extension of the distal phalanx of the great toe
19. Extensor Digitorum Brevis	Dorsal aspect of the foot, midway between the ankle and tarsometatarsal joints	Extension of the proximal phalanx of the toes
20. Gastrocnemius (lateral head)	Posterolateral aspect of the proximal third of the tibia, 5 to 10 cm distal to the head of the fibula	Ankle plantar flexion
21. Gastrocnemius (medial head)	Posteromedial aspect of the tibia 15 to 20 cm distal to the popliteal space	Ankle plantar flexion
22. Soleus	Posterior calf, 10 to 15 cm proximal to either the lateral or medial malleolus	Ankle plantar flexion
23. Flexor Hallucis Longus	Posterior to the lateral malleolus	Flexion of the distal phalanx of the great toe

24. Flexor Digitorum Longus	Posterior to the medial malleolus	Flexion of the distal phalanx of the four lesser toes

D. Facial Muscles

Muscle	*Location*	*Action*
1. Frontalis	3 to 5 cm superior to the medial third of the eyebrow	Horizontal wrinkling of the forehead skin
2. Corrugator	1 cm superior to the medial border of the eyebrow	Draws the eyebrow toward midline and causes vertical wrinkling of the forehead skin
3. Orbicularis Oculi Superioris	1 cm superior and slightly lateral to the lateral corner of the eyelid	Raises the upper eyelid
4. Orbicularis Oculi Inferioris	1 cm inferior to the midline of the lower eyelid	Opens the lower eyelid
5. Nasalis	At the junction of the nostril and face	Nostril flares
6. Zygomaticus	1 to 2 cm inferior and medial to the angle of the mandible with the zygomatic arch when the mouth is closed	Upper lip moves laterally and superiorly

Appendix A (cont'd.)

C. Lower Extremity (cont'd.)

Muscle	Location	Action
7. Quadratus Labii Superioris	Midway between the nostril and upper lip	Upper lip closes
8. Quadratus Labii Inferioris	1 cm inferior to the lower lip, closer to the corner than to the midpoint of the mouth	Lower lip closes
9. Orbicularis Oris	1 to 2 cm lateral to corner of the mouth	Upper and lower lips close simultaneously
10. Mentalis	1 cm lateral to the point of the chin	Vertical wrinkling of the skin of the chin

APPENDIX B
MOTOR POINT AND DERMATOME CHARTS

* * *

As there are many anatomical variations, the charts are standardized in reasonable manner.

Segmental innervation of muscles is taken from *Gray's Anatomy* published by Lea and Febiger.

The following abbreviations are used:

M — Muscle
N — Nerve
B — Branch of Nerve
C — Cervical Nerve Roots
T — Thoracic Nerve Roots
L — Lumbar Nerve Roots

* * *

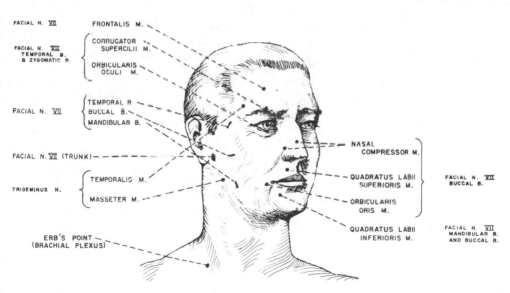

MOTOR POINTS OF FACE
Figure 3-B-1

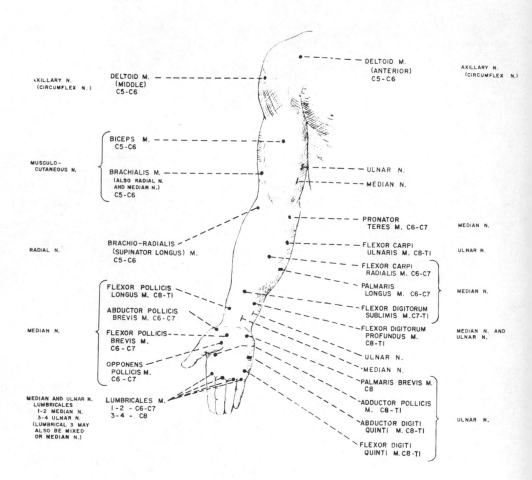

MOTOR POINTS OF ANTERIOR ASPECT OF UPPER EXTREMITY

Figure 3-B-2

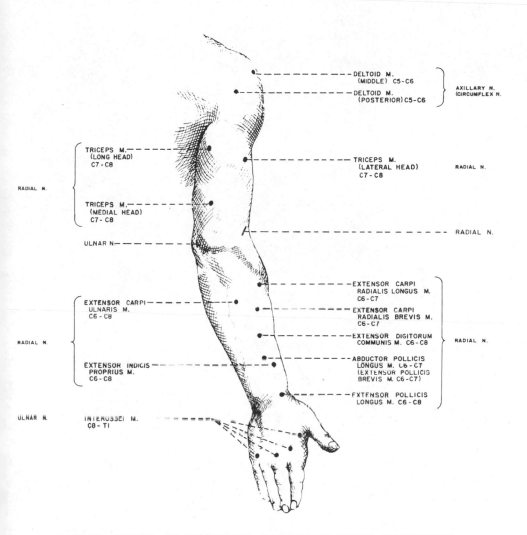

MOTOR POINTS OF POSTERIOR ASPECT OF UPPER EXTREMITY

Figure 3-B-3

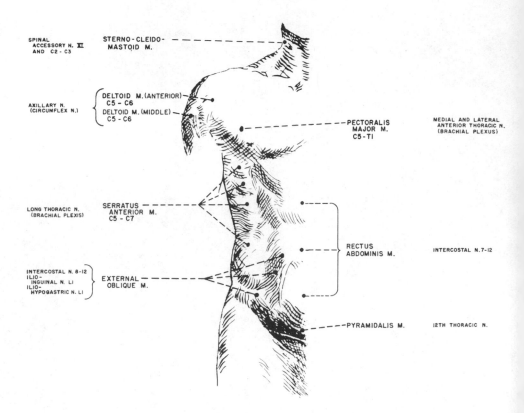

SPINAL
ACCESSORY N. XI
AND C2 - C3

STERNO-CLEIDO-
MASTOID M.

AXILLARY N.
(CIRCUMFLEX N.)

DELTOID M. (ANTERIOR)
C5 - C6
DELTOID M. (MIDDLE)
C5 - C6

PECTORALIS
MAJOR M.
C5 - TI

MEDIAL AND LATERAL
ANTERIOR THORACIC N.
(BRACHIAL PLEXUS)

LONG THORACIC N.
(BRACHIAL PLEXIS)

SERRATUS
ANTERIOR M.
C5 - C7

RECTUS
ABDOMINIS M.

INTERCOSTAL N. 7-12

INTERCOSTAL N. 8-12
ILIO-
INGUINAL N. LI
ILIO-
HYPOGASTRIC N. LI

EXTERNAL
OBLIQUE M.

PYRAMIDALIS M.

12TH THORACIC N.

MOTOR POINTS OF ANTERIOR ASPECT OF TRUNK

Figure 3-B-4

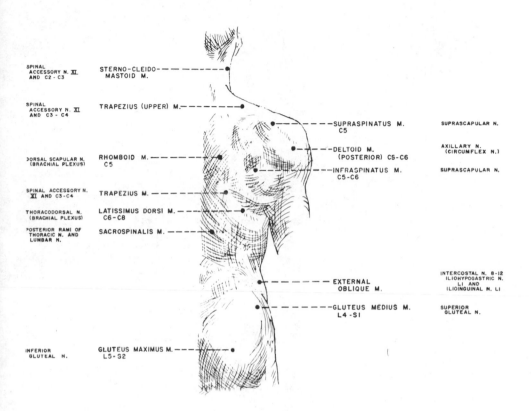

MOTOR POINTS OF POSTERIOR ASPECT OF TRUNK

Figure 3-B-5

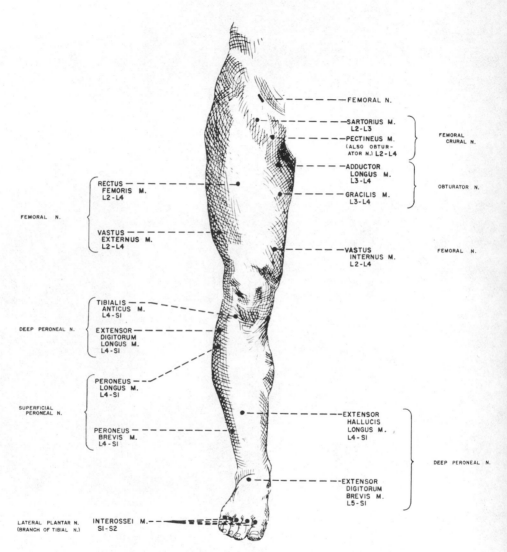

FEMORAL N.

SARTORIUS M.
L2-L3

PECTINEUS M.
(ALSO OBTUR-
ATOR N.) L2-L4

FEMORAL
CRURAL N.

ADDUCTOR
LONGUS M.
L3-L4

RECTUS
FEMORIS M.
L2-L4

GRACILIS M.
L3-L4

OBTURATOR N.

FEMORAL N.

VASTUS
EXTERNUS M.
L2-L4

VASTUS
INTERNUS M.
L2-L4

FEMORAL N.

TIBIALIS
ANTICUS M.
L4-SI

DEEP PERONEAL N.

EXTENSOR
DIGITORUM
LONGUS M.
L4-SI

PERONEUS
LONGUS M.
L4-SI

SUPERFICIAL
PERONEAL N.

EXTENSOR
HALLUCIS
LONGUS M.
L4-SI

PERONEUS
BREVIS M.
L4-SI

DEEP PERONEAL N.

EXTENSOR
DIGITORUM
BREVIS M.
L5-SI

LATERAL PLANTAR N.
(BRANCH OF TIBIAL N.)

INTEROSSEI M.
SI-S2

MOTOR POINTS OF ANTERIOR ASPECT OF LOWER EXTREMITY

Figure 3-B-6

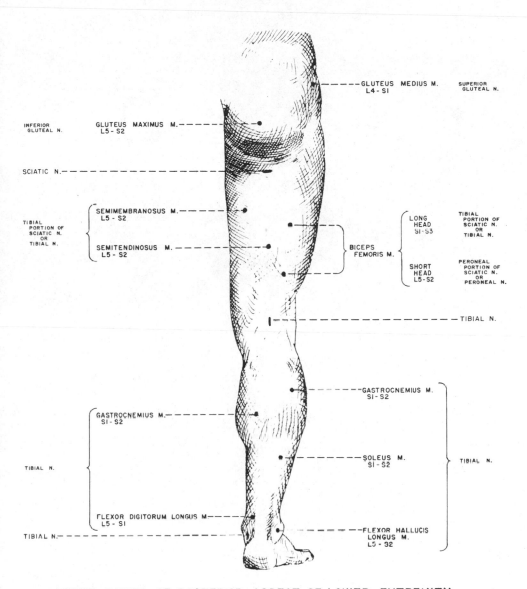

MOTOR POINTS OF POSTERIOR ASPECT OF LOWER EXTREMITY

Figure 3-B-7

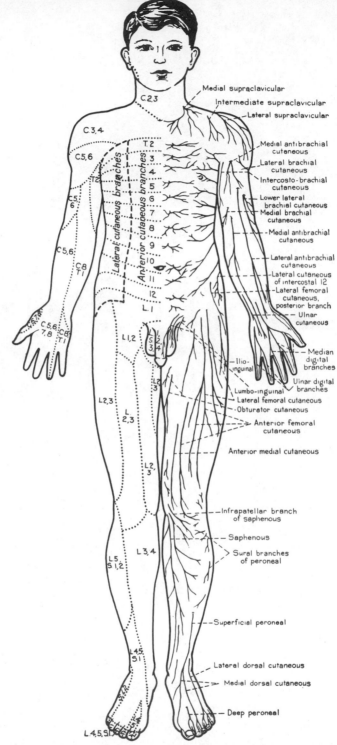

Figure 3-B-8. Diagram to show distribution of spinal cutaneous nerves on the ventral surface of the body. The position and course of the nerves are shown on the left side of the body and the segmental distribution of each as numbered is shown on the right side. By Permission from Morris' Human Anatomy, by J. Parsons Schaeffer, M.D. Copyright, 1953, McGraw-Hill Book Co., Inc.

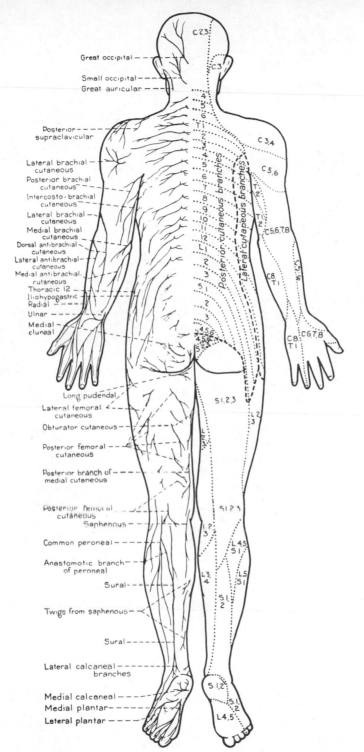

Figure 3-B-9. Diagram to show distribution of spinal cutaneous nerves on the dorsal surface of the body. The position and course of the nerves are shown on the left side of the body and the segmental distribution of each as numbered is shown on the right side. By permission from Morris' Human Anatomy, by J. Parsons Schaeffer, M.D. Copyright, 1953, McGraw-Hill Book Co., Inc.

REFERENCES

1. Levine, M. et al.: Relaxation of spasticity by electrical stimulation of antagonistic muscles. *Arch Phys Med Rehabil, 33:*668-73, 1952.
2. Vogel, M. et al.: Use of tetanizing currents for spasticity. *Phys Ther, 35:*435-7, 1955.
3. Covalt, N. K. and Griffin, J. E.: The place of low volt currents in hydrotherapy. *Phys Ther, 36:*99-105, 1956.
4. Bouman, H. D. and Shaffer, K. J.: Physiological basis of electrical stimulation of human muscle and its clinical application. *Phys Ther, 37:*207-23, 1957.
5. Liberson, W. et al.: Functional electrotherapy in cerebrovascular accidents. *Arch Phys Med Rehabil, 42:*101-5, 1961.
6. Glanville, H. J.: Electrical control of paralysis. *Proc R Soc Med, 65:*233-5, 1972.
7. Rebersek, S. and Vovodnik, L.: Proportionally controlled functional electrical stimulation of the hand. *Arch Phys Med Rehabil, 54:*378-82, 1973.
8. Harris, F. A. et al.: Electronic sensory aids as treatment for cerebral palsy children. *Phys Ther, 54:*354-65, 1974.
9. Illis, L. S. and Sedgwick, E. M.: Spinal cord stimulation. *Brit J Hosp Med, 20:*682-7, 1978.
10. Cook, A. W. et al.: Functional stimulation of the spinal cord in multiple sclerosis. *J Med Eng Technol, 3:*18-23, 1979.
11. Brindley, G. S. et al.: Electrical splinting of the knee in paraplegia. *Paraplegia, 16:*428-37, 1979.
12. Baker, L. L. et al.: Electrical stimulation of wrists and fingers for hemiplegic patients. *Phys Ther, 59(12):*1495-99, 1979.
13. Kelly, J. L. et al.: Procedures for EMG biofeedback training in involved upper extremities of hemiplegic patients. *Phys Ther, 59(12):*1500-07, 1979.
14. Bowman, B. R. et al.: Positional feedback and electrical stimulation: An automated treatment for the hemiplegic wrist. *Arch Phys Med Rehabil, 60:*497-501, 1979.
15. Meyer, G. A. and Fields, H. L.: Causalgia treated by selective large fiber stimulation of peripheral nerve. *Brain, 95:*163-8, 1972.
16. Fordyce, W. E.: Operant conditioning for pain. *Arch Phys Med Rehabil, 54:*399-408, 1973.
17. Fordyce, W. E.: Office management of chronic pain: Learning factors. *Minn Med, 57:*185-8, 1974.
18. Melzack, R.: Prolonged relief of pain by brief intense transcutaneous somatic stimulation. *Pain, 1:*357-73, 1975.
19. Sarno, J. E.: Chronic back pain and psychic conflict. *Scand J Rehabil Med, 8:*143-53, 1976.
20. Fox, E. J. and Melzack, R.: Transcutaneous electrical stimulation and acupuncture: Comparison of treatment for low back pain. *Pain, 2:*141-8, 1976.

21. Thorsteinsson, G. et al.: Transcutaneous electrical stimulation: A double blind trial of its efficacy for pain. *Arch Phys Med Rehabil, 58:*8-13, 1977.
22. Callaghan, M. et al.: Changes in somatic sensitivity during transcutaneous electrical analgesia. *Pain, 5:*115-27, 1978.
23. Mannheimer, J. S.: Electrode placements for transcutaneous electrical stimulation. *Phys Ther, 58:*1455-62, 1978.
24. Wolf, S. L. et al.: Relationship of selected clinical variables delivered during transcutaneous electrical nerve stimulation. *Phys Ther, 58:*1478-85, 1978.
25. Hiedl, P., et al.: Local analgesia by percutaneous electrical stimulation of sensory nerves. *Pain, 7:*129-34, 1979.
26. Thomson, J. D.: Effects of electrical stimulation on denervated muscle. *Am J Phys Med, 36:*16-20, 1957.
27. Kinnen, E.: Electrical impedance of human skin. *Med Electron Biol Eng, 3:*67-70, 1965.
28. Farmer, W. C.: Electrophysiological bracing in radial nerve compression injury. *Phys Ther, 46:*857-61, 1966.
29. Smith, E. and Steinberger, W.: Direct electrical stimulation of denervated rabbit muscle. *Arch Phys Med Rehabil, 49:*566-73, 1968.
30. Stanwood, J. E. et al.: Diagnosis and management of brachial plexus injuries. *Arch Phys Med Rehabil, 52:*52-60, 1971.
31. Wakim, K.: Influence of frequency of electrical stimulation on circulation. *Arch Phys Med Rehabil, 34:*291-95, 1953.
32. Martella, J. et al.: Prevention of thromboembolic disease by electrical stimulation of leg muscles. *Arch Phys Med Rehabil, 35:*24-29, 1954.
33. Gault, W. R. and Gatens, P. F.: Use of low intensity direct current in management of ischemic skin ulcers. *Phys Ther, 56:*265-69, 1976.
34. Pollock, A. V.: Electrical stimulation of the calf. *Scott Med J, 23:*332-3, 1978.
35. Davson, H.: *A Textbook of General Physiology,* 4th ed., Vol. II. Baltimore, Williams & Wilkins, 1970, pp 1041-44.
36. Bouman, H. D. and Shaffer, K. J.: Physiological basis of electrical stimulation of human muscle and its clinical application. *Phys Ther, 37:*207-23, 1957.
37. Abramowitsch, D. and Neousskine, B.: *Treatment by Ion Transfer.* New York, Grune, 1946.
38. Bishop, B.: Vibratory stimulation. III. Possible applications of vibration in treatment of motor dysfunctions. *Phys Ther, 55:*139-43, 1975.
39. Woo-Sam, J. et al.: Sex differences in adaptation to peripheral electro-stimulating surgical implants. *Arch Phys Med Rehabil, 53:*425-9. 1972.
40. *Clinical Evaluation of the Ljubljana Functional Electrical Peroneal Brace.* Report E-7, National Academy of Sciences, 1973.
41. Shriber, W.: *A Manual of Electrotherapy,* 4th ed. Philadelphia, Lea & Febiger, 1975.
42. Thomson, J. D.: Effects of electrical stimulation on denervated muscle. *Am J Phys Med, 36:*16, 1957.

43. Stillwell, G. K. and Wakim, K. G. Electrical stimulation of muscle. *Arch Phys Med Rehabil, 43:*95-8, 1962.

44. Smith, E. and Steinberger, W.: Direct electrical stimulation of rabbit muscle. *Arch Phys Med Rehabil, 49:*566-73, 1968.

45. Reed, J. and Jarrett, A.: Enzymatic and histologic effects of a standard stimulus to the skin of psoriatic patients. *Arch Dermatol, 95:*632-41, 1967.

46. Shepard, J. T.: *Physiology of the Circulation in Human Limbs in Health and Disease.* Philadelphia, Saunders, 1963.

47. Abramson, D. I.: *Circulation in the Extremities.* New York, Acad Pr, 1967.

48. Bishop, B.: Pain: Its physiology and rationale for management. *Phys Ther, 60:*13-37, 1980.

49. Nelson, H. E. et al.: Electrode effectiveness during transcutaneous motor stimulation. *Arch Phys Med Rehabil, 61:*73-77, 1980.

50. Kahn, J.: *Low Volt Technique.* Syosset, N. Y., Kahn, 1973, pp. 1-10.

51. O'Malley, E. & Oster, Y.: Influence of some physical chemical factors on iontophoresis using radio-isotopes. *Arch Phys Med Rehabil, 36:*310-6, 1955.

52. Murray, W. et al.: The iontophoresis of C_{21} esterified glucocorticoids: Preliminary report. *Phys Ther, 43:*579-83, 1963.

53. Griffin, J. et al.: Patients treated with ultrasonic driven hydrocortisone and ultrasound alone. *Phys Ther, 47:*595-601, 1967.

54. Nowak, E. J.: Experimental transmission of lidocaine through intact skin by ultrasound. *Arch Phys Med Rehabil, 45:*231, 1964.

55. Wanet, G. & Dehon, N.: Clinical study of ultrasonophoresis with a topical application of phenylbutazon and *Alphakadol. J Belge de Rhum Med Phys, 32#2,* 1976. (In French)

56. Smorto, M. P. et al.: *Clinical Electroneurography: An Introduction to Nerve Conduction Tests,* 2nd ed. Baltimore, Williams & Wilkins, 1980.

57. Cromwell, L. et al.: *Biomedical Instrumentation and Measurements.* Englewood Cliffs, N. J., P-H, 1973.

58. Davis, J. F.: *Manual of Surface Electromyograph.* W.A.D.C. Technical Report 59-194 (Project 7184: Task 71580) McGill University, Allen Memorial Institutes of Psychiatry, Montreal, 1959.

59. Currier, D. P.: Motor conduction velocity of axillary nerve. *Phys Ther, 51:*503-509, 1971.

60. Carpendale, M. T. F.: Conduction time in the terminal portion of the motor fibers of the ulnar, median and peroneal nerves in healthy subjects and in patients with neuropathy. Thesis, University of Minnesota, 1956.

61. Currier, D. P. et al.: Sensory nerve conduction: Effect of ultrasound. *Arch Phys Med Rehabil, 59:*181-185, 1978.

62. Currier, D. P. et al.: Sensory nerve conduction: Heating effects of ultrasound and infrared. Submitted for publication.

63. Currier, D. P. et al.: Changes in motor nerve conduction induced by exercise and diathermy. *Phys Ther, 49:*146-152, 1969.

64. Kaeser, H. E.: Nerve conduction velocity measurements. In Vinken, P. J. and Bruyn, G. W. (Eds.): *Handbook of Clinical Neurology*, Vol 7. New York, Am Elsevier, 1970.

65. Thomas, J. E. et al.: Ulnar nerve conduction velocity and H-reflex in infants and children. *J Appl Physiol, 15:*1-9, 1960.

66. Wagman, I. H. et al.: Maximum conduction velocities of motor fibers of ulnar nerve in human subjects of various ages and sizes. *J Neurophysiol, 15:*235-244, 1952.

67. Buchthal, F. et al.: Evoked action potentials and conduction velocity in human sensory nerves. *Brain Res, 3:*1-122, 1966.

68. Guld, C. et al.: Report of committee on EMG instrumentation. *Electroencephalogr Clin Neurophysiol, 28:*399-413, 1970.

69. Cohen, H. L. et al.: *Manual of Electroneuromyography*, 2nd ed. New York, Harper & Row, 1976.

70. Buchthal, F. et al.: Volume conduction of the spike of the motor unit potential investigated with a new type of multielectrode. *Acta Physiol Scand, 28:*331-354, 1957.

71. Buchthal, F. et al.: Motor unit territory in different human muscles. *Acta Physiol Scand., 45:*72-87, 1959.

72. Goodgold, J. et al.: *Electrodiagnosis of Neuromuscular Diseases*, 2nd ed. Baltimore, Williams & Wilkins, 1980.

73. Marinacci, A. et al.: Electromyogram in neuromuscular re-education. *Bull Los Angeles Neurol Soc, 25:*57-71, 1960.

74. Basmajian, J. V.: Conscious control of individual motor units. *Science, 141:*440-441, 1963.

75. Brown, B. B.: *New Mind, New Body*. New York, Harper & Row, 1974.

76. Jacobson, E.: *Progressive Relaxation*. Chicago, U of Chi Pr, 1938.

77. Wolf, S. L.: Anatomical and physiological basis for biofeedback. In Basmajian, J. V. (Ed.): *Biofeedback: Principles and Practice for Clinicians*. Baltimore, Williams & Wilkins, 1979, Chapter 2.

78. Brown, B. B.: *Stress and the Art of Biofeedback*. New York, Harper & Row, 1977, Chapters 2, 3.

79. Bishop, B.: Spasticity: Its physiology and management. *Phys Ther, 57:*371-401, 1977.

80. Brown, D. R.: *Neurosciences for Allied Health Therapies*. St. Louis, Mosby, 1980, Chapter 10.

81. Harris, F.: Inapproprioception: A possible sensory basis for athetoid movements. *Phys Ther, 51:*761-770, 1971.

82. DeBacher, G.: Biofeedback in spasticity control. In Basmajian, J. V. (Ed.): *Biofeedback: Principles and Practice for Clinicians*. Baltimore, Williams & Wilkins, 1979, Chapter 6.

83. Griffin, J. E.: An active relaxation technic for pain relief. *Phys Ther Rev, 38:*675-678, 1958.

84. Wolf, S. L.: Essential considerations in the use of muscle biofeedback. *Phys Ther, 58:*25-31, 1978.
85. Koppman, J. W. et al.: Voluntary regulation of temporal artery diameter by migraine patients. *Headache, 14:*133-138, 1974.
86. Green, E. et al.: General and specific applications of thermal biofeedback. In Basmajian, J. V. (Ed.): *Biofeedback: Principles and Practice for Clinicians.* Baltimore, Williams & Wilkins, 1979, Chapter 11.
87. Jacobson, E.: Electrophysiology of mental activity. *Am J Psychol, 44:*677-694, 1932.
88. Jacobson, E.: *You Must Relax.* New York, McGraw, 1957.

Chapter 4

THE DIATHERMIES

INTRODUCTION

DIATHERMY MAY BE DEFINED as the generation of heat in the body tissues due to the resistance offered by the tissues to the passage of high frequency electric currents. There is medical diathermy, wherein the anticipated tissue temperature rise is within physiological limits, and surgical diathermy, wherein the anticipated tissue temperature rise is destructive.[1] This volume is concerned only with medical diathermy.

Any device that generates an electric current will simultaneously generate an electric field and a magnetic field.[2] Tissues will selectively absorb more of the electric or more of the magnetic field depending upon their chemical composition. Tissues with a high fat content will tend to act as insulators and resist the passage of electric field energy. In the process of resisting the penetration of the electric field, the tissue temperature will rise.

Fat does not resist the passage of the magnetic field. Tissues of high electrolyte content will tend to oscillate in the presence of a high frequency magnetic field. The degree of oscillation, at the intraatomic level, will be in direct proportion to the polarity of the absorbing molecule. Water is the most polar molecule present in tissues in large quantity and is the major constituent of normally occurring electrolytes. Thus, it is the reaction of absorbing tissues to both the electric and magnetic field which causes the tissue temperature rise (TTR). The objective of treatment by medical diathermy is to cause vasodilation and/or skeletal muscle relaxation, with subsequent pain relief.

HISTORICAL BACKGROUND

In the early twentieth century, as the then infant science of electronics developed practical ways to generate high frequency oscillating currents (f > 1 Mc), radio came into existence. It was soon discovered that if living tissue was exposed to practical quantities of this high frequency energy, its resistance to penetration of the energy caused the absorbing tissue to get hot. This form of energy caused less rise in skin temperature and more rise in subcutaneous fat and underlying muscle temperature as compared to infrared lamps, bakers, and whirlpools.

The first commercially available clinical diathermy units appeared in the late 1910s and early 1920s. The high frequency energy was generated by multiple spark gaps. The frequencies were unstable but within the range of 1 to 10 million Hertz (MHz). The electrodes were flexible bare metal plates. A layer of conducting jelly was placed between the plate and the skin. Electrical burns were a frequent occurrence, especially when the electrodes were applied to a surface of irregular contour. Maintenance of adequately functioning spark gaps was a nuisance. As radio came into widespread use, the spark gap diathermies caused many problems, particularly because of generation of an unfilterable static in both nearby and remote radios, but these diathermy machines were capable of causing a deeper TTR than any form of conductive heating.

In the late 1920s and the 1930s, advances in electronics permitted generation of still higher frequencies on a practical scale. Most importantly, spark gap generation of high frequencies became obsolete, and frequency control on the order of $\pm$ 1 percent became possible. To distinguish between the older and newer diathermy machines, the older was designated as long wave and the newer as short wave (SWD) diathermy. Reasonably close frequency tolerance became possible in the 10 to 100 MHz range. Because radio broadcasting was playing an ever-increasing role in society, with the number of broadcasting stations steadily increasing, authority to regulate the frequency and power output of each station was granted to the Federal Communications Commission (F.C.C.), along with the capability and resources to closely monitor the airwaves.

Any medical diathermy unit is actually a radio transmitter. Although the power output of such units rarely exceeds 200 watts, this is sufficient to cause nearby radio and television reception to be garbled, because of frequency interference. In the late

1930s, the Federal Communications Commission assigned certain short wave frequencies for medical diathermy. Medical use of long wave diathermy was banned, since adequate frequency control was not feasible at competitive cost. To give manufacturers time to adjust production to the new standards and to give purchasers of the older style of equipment a reasonable chance to recover their investment, 1947 was set as the year when long wave diathermy could no longer be used. Under the F.C.C. regulations, SWD design had to be tested and approved for frequency stability and other performance characteristics before the unit could go into production. The F.C.C. assigned as primary frequency 27.12 MHz ± 0.6 percent. Allowable secondary frequencies were 13.56 and 40.68 MHz, each with a permitted fluctuation of ± 0.05 percent.[4] Calculations based on frequency and wavelength relationships discussed in Chapter 2 yield a wavelength of 11 m for the primary frequency, 22 m for the lower frequency, and 7 m for the highest allowed frequency. No American manufacturer uses the high frequency, since it cannot be manufactured competitively. Only one uses the lower allowed frequency,* since frequency toleration of ± 0.6 percent is easier to design than toleration of ± 0.05 percent.

The lower frequency has one significant advantage. Any electrical engineer will confirm that with generation of a high frequency current, at any given intensity the magnetic field will become stronger as the frequency is increased, up to a frequency of between 10 and 15 MHz. Beyond this frequency the magnetic field strength steadily decreases while the electric field increases in strength. Hence, a clinical SWD unit that operates at 13.56 MHz will produce a stronger magnetic field as compared to generators whose principal operating frequency is 27.12 MHz. It has been known since the 1940s that it is the tissue reaction to the magnetic field that causes a temperature rise in tissues of high electrolyte content, and reaction to the electric field that heats subcutaneous fat.[5] Thus the use of a low frequency SWD generator permits a greater amount of deep heating with a lesser risk of overheating the subcutaneous fat.

---

* The Birtcher Crystal Bandmaster, Model 802. The Birtcher Corporation, Los Angeles, California.

The problem of how to obtain a stronger magnetic field as compared to electric field at the allowed frequency of 27.12 MHz has been at least partially solved with the evolution of solid state circuits as an alternative to vacuum tube oscillating circuits. As improvements in transistorized and integrated circuits have moved out of the laboratory and into the marketplace, it has become possible to have high current as opposed to high voltage shortwave diathermy units. Available *high current*, high frequency (27.12 MHz) units can develop a strong magnetic field at the 11 meter wavelength. The first of the units for clinical use appeared in the 1960s.† A second company was able to arrive at a useful design in the 1970's.‡ Comparative testing data, which will be published early in the 1980s, has shown that with this new generation of SWD units it is possible to produce a clinically useful magnetic field effect with less risk of overheating subcutaneous fat.[6]

Other advances in electronic circuitry, especially the development of the multiple cavity anode, permitted generation of frequencies called microwave. These are in the range of 100 to 10,000 MHz. Microwave diathermy came into clinical use in the late 1940s. Until 1972, the only microwave frequency allowed for medical use was that of 2,456 MHz with a ± 2 percent toleration. Yet early in the 1950s, it was clearly demonstrated that lower microwave frequencies would be much more effective in causing a significant TTR in soft tissues at a depth of 3 to 5 cm.[3] The wavelength of electromagnetic energy having a frequency of 2,456 MHz is approximately 12 cm. For a frequency of 900 MHz, the wavelength is about 33 cm.[3-6]

Neither short wave nor microwave diathermy is in as widespread demand now as it was in the 1950s. A major factor in the decline of use is that, in the presence of a subcutaneous fat layer more than 1 cm thick, the fat temperature is likely to rise to dangerous levels (above 45°C) while the underlying muscle temperature rise is insignificant or may even drop.[7, 8] Subcutaneous fat is an excellent resistor to the penetration of an electric field, because of its low electrolyte content, and is not

---

† Autotherm®. Mettler Electronics Corporation, Anaheim, California.

‡ Magnetherm®. International Medical Electronics, Ltd., Kansas City, Missouri.

stimulated by penetration of the magnetic field. Both these factors, coupled with the low specific heat of fat (approximately 0.5, compared to 1.0 for water) can give rise to a serious burn in fat even though there is little visible evidence of temperature rise in skin.

Furthermore, efficient and effective electrode placement takes time, and selection of the right type of electrode for the area to be treated can make the difference between a placebo and a physiologically effective treatment. Lastly, evolution of the use of ultrasonic energy, which does produce a significant deep tissue temperature rise without the danger of overheating of subcutaneous fat, and within a much shorter treatment time, has diminished demand for utilization of the diathermies.

SHORT WAVE DIATHERMY ELECTRODES

The 1930s saw the development of four types of short wave diathermy (SWD) electrodes. In order of development, they are as follows:

1. pads and cuffs
2. air-spaced plates
3. the drum
4. the induction field cable

Pad Electrodes

Two pad electrodes are required to complete the electrical circuit. The pad electrode is nearly equal in length and width. It consists of a flexible metal plate about 1 mm thick, covered with rubber or other insulating material several millimeters thick, on all surfaces. For uniform distribution of energy transfer from electrode to patient, contact pressure should be uniform throughout the electrode surface. Consequently, in standard application, a 1 to 2 cm layer of soft insulating material is placed between the electrode and the skin. Frequently, the electrode is supplied with a loose cotton sack plus soft felt pads having an area slightly larger than the metal plate. This padding is held in place by the loose sack and serves to minimize small areas of firm versus light pressure when the pad is held in place by body weight or a sandbag. Such dielectric spacing helps to insure that the skin temperature will not rise to injurious levels even though enough energy is used to raise subcutaneous tissue temperature.

The pad electrodes should not be placed closer together than about 5 cm and may be positioned a meter or more away from each other. If they are too close together, most of the energy will travel from pad to pad through air or across skin surface rather than from one pad into the patient and then to other pad. This will not cause a deep tissue temperature rise. When pad electrodes are used, the patient becomes a part of the electrical circuit.

The cuff electrode is similar in construction and use to the pad electrode, except its length is much greater than its width. It is intended for use as a "wrap-around" electrode. Two are required to complete the electrical circuit. When the electrical insulation covering the cuff is in good condition, the ends of the metal plate may be overlapped with safety, but for longer cuff electrode life it is recommended that several layers of toweling or felt be inserted between the overlapping ends.

Neither the pad or the cuff electrode will cause a significant deep tissue temperature rise unless contact pressure is uniform throughout the electrode surface. For this reason, their use when a deep TTR is desired was banned by the Council on Physical Therapy equipment of the American Medical Association in 1952.[3] They are as effective as hot packs or other sources of infrared energy for causing a superficial TTR, and since the diathermy generator with its electrodes can be awesome in appearance, some patients will undoubtedly perceive more pain relief from a TTR caused by this form of diathermy as compared to relief gained from exposure to hot packs.

Air-Spaced Plate Electrodes

The next development in short wave diathermy electrodes was the air-spaced plate. Two are needed to complete the electrical circuit. The patient becomes a part of the electrical circuit. All these electrodes have a rigid metal plate. In older designs, this was covered on all surfaces with a layer of Bakelite® several millimeters thick. This is a good electrical insulator. The plate is surrounded by an adjustable plate guard, one surface of which is placed in contact with a single layer of bath toweling, which should always be on the skin. The guard adjustment permits the plate to be placed 1 to 6 cm from the skin, thus permitting variation in depth of penetration of energy.

Newer designs consist of a bare metal plate enclosed in a transparent electrical insulator. The insulator (guard) is not adjustable, but the plate is adjustable within the guard, through a range of 1 to 3 cm. Figure 4-1 illustrates the arrangements of the essential components of an air-spaced plate electrode. The purpose of the plate guard is to prevent touching of the electrode plate when the patient circuit is energized. A severe electrical burn could result, especially if the contacting skin is moist.

Depth of penetration of energy from air-spaced plate electrodes is *inversely proportional to the distance from plate to skin, as long as the plate guard is in contact with the single layer of toweling on the skin.* Conversely, the sensation of heat produced within the absorbing tissues is in *direct proportion* to the distance from the plate to the skin.

There are far more thermal receptors in the skin than in subcutaneous fat or muscle. Hence, it is simple to demonstrate the relationships between sensation and penetration with use of

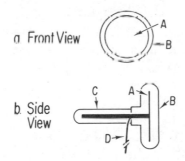

Figure 4-1. A typical air-spaced plate designed in the 1950s.

A. Bare metal plate about 15 cm in diameter and 2 mm thick.

B. Clear plastic plate guard, allowing adjustment of plate through a range of 3 cm.

C. Adjusting handle, with a pin lock so that electrode will not change position while in use.

D. Lead cord from plate to apparatus terminal. One lead is required for each plate.

air-spaced plates. With a subject sitting on a wooden or plastic stool (*not* metal), expose a shoulder. Place a small towel roll in the axilla to absorb perspiration. Place a single layer of toweling over all surfaces of the shoulder. Place one plate anterior and the other posterior to the shoulder. Each plate *guard* should be in firm contact with the toweling. Adjust the plates within their guards so that they are visually equidistant from the skin. Turn up the intensity until the subject reports a gentle sensation of warmth. This will usually require an intensity of 30 to 50 percent of available power. Treat for five minutes. It is anticipated that the subject will report equal sensation of warmth posteriorly and anteriorly. If either the clavicle or the spine of the scapula has minimal soft tissue covering, the subject may report more warmth on one side or the other, as the case may be. Turn the intensity to zero. Adjust the distance of *one* of the plates so that it is different from the other by one or more centimeters. Return the intensity to the previous level. In two or three minutes, the subject will volunteer that the sensation of heat is now different on the anterior as compared to the posterior aspect of the shoulder. If the plate was moved away, *sensation* of heat will have decreased in that area. If the plate was moved closer, the *sensation* will have increased.

The closer a plate is to the skin, the greater the chances that more energy will be directed perpendicularly toward the skin. Hence, there will be more absorption and less reflection. If more than 700 to 800 microwatts per cm^2 per second are absorbed by the skin, hyperemia or erythema and finally skin destruction (burn) will occur.[9] When the plate is further away, the chances are increased for reflection of energy from the skin. However, the chances of that reflected energy hitting the plate and being redirected back toward the skin are less. Hence, the closer the plate, the greater the chances for absorption. If the plate *guard* is not in contact with the toweling and the plate is at maximum distance from the guard, then there is so much reflection and scattering that an insignificant quantity of energy is absorbed, and little or no temperature rise will occur in the skin or underlying tissues.

Air-spaced plates function much like a capacitor. A capacitor by definition consists of conducting plates separated by a dielectric. The opposing plates are oppositely charged by a source of voltage, and the electrical energy of the charged system is stored in the polarized dielectric.[1, 2] For clinical purposes, a dielectric is any material, including dry air, that is an electrical insulator. The presence of such an insulator between plates of opposite charge forces transfer of energy by induction rather than conduction. In normal clinical usage, a part of the patient is placed between the two plates. The skin acts as a dielectric, since dry skin is a poor conductor. High voltage (3,000 to 15,000 volts), low amperage (microamperes) current is passed by the high frequency oscillating circuit to each plate millions of times per second. When the plate that is storing energy is filled to capacity, it discharges, transferring energy through and around the patient to the plate of low potential, which returns much of the energy to the apparatus. The net effect of the resistance to passage and absorption by intervening tissue is a rise in tissue temperature.

Certain precautions must be exercised in the use of air-spaced electrodes or there will be insignificant penetration of energy through the skin and hence no deep temperature rise. Thus, if 10 cm diameter plates are used, one on the anterior and the other on the posterior forearm, the plates will need to be at least 10 cm apart to achieve significant penetration. Otherwise, 90 percent or more of the energy will go directly from plate to plate or across the skin. This is especially true on a humid day. However, if one plate is placed on the distal volar forearm and the other on the proximal posterior forearm, the distance between the plates will be more than 10 cm and good deep heating would occur.

Most plates presently in use have a diameter more on the order of 20 cm. This limits the areas of the body that may be treated by this type of electrode. The usual procedure is to center the area to be treated between the electrodes. Thus, if a TTR is desired among tissues in and around the knee, one electrode could be applied to the medial or anterior midthigh and the other to the posterior midcalf. When the patient circuit is energized, for the first few minutes s/he will have a greater sensation of heat under one of the electrodes. Then s/he will note this sensation gradually moving toward the knee. Within ten minutes of treatment, s/he will note a greater sensation at the knee than on the skin under either of the plates. Skin temperature measurements before and after treatment will confirm this point.

As a general rule, when using air-spaced plates, the area to be treated should be centered between the plates in order to assure that the distance between the plates is greater than their diameter. If the distance is significantly less, there will be little deep tissue temperature rise, even though the sensation of heat is great.

Because air-spaced plates can function when they are 75 to 100 cm apart, the resultant thermal effect is superior to that of other SWD electrodes and to other forms of energy available to the physical therapist when a mild TTR is desired in a large volume of tissue. Thus, in the early stages of a chronic organic occlusive peripheral vascular disorder, when vasospasm is a larger factor than actual decrease in arterial lumen, air-spaced plates can be more effective, and safer, than multiple hot packs or infrared lamps. When the electrodes are far apart, the quantity of energy available for absorption per volume of tissue is lower than it would be for an equivalent energy source covering a smaller area, such as a hot pack or whirlpool.

The Drum Electrode

The drum electrode consists of one or more monoplanar coils of thick (3 to 4 mm) single-strand copper wire, which is rigidly positioned inside a Bakelite housing (Fig. 4-2). The housing has a dead-air space of 1 to 2 cm in all directions from the coil. For treatment of small, flat areas, a single coil drum may be used. For treatment of larger areas, two or three coils are linked together in series, with hinged sections so that some attempt may be made to follow contour. Still other types of drums are intended only for use on extremities. These will have a fixed curve built into the coils and their housings to accommodate the roughly cylindrical circumference of a segment of an extremity.

When a drum electrode is utilized, the patient is *not* a part of

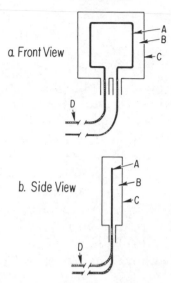

a. Front View

b. Side View

Figure 4-2. A typical drum electrode. Two or three drums, with hinge joints between each unit, are usually linked in series.

A. A single strand of copper wire, 3 or 4 mm thick, shaped into a rectangle of approximately 5 × 15 cm.
B. Dead air space of about 1 cm in all directions.
C. Bakelite housing 2 to 3 mm thick.
D. Lead cord from plate to apparatus terminal. The lead is of woven copper, with a diameter of 4 to 5 mm, covered by a loosely fitting rubber or plastic insulation several millimeters thick. Two leads are required, irrespective of whether one or more than one drum is linked together.

an electrical circuit as is the case with air-spaced plates. When the drum is energized, the nearby body segment is within the magnetic field but much less within the electric field created by the diathermy generator. Tissues of high electrolyte content, i.e. tissues with a good blood supply, respond to the presence of a strong magnetic field with the formation of "eddy currents" through intramolecular oscillation. This attempt to follow the rise and fall of the magnetic field millions of times per second causes rise in tissue temperature. When the subject feels a gentle sensation of warmth (skin temperature rise), a significant quantity of magnetic field energy has penetrated to a depth of 2 to 3 cm, provided that the skin is no more than 1 to 2 cm distant from the coil. Good technic requires that the coil *housing* be in light contact with the single layer of bath toweling that should always cover the skin in the area of the electrode.

Subcutaneous fat has a poor blood supply and hence a low electrolyte content. Thus, it is not stimulated by passage of the magnetic field. It does respond, however, to the concomitant electric field which also radiates from the coil. When the drum electrode is efficiently applied, it can be anticipated that approximately 50 percent of the absorbing tissue response will be due to the electric field and 50 percent due to the magnetic field.[3, 4] With poor drum positioning, the magnetic field effect will be diminished. Then the patient will perceive a stronger *sensation* of warmth but is likely to have an insignificant temperature rise except in the skin and subcutaneous fat.

The coil is fixed within a rigid housing. The patient surface of the housing should be as close to the single layer of toweling as possible without indenting the skin. If a corner of the housing actually does indent the skin, a "hot-spot" may occur. The electric field does not radiate strongly as far as the magnetic field. If the housing is too close to the skin, fat temperature may rise enough to cause enough perspiration formation to concentrate the electric field at that point, since the electric field will always follow the path of least resistance.

When the drum is energized, the patient is actually absorbing both electric and magnetic field energy. Any high voltage, high frequency current flow through a metallic conductor will generate a substantial electrical field in the area close to the conductor and a significant magnetic field through a greater distance. With the frequencies and voltages used in short wave and microwave diathermy, the magnetic field will be significant up to 5 cm away from the metallic conductor. The magnetic field actually extends much farther, but it is only strong enough to cause a substantial TTR a few centimeters away at patient circuit power levels that the skin can tolerate without damage.[3]

It is the living tissue reaction to the magnetic field which causes the beneficial temperature rise when the drum electrode is used. The magnetic field penetrates the subcutaneous fat without causing a significant fat temperature rise. The magnetic field is absorbed by the deeper tissues with a high electrolyte content. Blood has the highest electrolyte content (approximately 154 mEq/liter) of all normal body tissues. Although not classified as a tissue, urine can have a much higher, the same, or a much lower electrolyte content as compared to blood, depending upon the concentration of the urine at any given time.

Penetration of the electric field is resisted by the subcutaneous fat because fat is an electrical (but not magnetic) insulator. Fat has a low water and salt content. The net result is that the temperature of the subcutaneous fat is raised rapidly by exposure to an electric field. Because fat has a lower specific heat than water (about 0.5 to 1.0), it is very easy to cause a dangerous fat temperature rise with little or no rise in temperature of underlying tissues.

In contrast with the drum electrode, the air-spaced plate electrode system generates a much stronger electric field and weaker magnetic field. This is in large part due to the fact that there is a stronger dielectric inherent in the capacitor system.[3, 4, 10, 11]

The drum electrode, whether it consists of one or more than one coil linked in series, cannot cause a TTR in as large a volume of tissue as can widely separated air-spaced plates, but it can cause a deeper TTR because of its greater magnetic field generation.[4, 5, 10]

In almost all clinical usage, the drum is the easiest electrode to apply. However, if the subcutaneous fat is more than about 2 cm thick, there will be no TTR of any consequence in any underlying tissue at any intensity the subcutaneous fat will tolerate. Only in unusual circumstances can one anticipate a useful TTR more than 3 cm deep to the skin with short wave diathermy, regardless of the type of electrode used.[3, 8, 9, 11, 12]

The Cable Electrode

When a cable electrode is used, as is the case with the drum electrode, the patient is not a part of the electric circuit, but the absorbing tissues do react to the electric and magnetic fields that surround the energized patient circuit. The cable electrode consists of a multistranded woven copper wire cable about 1 cm in diameter and varying in length from 2.5 to 4.5 m as supplied for different short wave generator units. The cable is covered, except at its terminals, by a flexible rubber insulating material 3 to 5 mm in thickness (Fig. 4-3).

The cable is much more flexible than either the air-spaced plate or the drum electrode. It can follow the contour of any body segment readily and hence can be used to cause a relatively deep TTR in more areas of the body. However, there is no question that it takes more time, skill, and linen to apply the cable electrode safely and effectively.

Since the cable is not enclosed within a plate guard (air-spaced plate) or in a rigid housing (drum), the therapist must place a dielectric material between the patient and the cable to insure an adequate dielectric space between skin and cable. Bath toweling should always be placed next to the skin, as the toweling is a good absorber of perspiration. The layer of toweling should be followed by more toweling or other standard linen. If the cable is to lie on the patient, the total dielectric space should be approximately 1 cm. If the patient is to lie on the cable, his body or extremity weight will compress the dielectric material so that an additional 1 to 2 cm of soft insulating material must be added. The hazard of an electrical burn increases markedly when the dielectric space is less than 1 cm, especially on a humid day.

It is imperative that turns of the cable never touch each other when the patient circuit is energized. If cable surfaces touch, a short circuit can result, which can ruin the cable. More seriously, the short circuit can cause nearby linen to catch on fire. Rubber sleeves or other insulating material should be placed between turns where they must cross. Stiff spacers of any insulating material should be used to establish and maintain a uniform distance between turns when the cable is wound as either a two- or a three-dimensional coil. All winding and other preparations should be completed and not modified while the patient circuit is energized.

After each treatment, the cable should be unwound and stored as nearly linearly as possible. If the cable is left wound in a pattern for a prolonged period of time, it will be more difficult to adjust it for a different coil size or shape. The time and care needed to prepare a cable electrode for safe and effective use is a major reason why it is no longer commonly used.

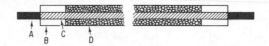

Figure 4-3. A typical cable electrode.

A. Solid metal tip 5 to 10 mm in diameter and 3 to 5 cm in length.
B. Rigid plastic or ceramic hollow insulator 10 to 15 mm in diameter and 5 to 10 cm in length.
C. Multistranded woven copper wire about 5 mm in diameter and 2.5 to 4.5 m in length.
D. Flexible rubber or plastic insulation, 2 to 5 mm thick, throughout the length of the cable.

When properly applied, the cable produces as much magnetic field as the drum electrode. It has the added advantage that it can cause a TTR deep to *all* surfaces of an extremity simultaneously and with great uniformity, since it follows contours readily. The monoplanar drum can add energy to only one surface at a time. When the drum is applied in a biplanar fashion, as many as three surfaces can be treated simultaneously, but the drum is hard to position for uniform energy absorption because few body segments are of a regular contour.

When the cable is improperly applied (turns too close together), both the electric and magnetic fields are apt to jump from turn to turn of the cable. This will shorten the useful life of the cable. More importantly, if turns are too close, there will be only superficial heating of the patient. In apparatus designed specifically for the cable electrode, the turns can be 10 cm or more apart and still add enough magnetic field energy to the patient to cause a significant deep TTR. The cable then becomes the ideal electrode to generate a mild tissue temperature rise throughout an extremity with greater uniformity of energy absorption than with any other SWD electrode.

GENERAL PRECAUTIONS WITH SHORT WAVE ELECTRODES

There are several points about use of SWD electrodes which, if followed faithfully, will minimize the risk of burning the patient and increase the life expectancy of the electrode.

Whenever diathermy is applied, there will be accumulation of perspiration on the skin. Perspiration is composed largely of water and various salts. It is an excellent conductor of electricity. Hence, a single layer of bath toweling should always cover the skin in the area being treated. Bath toweling is an excellent absorber of perspiration and will prevent its pooling in skin hollows or where skin surfaces ordinarily touch one another. Its regular and faithful use will make the risk of the patient receiving a severe and painful electrical burn negligible.

The lead cables from the generator to the electrode should never be allowed to touch each other when the unit is in operation. High voltage *or* high current, high frequency electrical energy is transmitted into the metallic part of the patient circuit. If the lead cables touch, a short circuit is likely. In the case of the cable electrode, the entire cable is the "lead" as well as the electrode. Therefore, the physical therapist should utilize spacing of any insulating material as indicated when inspecting the setup prior to energizing the circuit. A 1 to 2 cm separation is adequate.

Living tissue should never be permitted to touch either the lead cable or the electrode when the patient circuit is energized. This can result in a severe electrical burn, especially if the contacting skin is moist.

Three demonstration experiments are outlined at the end of this chapter. These procedures will simply and readily confirm the differences in heating patterns with the air-spaced plates, the drum, and the cable electrodes.

MICROWAVE DIATHERMY ELECTRODES

With *short wave* diathermy generators, much of the energy is lost within the machine circuit and/or patient circuit before there can be energy transfer to the patient. This is because the oscillating circuit that converts line current into the requisite high frequency radiates energy in all directions and because the lead cables that carry energy from the machine circuit to the electrodes are not shielded against loss of electric field energy. At any given intensity, at least one third of the generated high frequency energy never comes close to the area to be treated.

With *microwave* transmission, essentially no energy is lost between the oscillating circuit and the transmitting antenna, and because these wavelengths (12 or 33 cm) can be focused toward the patient, loss between the antenna and patient rarely exceeds 10 percent, even though the antenna may be as far away as 15 cm. The microwave antenna is commonly referred to as a director because it beams energy toward the patient. Such focusing is possible because microwave wavelengths are short enough to have some of the properties of visible light. On the other hand, the shortest short wave diathermy wavelength in clinical use is 11 m. This and longer wavelengths cannot be adequately focused for efficient clinical use at a practical cost.

In order to meet the FCC regulation for frequency tolerance at microwave frequencies, approximately ± 2 percent, the insulation between the metallic conductors that transfer this extremely high frequency energy from generator to antenna must be far superior to the insulation needed for similar transfer of the lower frequency shortwave energy. Furthermore, because of the higher voltages needed to drive the microwave oscillating

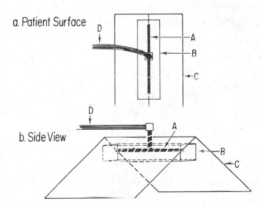

Figure 4-4. Typical microwave director for uniform output throughout the patient surface.
    A. Bare metal antenna 5 to 10 cm in length, 3 to 4 mm in diameter.
    B. Solid block of clear plastic completely enclosing the antenna.
    C. Patient surface of the metal reflector. The two large dimensions make a nonadjustable 90° angle. Dimensions are approximately 1 mm thick × 10 cm wide × 15 cm long.
    D. Coaxial cable lead from antenna to generator.

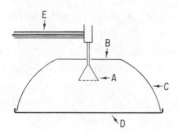

Figure 4-5. A typical microwave director for maximum focusing of energy midway between the center and the periphery.
  A. Bare metal antenna 1 to 2 cm in diameter.
  B. Flat surface of metal reflector (5 to 10 cm in diameter) Distance from B to D is 2 to 5 cm.
  C. Curved surface of reflector (10 to 15 cm).
  D. Detachable translucent plastic covering 1 mm thick.
  E. Coaxial cable lead from antenna to generator.

frequency circuit, 15,000 to 30,000 volts, the insulation between the outer conductor and any living tissue that could touch the lead cable must also be superior. The only practical way to meet these transmission requirements is to use a coaxial cable to deliver energy from the machine circuit to the patient. In order to deliver a significant quantity of energy, i.e. enough to cause a TTR, the insulation must be relatively rigid. The net result is that the lead cable from the machine to the antenna is far less flexible than that which is used for shortwave transmission. This can make ideal positioning of the director a problem. Figures 4-4 through 4-6 illustrate various aspects of director design.

In microwave treatment, the antenna is aimed at the surface of the body segment to be treated. The closer the antenna is to the skin, the greater the amount of energy available for absorption, but the smaller the area that can be treated at one time. Most clinical directors will have labeling clearly affixed indicating the approximate percent of power that can safely be used at any given distance from the typical patient. If this restriction is followed, the patient with normal sensation will perceive a comfortable *sensation* of warmth without risk of causing a dangerous deep tissue temperature rise. For directors in common clinical use, the closest distance is 2.5 cm and the greatest about 15 cm, with the director perpendicular to the skin surface. These dis-

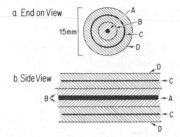

Figure 4-6. Microwave coaxial cable.

A. Inner conductor wire.
B. Layer of insulation surrounding inner conductor.
C. Outer conductor wire (a slightly flexible hollow cylinder).
D. Outer insulation surrounding outer conductor.

tances permit safe use of 20 to 75 percent of available power if sensation and circulation in the tissues being exposed are within normal limits and there are no contraindications for utilization of diathermy.

Only one surface and one area can be treated at one time. A number of director sizes and shapes have been developed and used over the years. Perhaps the most widely used antenna at this time is one that is enclosed in a rectangular metallic reflector which focuses the energy over an effective area of about 215 cm^2. If placed 2 to 3 cm from the skin, one should anticipate that approximately the same skin area will absorb a significant amount of the radiated energy at an approximately uniform level if the contour of the skin is flat. If the director is farther away, a slightly larger area can be treated. To produce an equal temperature rise in skin or in subcutaneous tissues, the power used must be increased as distance from antenna to skin is increased.

Other directors have effective areas as small as 54 cm^2 or as large as 470 cm^2. Some are designed for low energy transfer at the center and periphery as compared to the area in between. Such directors are usually hemispherical in shape, in contrast with the square or rectangular appearance of those designed for uniform energy transfer. The hemispherical directors are intended to be centered over a bony prominence. Because of its density, bone will absorb more of any diathermy wavelength energy as compared to any soft tissue. This design of the reflector is intended for use when a rise in soft tissue temperature is needed without causing a dangerous rise in temperature of bone that is close to the surface.

Energy of clinical microwave wavelengths (12 or 33 cm) causes a TTR in living tissue largely through stimulation of polar molecules. The more asymmetric a molecule, the more polar. Water is the most polar molecule present in the body in large quantity. Polar molecules attempt to spin or oscillate in response to the alternate buildup and collapse of high frequency electric and magnetic fields.[3, 10] In microwave diathermy application, the buildup and collapse occurs hundreds of millions of times per second. Molecular oscillation cannot occur under such conditions, but intraatomic vibration can. The increase in intraatomic vibration has a net effect of tissue temperature rise. The same response takes place upon absorption of short wave diathermy wavelengths of energy, but since the frequency is so much lower, the polar molecule vibration is not the dominant factor in producing a rise in absorbing tissue temperature.

Blood has the highest water content of all normally occurring tissues. Tissues with a good blood supply will exhibit a useful TTR upon absorption of microwave energy. However, if the subcutaneous fat layer is more than 1 cm thick, the fat temperature will rise to dangerous levels (above 45°C) before there can be adequate underlying soft tissue temperature rise. If the fat layer is 2 or more cm thick, there can be no deep temperature rise at intensities that a patient can safely tolerate.

Because of its low specific heat and because of its resistance to penetration of electric field energy, subcutaneous fat is a very real obstacle to practical utilization of *any* form of diathermy. This is especially true for microwave energy at the originally assigned frequency of 2,450 MHz.[3] It is somewhat less of an obstacle with the newer allowed frequency of 900 MHz.[3, 5, 6] However, very few microwave diathermies of this lower frequency are in clinical use, since this lower frequency was not approved for clinical practice until 1972.

INDICATIONS FOR APPLICATION OF THE DIATHERMIES

Utilization of diathermy is indicated for treatment when

chronic pain is a problem and when causing a transient local relaxation of skeletal muscle or a local increase in circulation is likely to relieve that pain. SWD and MWD will relieve pain significantly only if a rise in temperature in tissues 1 to 3 cm deep to the skin will be effective in interrupting or arresting muscle spasm or in causing vasodilation for brief periods of time. The TTR induced in muscle by diathermy will rarely last more than one-half hour after treatment and will rarely exceed 2° to 3°C.[7, 8] The interrelationships between pain, muscle spasm, vascular insufficiency, and chronic edema are discussed in Chapter 1.

SWD or MWD may be preferred to other means of causing a TTR in the following situations:

1. When a concomitant dermatological lesion is exacerbated by skin hydration
2. When tissues cannot tolerate a significant increase in weight or pressure applied externally
3. When a patient cannot or will not stay in a position necessary for application of other forms of energy
4. When a mild rise in temperature within a volume of tissue deep to subcutaneous fat is desirable
5. When the muscular or vascular malfunction lies sufficiently deep to the skin so that conductive heating cannot bring about the desired change
6. When the patient's psychological response to his medical problem(s) is intolerant of simple treatment — when only a complicated-appearing treatment is adequate for his emotional needs.

In regard to skin hydration, although the patient who receives any diathermy treatment will usually perspire in the area being treated, it is quite rare that the perspiration will be present in sufficient quantity to cause hydration of the skin. Exposure to whirlpool, Hubbard tank, paraffin bath, or to hot packs would be more likely to raise skin temperature to the point where the skin would become transiently edematous.

Patients with subacute or chronic orthopedic lesions may become less comfortable during or after treatment with hot packs or immersion in large volumes of water because of the weight and pressure of the direct contact with the energy source. Diathermy electrodes or directors are never in direct contact with the skin and hence do not cause discomfort through weight or pressure. Although the patient needs to be willing and able to stay reasonably immobile during treatment with diathermy, minor movement of the part would require less readjustment or correction than could be the case with hot packs or paraffin. Utilization of either air-spaced plate electrodes or the induction field cable makes it possible to raise tissue temperatures over a larger area and volume than is practical with hot packs, infrared lamps, paraffin, or ultrasound, within the same time period. The whirlpool or Hubbard tank can be used for areas as large or larger than can be done with diathermy, but their effects do not penetrate as deeply. None of the conductive heat sources available to the physical therapist can be as effective in causing a deep TTR.

Lastly, there are some patients who cannot accept the fact that treatment with anything so common and obvious as hot packs or whirlpool can be significant in relieving their pain. However, if exposed to what is so visibly a complicated and mysterious device as a diathermy, the patient may perceive considerable pain relief.

CONTRAINDICATIONS FOR APPLICATION OF THE DIATHERMIES

There are several major contraindications for use of the diathermies. They should never be used in the presence of any metal in the area to be treated, regardless of whether the metal is internal or external to the patient. The diathermy generator transmits high frequency, high voltage electric and magnetic field energy into the patient, which is absorbed by various tissues and hardware within its depth of penetration. The transmitted energy is converted into heat by the absorbing tissues. Any metal within the field will concentrate this energy at points (screws) or edges (plates). This will cause adjacent tissues to get very hot. Consequently, the patient should *never* be treated with diathermy while sitting on a metal stool, lying on an innerspring mattress, or touching a zipper on a pillow, nor should there be any jewelry in or near the treatment area.

It is essential if there is any scar in or near the treatment area that the therapist check with the patient and with the patient's chart to determine if there is metal deep to the scar. With the current widespread use of internal fixation of fractures, joint replacements, and so forth, the presence of metal screws, wires, and plates deep to a scar is common. War veterans may have shrapnel buried in their soft tissues. It is the therapist's responsibility to avoid the use of any form of diathermy if it is suspected or known that metal is within the area to be treated.

Watches should not be worn by the patient or therapist while a treatment is being given. In addition to the possibility of a burn, the watch can become magnetized and will not keep accurate time until it has been demagnetized. This can happen even with watches that are labeled "antimagnetic."

The most important contraindication for treatment with any diathermy unit anywhere on the body is when the patient's cardiac status is such that any kind of a cardiac pacemaker is used. The high frequency, high voltage electric field can cause the pacemaker to become erratic or to stop. It is the therapist's responsibility to know if the patient utilizes a pacemaker. The presence of a pacemaker anywhere in the treatment area, i.e. on another patient, is an absolute contraindication for the use of any form of diathermy.[13] There is strong evidence that no one wearing a cardiac pacemaker should be within 15 feet of any working SWD or MWD unit.[13] Although no reports have been published, it would seem logical that the same constraint would hold true for any patient using an electrically driven cord, cerebellar, or cortical implant.

SHORT WAVE DIATHERMY TECHNIQUES

Electrode Terminals

Some models of short wave diathermy (SWD) generators are designed to use any of the common electrodes: air-spaced plates, the drum, or the cable. Others are designed for use with only one or two types of electrode. The machine terminals are commonly designed so that leads from one type of electrode cannot be inserted into an oscillating circuit designed for another type of electrode. There will always be at least two machine circuit terminals to which the two electrode leads must be attached unless the apparatus is designed for only one kind of electrode, in which case there will be a permanent connection between the machine and patient circuit. Lead cables from one manufacturer will not fit the terminals of another make of generator, although usually the electrode leads are interchangeable among the various models provided by one manufacturer. The therapist must then know which electrodes belong to which diathermy generator.

Support Arms

Most models of SWD are designed for use with several types of electrodes. Air-spaced plates and the drum electrode must be supported away from the generator and close to but not in contact with the patient surface. Since there must be two air-spaced plates to complete the circuit, there must be two support arms. Each is manually adjustable as to height, angulation, and rotation at several joints. The drum electrode requires only one support arm. The cable electrode does not utilize a support arm. The electrodes are detachable from their support arms, and their respective leads from the machine terminals, by snap-fit or by spring-loaded locking mechanisms. Electrodes should never be removed from their support arms or from the machine circuit terminals while the patient circuit is energized. The patient circuit should never be energized unless electrodes have been properly positioned over a patient. If the patient circuit is energized without a subject in the circuit, the life expectancy of the machine and patient circuits will be shortened, since both circuits are designed to work within a certain impedance range.[4] Any diathermy apparatus and its accessories are expensive. With reasonable care and with daily use, such a unit should last for at least ten years.

Treatment Time

The generally accepted treatment time for exposure of one body area to SWD is twenty to thirty minutes.[9-12] There is ample documentation that significant vasodilation will have reached its peak within this length of time if the patient's circulatory system is capable of normal function. If treatment is continued for a longer period, i.e. forty-five to sixty minutes, the risk of rebound increases. Rebound is a phenomenon that may occur within the vasular tree when living tissues are exposed to energy addition or withdrawal which causes a marked rise or fall in tissue temperature. The known mechanisms are discussed in Chapter 5. The rebound phenomenon is not a desirable effect of treatment. Its occurrence is unusual in a person whose nervous and circulatory systems are capable of normal function unless treatment time exceeds thirty minutes. Before and after treatment, digital temperature measurements will provide objective evidence as to whether rebound occurred. If digital skin temperature drops after treatment, a significant amount of vasoconstriction has taken place.[8, 9]

Tuning the Oscillating Circuit

Most models of SWD designed after the 1940s have automatic control of the oscillating circuit such that it permits variation in machine circuit frequency as the patient impedance changes. Change in impedance is to be expected as skin temperature rises. Several mechanisms which are used for the automatic tuning, or resonance, of the machine circuit to the patient circuit are discussed in Chapter 8. Suffice here to say that manual or automatic tuning permits more efficient energy transfer from the oscillating machine circuit to the patient. Many SWD units that have to be manually tuned are still in clinical use.

When manual tuning is necessary, after the patient and the electrodes are in position for treatment, the intensity is turned up to 30 to 40 percent of available power. Next, the control labeled "Tuning" (or "Resonance") is rotated until a maximum swing to the right occurs by the *power indicator needle*. The patient will almost always indicate he feels a sudden surge of warmth when the machine circuit is in tune. In any diathermy treatment, the patient with normal sensation should have only a mild sensation of warmth. Therefore, if after tuning the patient states the area being treated feels hot, the intensity *(not the resonance)* control should be turned down. If the patient reports only a vague sensation of warmth after the power indicator needle indicates that tuning has been accomplished, the intensity *(not the resonance)* control should be turned up. If more than 50 to 60 percent of available power is needed to produce a comfortable sensation of warmth, something is wrong with the patient circuit setup — too much or too little dielectric is a common error — or something has deteriorated within the machine circuitry, or the electrodes or their leads are malfunctioning. If the therapist is satisfied that electrode positioning is proper and that the machine circuit has been tuned, and the patient is still not perceiving energy input, then professional servicing of the apparatus is indicated.

When using manually tuned apparatus, it is important to remember to check the tuning again after treatment has proceeded for about five minutes. Most of the skin temperature rise that is going to occur will have taken place within a five-minute period. As skin temperature increases, impedance decreases, and the machine circuit may have to be readjusted as to frequency. If the machine circuit is not tuned and retuned, no significant amount of energy will penetrate the skin and no appreciable deep TTR will occur.

Skin Inspection

No clothing should be permitted to remain in the area to be treated. The skin should be inspected for scars or other blemishes before treatment. Any and all blemishes should be described in writing at the time of initial treatment. If there is traumatic or surgical scar tissue in the area, it is the therapist's responsibility to find out if there is any metal in or deep to the skin. If so, diathermy should not be used. Any change in appearance of any blemish after a treatment should be recorded. If this is done, the patient cannot return a week or a month later and claim the treatment caused damage. Since vasodilation is likely to occur during and after treatment, and is desirable, constricting clothing proximal to the treatment area should be loosened or removed. Likewise, the treated part should be horizontal or elevated rather than dependent, to permit the effects of gravity to aid venous return. If the treated part is dependent, edema present may be increased rather than diminished.

After skin inspection, the area to be treated should be covered with a single layer of bath toweling. This is to prevent accumulation of perspiration. If skin folds in or near the area are touching, the part should be positioned so that the folds are completely separated or additional toweling inserted so that perspiration cannot pool or accumulate.

Air-Spaced Plate Electrodes

Two plates must be used, with a segment of the patient between them, if the patient circuit is to be complete. Each plate is attached to a support arm. Each plate has its own lead cord for connection to an apparatus terminal. The lead cords should never touch each other when the patient circuit is energized. The area to be treated should be covered with a single layer of bath toweling and the plate guard placed in contact with it. Either the plate can be manually adjusted within the fixed plate guard or the plate guard can be adjusted around a fixed plate. For deepest *penetration,* the further the plate from the skin the better. For strongest *sensation* of heat, the closer the plate to the skin the better. Reasons for this fact were discussed earlier in this chapter. The plates may be equidistant or at different distances from the skin, depending upon treatment and patient needs. The plate itself should never be touched when energized. A severe electrical burn can result, especially if the contacting skin is moist.

Air-spaced plate electrodes are especially useful if one wishes to cause a TTR in both upper or both lower extremities simultaneously. Because the *circumference* of most forearms is not much larger than the *diameter* of most plates, it is usually better to position the plates on the upper arms. With a standard twenty-minute treatment, such positioning will induce transient muscle relaxation and vasodilation throughout both upper extremities and the upper trunk. Axillary skin folds must not be permitted to touch. This treatment is contraindicated in the presence of significant cardiac pathology.

Placement of one electrode on each calf or thigh will produce similar results in the lower extremities and pelvis. Care must be taken that the thighs do not touch, by positioning or by use of additional toweling. This treatment should not be used during or immediately preceding the menstrual period, since there may be a pelvic temperature rise.

Very occasionally, there is need for use of air-spaced plate electrodes to encourage liquifaction of a consolidated area of lung tissue that has not been resorbed with the use of antibiotics. In this case, one plate would be applied over the anterior thorax and the other over the posterior thorax, in the area of consolidation. This treatment would be contraindicated in the presence of cardiac pathology or a history of pulmonary hemorrhage or infarct.

Most other areas of the body can be better treated with other electrodes or with other physical agents. Therefore, unless air-spaced plate electrodes are the only ones available, they are not as widely used as they were twenty years ago. If they are used, the best deep TTR will usually be obtained when the plates are as far away from the face of the plate guard as possible.

The Drum Electrode

This is probably the most commonly used of all diathermy electrodes. It is by far the easiest to apply and can be used to treat most areas of the body so long as the area to be treated is not large. Most drums can adequately treat an area from 10 to 15 by 30 to 35 cm in size.

For reasons presented earlier, a single layer of bath toweling should always be placed between the skin and the patient surface of the drum. The drum should be adjusted to follow contour as much as possible and should be as close to the toweling as possible without touching the toweling. This positioning will allow the most nearly uniform TTR and will minimize the risk of "hot-spot" formation.

The drum electrode is frequently used in treatment of chronic low back pain. The setup most often used calls for the patient to be lying prone, with the lumbar area flattened as much as possible. In the thin individual, this flattening can be accomplished by the addition of one or more pillows underneath the abdomen (*not* underneath the hips). After the toweling is in place, the hinged drum is placed so that its long dimension is at right angles to the vertical axis of the trunk. Care should be taken that the edges of the drum do not touch the pelvic brim, sacrum, or inferior ribs. Because bone is more dense than soft tissue, it will absorb more electromagnetic energy than surrounding soft tissue if the bone is within the limits of depth of penetration of the energy (2 to 3 cm deep to the skin). The spinous processes of vertebrae are rarely a hazard because only a small volume and surface of the process will be close to the patient surface of the electrode. If bone is too close, it is likely the patient will report a stronger sensation of warmth there than elsewhere. This is because both skin and periosteum are more richly supplied with thermal receptors than are other body tissues. The visible warning sign of a "hot-spot" is a discrete area of marked hyperemia. If electrode placement is not altered when this occurs, the "hot-spot" will usually evolve into a burn. Diathermy burns usually have an iceberg effect, i.e. much less shows on the surface as compared to major damage deep to the skin.

It is then apparent that the therapist must orient the patient prior to treatment that the sensation of warmth that should evolve within a treatment should be uniform rather than spotty, and that the patient should inform the therapist of any irregularity of sensation rather than try to tolerate it. Such uneven sensation is more apt to occur with either the drum or cable electrode as compared to air-spaced plates. This is because the plates are more often positioned so as to cause a TTR in a larger volume of tissue than may be the case with the drum or cable electrode.

The drum is frequently used to treat a segment of an extremity. Most often, the drum is positioned so that any three contiguous surfaces of the extremity are close to the patient surface of the drum. Thus, if a thigh were to be treated with the patient supine, the center of the drum would be facing the anterior aspect while one wing would be close to the lateral and the other wing close to the medial thigh. When any part of a lower extremity is treated with a drum, care must be taken that the non-patient surface of the electrode does not touch nearby tissue. The drum radiates energy in all directions.

Since extremity circumferences tend to be conical as well as cylindrical, it may be difficult to follow contour evenly. Because joints have bony masses near the surface, as well as numerous protuberances, it can be very difficult to avoid "hot spots" with the drum electrode. Either air-spaced plates or the cable electrode can be utilized for a greater uniformity of TTR in an area that includes a major joint. An equal or better TTR can be produced in distal joints, i.e. ankle or wrist, with conductive heating, as discussed in Chapter 5.

Treatment of the hip area by short wave diathermy is of doubtful benefit. The hip joint is deep — about 10 to 12 cm in the average adult. This is well beyond the depth of penetration of SWD under optimal conditions. Additionally, the posterior aspect is covered by 3 cm or more of subcutaneous fat, even in a slender adult. Hence, little hip muscle or joint temperature rise can be achieved with SWD. Fortunately, there are more deeply penetrating physical agents, i.e. ultrasound, which can achieve a significant TTR at the desired depth.

The Cable Electrode

When using a cable electrode, it may be wound in either a two-dimensional or three-dimensional form. The two-dimensional form most often used is the pancake coil. The pancake consists of three or four circular turns in one plane, with a uniform spacing of 1 to 3 cm between each turn. Symmetry of the turns will minimize "hot-spot" formation as well as assure long life of a cable electrode. Symmetry is readily achieved by use of spacers at several points throughout the pancake. Spacers are usually not interchangeable among cables for different brands of SWD units, since manufacturers will differ in the thickness of the insulation covering the woven copper wire by as much as 5 mm. The lead end of that segment of the cable which makes the innermost turn must cross over other turns en route to its machine terminal. Utilization of additional insulating material at least 5 mm thick is mandatory at the point of crossover. If not used, when the patient circuit is energized, a short circuit will develop. This will damage the cable beyond repair and can cause a burn in nearby living tissue. A hollow rubber sleeve is furnished, as are spacers, with each cable. The sleeve is slit lengthwise for ease of application. Any insulating material, i.e. bath toweling, may be substituted. It follows that the cable leads going from the wound cable to the machine terminals should never be allowed to touch because of the risk of causing a short circuit.

For the pancake coil to function most effectively, the innermost turn should have a diameter not to exceed 15 cm (6 inches). Apparatus not designed for use with cables may not have adequate provision for tuning, automatic or manual, if the innermost turn is larger in diameter. For the same reasons, the leads from the two ends of the turns should be approximately equal in length. A difference in lead length of up to 15 cm will usually present no problem. With practice in using the cable electrode, attention to these points will become habitual.

The pancake coil is frequently used in treatment of chronic lumbar and/or thoracic back pain. Application of a drum electrode would be less time consuming. However, the pancake coil can be applied with the patient in the hook-lying position, whereas the drum cannot. In the hook-lying position, the patient lays on his back with hips and knees sufficiently flexed so that his feet are flat on the plinth. This position minimizes lumbar lordosis. Supine or prone positioning will tend to increase lordosis, especially in the thin individual. Patients with low back pain almost always benefit from a decrease in lordosis. The drum electrode cannot be used for treatment of the back if the patient is supine or in the hook-lying position. The pancake cable is well tolerated.

The other commonly used cable winding is three dimensional. It is used in the technique with the clinical designation of "wraparound" application. This is useful in the treatment of a segment of an extremity. Since the cable is literally wrapped around the extremity with three to five turns, good uniformity of TTR can be achieved up to a depth of about 3 cm. The turns should be at least 3 cm apart. When used with apparatus specifically designed for cable (or drum) electrodes (operating frequency = 13.56 MHz), the turns can be as much as 10 cm apart. When applied in this manner, very large areas and volumes of tissues can be treated with excellent uniformity of tissue temperature rise. Bony protuberances are no problem, since additional dielectric material can be easily added between cable and skin where the cable must be positioned close to bone. Spacers should be used to insure uniform distance between turns if they are only 3 to 5 cm apart.

A major problem with use of the cable electrode, with both the pancake coil and the wrap-around technic, is the amount of linen that must be used to provide an adequate dielectric between the cable and the skin. For best depth of penetration of energy the cable, the dielectric thickness should be at least 1 cm (cable on body), or 1.5 to 2 cm if body weight is compressing the dielectric on the cable. Bath toweling should always be placed next to the skin, just as for any SWD treatment. The rest of the necessary space can be filled with any dry linen. Only the innermost layer needs to be changed with each treatment. Purchase and maintenance of the requisite linen can be a major cost if use of the cable electrode is high. Also, it takes time and patience on the part of the therapist to properly position the linen and to effectively wind the cable to fit the area to be treated. Many therapists will not take the time to do a good job, especially if they do not realize that at times the cable electrode can be more effective than any other means of causing a deep TTR in a large cylindrical volume of tissue.

Since the core of the cable consists of many small-diameter strands of copper wire, and since it is wound in many different shapes for treatment of various areas, it is wise to check the cable regularly for deterioration. One easy way to do this is to plug in both ends of the cable to the appropriate apparatus terminals and lay the cable on a plinth in the form of an elongated U. The distance between the arms of the U should not exceed their distance apart at the terminals. Place appropriate dielectric material on the cable so that a subject can sit or lie on a small segment of both arms of the cable at about the midpoint of the U. The subject should feel a mild sensation of warmth at 30 to 50 percent of available power when the apparatus is tuned to the subject's impedance (either manually or automatically, as the case may be). If more than 50 percent of available power is needed to produce the sensation, the cable is defective and should be replaced. Another and simpler way to check for early signs of deterioration is to touch the cable, with no intervening dielectric, immediately *after* a full twenty-minute treatment. If it is hot to touch anywhere throughout its length, either the cable is becoming defective or the setup was less than optimal. If the cable tips are hot, they are no longer fitting properly into the machine terminals. Reasons for the overheating of the cable tips should be explored by the institution's electrician.

Thus, all three types of electrodes in common use with SWD have advantages and disadvantages. If diathermy is used daily, it is probably wise to have all three kinds of electrodes available, along with generators of each operating frequency (13.56 and 27.12 MHz).

MICROWAVE DIATHERMY TECHNIQUES

Microwave energy in medical use has a much higher frequency and shorter wavelength as compared to short wave diathermy. On the basis of physical laws discussed in Chapter 2, one might expect the depth of penetration would be less for microwave energy. This is *not* so for at least two reasons. First, the difference in wavelength (SWD at 22 and 11 m, MWD at 33 and 12 cm) is not great when one considers the wavelength range of the electromagnetic spectrum as a whole, from millions of kilometers to tenths of Angstrom units. Secondly, subcutaneous fat is as much or more of an obstacle for penetration of microwave as it is for shortwave energy. It is true, however, that because microwave energy can be beamed or focused toward the part to be treated, if the subcutaneous fat layer is 0.5 cm or less, MWD can cause a significant TTR up to a depth of 5 cm in soft tissue.[5, 6] The focusing allows more of the energy to strike the skin perpendicularly. This minimizes scatter and enhances absorption. Short wave energy cannot be focused with any practical clinical technic.

Areas to be Treated

Microwave energy can be beamed to only one surface at a time. For uniformity of TTR, the contour of that surface must be flat. Otherwise, that area closest to the director will exhibit a substantially greater rise in temperature as compared to those as little as 1 cm more distant. Bath toweling on the skin is not necessary because the energy transmitted to the patient is absorbed by a larger volume of tissue than is the case with SWD of equal intensity per unit area, provided the layer of subcutaneous fat is less than 5 mm in thickness. The deeper penetration of MWD under these conditions results in a smaller surface temperature rise and hence less perspiration production. Under optimal conditions, SWD will cause a significant TTR to a depth of 3 cm, whereas MWD will cause a rise to a depth of 5 cm.[3, 5, 6]

Machine Circuit Warmup

It takes considerably more time for an MWD generator to modify house current into useful quantities of microwave energy than it does for an SWD generator to convert line current into short wave energy. All commercially available microwave units require a minimum warmup time of at least two minutes. As the unit continues to be used, the warmup time gradually increases, up to five minutes. The control panel will usually have some sort of indicator light to let the operator know when the machine circuit is ready to deliver a significant amount of microwave energy. Only then should the patient circuit be energized. Most therapists will spend the 2- to 5-minute warmup time positioning the director and the patient for safe and effective treatment.

Intensity

Intensity needed should be governed by the patient sensation of warmth. This should be mild, *never hot*. No tuning, automatic or manual, is possible because of the physical characteristics of the multiple cavity anode, which is the heart of the oscillating circuit in microwave generators.

Positioning of the Director

Depending upon the volume of soft tissue that is to absorb microwave energy, the patient surface of the antenna will be placed 2 to 15 cm from the skin. Each director should be clearly labeled by the manufacturer as to the average percent of power that is safe to use (no risk of overheating any soft tissue) at any given distance within the recommended range. The metallic reflector should be visually aligned so as to be as nearly perpendicular to the skin surface as is practical. In general, rectangularly shaped reflectors are designed for nearly uniform energy output throughout the reflector area, being only slightly less at the periphery as compared to the center.[3] The hemispherically shaped reflectors are designed for minimal energy output in the center 2 to 3 cm, with a band of high energy output several centimeters wide circumscribing the center area and diminishing again toward the periphery.

Neither the antenna nor the reflector should ever be touched by any living tissue when the antenna is transmitting this very high voltage, very high frequency energy. A severe electrical burn can result, especially if the contacting skin is moist.

Indications and contraindications for application of microwave energy are the same as for short wave energy and were given earlier in this chapter.

SUMMARY

Short wave and microwave diathermy energy can cause a deeper tissue temperature rise than any form of infrared energy. Consequently, in the management of clinical problems where a deep temperature rise is more likely to give pain relief, diathermy may be the treatment of choice. Reasons for penetration of this kind of energy under optimal conditions to a depth of 3 to 5 cm are discussed.

Each type of electrode and each frequency available has advantages and disadvantages over the others, so that the most effective treatment for the individual problem may require thoughtful selection of the best treatment parameters.

There are more *contraindications* for the use of either short wave or microwave energy than for any form of infrared application. Operation of diathermy generators safely and efficiently is complex. The risk of causing a burn is greater because there is less of a skin temperature rise and more of a deep tissue temperature rise. There are more thermal receptors in the skin than in underlying tissue. Hence, neither the patient nor the therapist may be aware of a dangerous subcutaneous temperature rise until pathological heating has occurred.

Diathermy in any form should never be used when there is a cardiac pacemaker anywhere in the clinical area, nor should it be used when there is any external or internal metal within or close to the field of this penetrating high voltage energy.

DEMONSTRATIONS FOR STUDENTS

I. **To Demonstrate Differences in Temperature Rise of Oil and Water Depending Upon Type of Short Wave Diathermy Electrode Used**

   A. Procure one two-liter and one three-liter glass or other non-conducting beaker. *Do not use metal beakers.* Fill the smaller beaker with tap water. Insert it into the larger beaker, letting the bottom of the small beaker rest on a folded dry washcloth or other insulating material so that the two beakers cannot touch. Fill the larger beaker with either paraffin or mineral oil, allowing a centimeter or so margin between the top of the small beaker and the oil level in the large beaker.

   B. The beakers and their contents should be allowed to sit at room temperature for at least one hour. Then, measure and record the temperature of each liquid.

   C. Wrap a cable electrode snugly around the outside of the large beaker, using at least three turns with at least a 3 cm distance between each turn, holding this position with cable spacers.

   D. Energize the cable at 50 percent available power. Tune the cable circuit if the generator requires manual tuning. Let the current flow for twenty minutes. After turning the power off, remeasure the temperature of the oil and of the water. *Do not* attempt to measure temperature while the power is on. The reading will be erroneous because of the magnetic field, and if an electronic thermometer was used, the probe and measuring circuits could be damaged beyond repair. Record the "posttreatment" temperatures.

   E. The next day, repeat steps A through D, using a drum electrode designed for the same generator. Note the differences in temperature change. The change in water temperature will be smaller because the beakers were not exposed circumferentially. Likewise, the change in oil temperature will be smaller, for the same reason, but the difference will be greater for the water.

F. The next day, repeat steps A through D, using air-spaced plate electrodes designed for the same generator. It will be observed that the increase in oil temperature will be much greater and the increase in water temperature will be much less than was the case for either the drum or cable electrodes. This should help one to remember that where the energy coming from the electrode is primarily electric field, essentially no energy is transferred to the inner beaker as a primary process, whereas when the energy coming from the electrode is roughly 50-50 electric and magnetic, a significantly greater amount penetrates to the contents of the inner beaker and hence produces a greater deep tissue temperature rise.

G. Hence, one can conclude that when properly applied, the drum or cable electrode is more apt to give a greater deep tissue temperature rise as compared to air-spaced plates. The latter are more apt to heat subcutaneous fat layers to dangerous levels with a minimal rise in underlying muscle temperature.

II. To demonstrate Significant Differences in Deep Tissue Temperature Rise Depending Upon Whether the Frequency Used Is 27.12 MHz or 13.56 MHz

A. The phantom setup should be as described in Demonstration I, steps A through D.

B. Use only cable electrodes, one for a generator of each of the above-assigned operating frequencies.

C. It will be noted that the temperature rise in the two beakers will vary on the basis of operating frequency. The generator operating at the higher frequency and shorter wavelength will produce a greater oil temperature and a lower water temperature rise as compared to the results when the lower frequency, longer wavelength unit is used, *if the energy added per unit volume* is equal in the two cases.

D. To insure that energy added is equal in both cases, first apply a cable electrode to a human subject. The coil can be wrapped around an upper arm or thigh, utilizing the standard treatment technics detailed within the chapter. Turn up the intensity until the subject reports a mild sensation of warmth. Note the percent of available power needed to achieve that sensation. Repeat, using the other generator, on the contralateral area approximately one hour later. Note the percent of power needed to achieve equivalent sensation. Use these two power settings to achieve the most reliable results when measuring temperature change within the phantom.

E. A major reason for the difference in results observed when comparing the two frequencies is that the relationships among capacitance, inductance, and reactance vary with the SWD frequencies. The lower frequency achieves a more nearly 50-50 relationship between electric and magnetic field production. It is the magnetic field that is the major factor in water temperature rise and the electric field that is the major factor in oil temperature rise.

F. One can then conclude that if one wishes to achieve the best possible deep TTR with the cable (or drum) electrode, one should use the lower frequency.

III. To Demonstrate That with Both SWD and MWD Electrical Energy Is Transmitted to the Patient and That MWD Frequencies Can Be Focused Whereas SWD Frequencies Cannot

A. Position a subject for treatment of any area.

B. Use any SWD generator in the standard fashion outlined within the chapter. Turn up intensity until the subject reports a mild sensation of warmth.

C. Another individual should then hold a 20 to 40 watt incandescent bulb or fluorescent light tube close to but not touching the energized electrode. *Do not* touch any metal on the bulb or tube. The bulb will light up.

D. This should indicate that a strong electric and/or magnetic field is present in the air around the electrode. If intensity is varied, the amount of light will vary in direct proportion. Intensity should be controlled by a third individual.

E. Move the light source along the electrode leads and around the generator. The bulb will stay lit, indicating the SWD generator emits significant energy in all directions.

F. Repeat steps A through D with any MWD generator. Note that the bulb will light up only when the bulb is between the director and the subject. As soon as the light source is moved to the surface of the director that is away from the subject, the light goes out. If moved along the antenna lead toward the generator, the bulb will not light up.

G. One can then conclude that MWD energy can be focused whereas SWD energy cannot, and that the transmission lead from generator to antenna is superior in insulation quality as compared to SWD.

REFERENCES

1. *Dorland's Illustrated Medical Dictionary,* 24th ed. Philadelphia, Saunders, 1965.
2. *Webster's Seventh New Collegiate Dictionary.* Springfield, Mass., Merriam, 1971.
3. Licht, S.: *Therapeutic Heat and Cold,* 2nd ed. New Haven, Licht, 1965, Chapters 3, 11, 12.
4. Hall, E. L.: Diathermy generators. *Arch Phys Med Rehabil, 33:*28-36, 1952.
5. Glasser, O. (Ed.): *Medical Physics,* Volume I. Chicago, Year Bk Med, 1945, pp. 1091-2.
6. Warren, G. C., Department of Physical Medicine, University of Washington, Seattle, Washington, personal communication, 1980.
7. Lehmann, J. F. et al.: Modification of heating patterns with 2456 and 900 Mc energy. *Arch Phys Med Rehabil, 45:*555-63, 1964.
8. Lehmann, J. F. et al.: Muscle heating with 915 Mc microwave diathermy. *Arch Phys Med Rehabil, 51:*147-51, 1970.
9. Abramson, D. I. et al.: Change in blood flow, oxygen uptake and tissue temperature with shortwave diathermy. *Am J Phys Med, 39:*87-95, 1960.
10. Downey, J. A. et al.: Vascular response in the forearm to heating by shortwave diathermy. *Arch Phys Med Rehabil, 51:*354-7, 1970.

11. Pringsheim, P.: *Fluorescence and Phosphorescence.* New York, Interscience, 1949.
12. Scott, P.: *Clayton's Electrotherapy and Actinotherapy,* 5th ed. London, Balliere, Tyndall and Cassell, 1965.
13. Jones, S. L.: Electromagnetic field interference and cardiac pacemakers. *Phys Ther, 56:*1013-18, 1976.

Chapter 5

THE INFRARED ENERGIES

INTRODUCTION

THEORETICALLY, ANY OBJECT whose temperature is greater than 0° Kelvin (-273°C) is radiating energy of wavelengths classified as infrared. Practical clinical sources include cold and hot packs, the whirlpool (and Hubbard tank), paraffin baths, steam cabinets, and infrared lamps. The physiological effects are similar for all these forms of energy if the temperature of the energy reaching the patient is higher than that of the skin or subcutaneous tissue that absorbs the energy. If the temperature of the source is lower than that of nearby skin, a different pattern of reaction will take place because thermal energy always flows from a source of relatively high to relatively low temperature. Therefore, when the patient is exposed to an object whose temperature is lower than that of skin, energy in the form of heat will flow from the patient toward that object. The local and whole-body response to loss of heat is different from the response to addition of heat.

NORMAL TISSUE TEMPERATURES

Normal human core (whole-body) temperature is 37 ± 1°C.[1] Skin and other tissue temperatures in the head, neck, and trunk are usually quite close to those values except in extreme environments. However, more distally in the extremities, normal skin and subcutaneous temperatures steadily decline, to a greater extent in the lower as compared to the upper limbs. The normal difference in arm and leg temperature is largely the result of the greater effects of gravity on circulation in the lower extremities resulting in greater circulatory stagnation.

In the normal individual in a temperate environment, subcutaneous temperature will be 1° to 2°C higher than that of overlying skin. Tissue closer to bone has a higher temperature than that close to skin. Under baseline conditions (no clothing, horizontally at rest for at least thirty minutes in a room whose temperature is constant at 21° to 22°C with humidity stable at 50 percent) a fingertip temperature of 32° and a toetip temperature of 28° would be the lower limits of normal skin temperature.[2]

During a twenty-four-hour period, the normal individual experiences fluctuation in distal extremity temperature, especially in the skin, in response to ambient temperature, caloric intake, and degree of skeletal muscle activity. Fluctuation on the order of ± 5°C is common in the fingers. They are usually exposed and normally play a major role in release or conservation of heat in maintaining core temperature. Fluctuation on the order of ± 2°C is more common in toes. They are usually encased in shoes.

If *local* tissue temperature reaches 45°C for an appreciable length of time, necrosis occurs from thermal damage. If local tissue temperature reaches 13°, necrosis occurs from intracellular ice crystal formation. These limits can be reached with brief exposure to a great temperature differential or with prolonged exposure to a lesser differential. *Core* temperatures above 42° or below 25°C are likely to be fatal, even if that temperature is maintained for only a short period of time.[1] The normal human has many mechanisms of local, nervous system, and humoral control to avoid such drastic changes in both local and core temperatures.[3, 4]

Alteration in blood volume and flow rate are the major mechanisms by which the normal body strives to maintain core and peripheral temperatures within tolerable limits. The local reactions, nervous system, and humoral controls all have roles in variation of vasomotor tension. In general, when energy absorption causes a *local* tissue temperature rise (TTR), as would be the case with application of the diathermies, the infrareds, and ultrasound, vasodilation will occur transiently. If energy is withdrawn (cold application), vasoconstriction will occur transiently. A significant TTR occurs when the circulating blood does not dissipate energy as fast as it is being added. If the local temperature rises and then levels off, the blood flow is then adequate to disseminate the added energy as fast as it is absorbed. If the local temperature drops (cold application), thermal energy is being withdrawn from the area faster than warmer blood can flow in from other body areas.

CLINICAL SKIN TEMPERATURE PATTERNS

In the normal adult, when energy is absorbed at a comfortable rate, maximum dilation will be achieved with a twenty- to thirty-minute exposure to any form of infrared or the diathermies. The anticipated skin temperature curve is a rather rapid rise for the first ten minutes, followed by a plateau for another ten to fifteen minutes, and either a rise or a drop if treatment continues beyond thirty minutes.[7] The initial rise is due to energy being absorbed at a faster rate than the gradually dilating arteriolar vessels can bring cooler blood into the area. The plateau occurs when there has been enough dilation so that a sufficient amount of cooler blood is coming into the area being treated for energy to be carried away as fast as it is being added. If the arterial vessels continue to dilate further, they may reach the point at which absorbed energy is carried away faster than it is added, at which time local temperature will start to drop toward the resting level. More often, the local arteries will have reached their maximum capacity for dilation at some point between a ten- and twenty-minute exposure to thermal energy and will then undergo a rebound vasoconstriction. Because energy is no longer disseminated as efficiently as before, the tissue temperature will rapidly increase.

If an infrared source is applied to cause a TTR, another anticipated reaction is uniform cutaneous vasodilation due to local histamine release. This leads to a gradual change in skin color — hyperemia — which is readily apparent in Caucasian or Mongolian skin. If any form of diathermy is used to cause the TTR, one would not expect to see as striking an amount of hyperemia because a considerable amount of this energy should be absorbed deep to the skin. Because diathermy wavelengths are longer than those for infrared, less energy is absorbed per unit *volume* of tissue. Therefore, the visible reaction will not be as great (*see* Chapters 2 and 4 for details).

MOTTLING

If exposure to and absorption of energy that causes a TTR continues appreciably beyond thirty minutes, a rebound vasomotor reaction usually occurs. If it does, and if it is ignored, an injurious TTR is likely to take place. This is more likely to take place with any form of infrared than with any form of diathermy because more energy is absorbed by superficial tissues when infrared is applied.[7]

The first warning that such a harmful reaction may take place is the appearance of mottling. In this situation, the skin will become abnormally white in patches, interlaced with angry red blotches. If this reaction appears, energy addition should be discontinued for that treatment period, or the rate at which energy is being added should be diminished. If no adjustment is made after mottling appears, a burn is likely to result. Once mottling has occurred, the skin is apt to retain its unique appearance for one-half to several hours after removal from the energy source. The angry red and pallescent patches gradually return to normal color as skin temperature reaches normal limits.

When energy is added with the intent of causing a TTR, one of the first tissue reactions to that change in environment is local release of histamine or histaminelike substances. Histamine is a potent vasodilator. Its release is seen clinically as hyperemia — a reddening of the skin. If the temperature change is fast and drastic, histamine is released in large quantities. Its massive release can cause a transient paralysis of the nerve supply to arteriole-sized vessels, forcing them to stay in maximum vasodilation until the histamine has been partially resorbed or metabolized. Recovery from the vessel paralysis may take several hours. Cells in the temperature-threatened area do not release histamine at a uniform rate. When arterial muscle is paralyzed in dilation, the associated capillaries are patent and engorged, yielding an angry red color. If the energy absorbing cells do not release enough histamine to cause paralysis but the cutaneous blood supply has been maximally dilated for a prolonged period, the muscle in vessel walls can go into spasm. This leads to local vasoconstriction with subsequent closing of associated capillaries. When the vasoconstriction is extreme, patches of pallor are plainly visible. These reactions result in the mottled appearance of the skin.

CIRCULATORY IMPAIRMENT AND INFRARED

If the patient to whom energy is being added has a circulatory impairment, a TTR to safe limits may occur much more rapidly than would be the case if his circulation were normal. This is largely due to the fact that when flow is impaired and energy is added, the heated blood is not replaced with cooler blood as quickly as with normal circulation. Thus, when adding energy in the presence of known circulatory problem, the intensity should be lower than otherwise. A commonly used technic in the known presence of a circulatory problem is "reflex-heating." In this technic, energy is added in an area remote to the site where a TTR is desired. Since most chronic circulatory impairments are more severe in the distal portions of the extremities and more severe in the lower extremities, the low back is frequently the site of choice for "reflex-heating." The degree of TTR in the distal lower extremities is considerably less than if energy were added directly to the involved problem area. The distal arterial vessels are more likely to be able to achieve enough dilation under these conditions of remote heating to safely dissipate the energy being added. Conversely, if the local TTR is too great, the local arterial vessels could go into spasm, vasoconstriction would occur and serious tissue damage (burn) could be the result.

Since any form of infrared will be less penetrating than any form of diathermy, the risk of skin damage with the application of infrared can be greater than with diathermy. However, cutaneous sensation is much more sensitive than that of underlying fat or muscle, because of the greater number of sensory receptors of all kinds, so the patient is more apt to be aware of a dangerous TTR if it affects the skin.

HOT PACKS

Hot packs are a very widely used form of infrared, with transfer of energy from source to patient primarily by conduction. They are inexpensive, easy to apply, and highly effective in relieving pain caused by superficial muscle spasm.

Hot packs in their present form came into use in the 1940s, with development of suitable thermostatically controlled water heaters and development of the pack itself. Some kinds of silicon dioxide (SiO_2) are very hygroscopic. Each molecule of the "sand" used in these packs has the capacity to absorb approximately seventeen molecules of water. This sand is contained in a woven fabric that is tight enough to hold the sand, but loose enough to admit water. When immersed in water, the pack swells to several times its dry size. The affinity of this special sand for water is so great that, when removed from water, it takes from three days to a week for the pack to dry. The individual pack is divided into pouches of about 15 × 5 × 3 cm when dry. They are supplied in various sizes, having as few as six and as many as thirty-six pouches in one pack, for application to any and all neck, trunk, and extremity segments. The division into pouches gives a reasonable degree of flexibility so that the wet pack can approximate body contour. The pack will not leak sand unless the fabric is ruptured. With reasonable care in handling, the pack should last for five years or more.

The Water Heating Unit

The standard stainless steel container for heating the water comes in many sizes, from that needed to hold three standard size packs (twelve pouches, divided into two rows of six each) up to containers large enough to hold twenty-five packs, each with thirty-six pouches. Depending upon container size, there will be one or more heating units in the bottom of the container. The packs are stored in racks, which hold the packs vertically and are completely covered with water. When properly placed in the container, the pack never touches the heating unit. If it does, the fabric will scorch or burn and result in a sand leak. If this happens, the water becomes turbid, and the pack should be discarded.

The heating unit can be adjusted to maintain water temperature set for anywhere between 65° and 90°C. It is recommended that a good waterproof and relatively unbreakable thermometer be kept in the pack console. The heating unit can malfunction and cause the water temperature to go up or down beyond the practical temperature range. The thermometer should be read at least twice daily.

Precautions When Using Hot Packs

No one can tolerate direct contact with water at 65°C without tissue damage. Consequently, insulating bath toweling is standardly used between skin and pack. Toweling on the side of the pack away from the patient will also help to minimize heat loss from pack to room air. If initial pack temperature is lower than 65°C, by the end of the standard twenty-minute treatment the patient is likely to have a cold, clammy sensation, which will not encourage muscle relaxation. A reasonable rule of thumb for a first exposure to hot packs, if stored at that temperature, is three layers of bath toweling between packs and skin. If initial storage was at 90°C, there should be at least six layers of insulating toweling. The above suggestions are for when the pack is lying on the patient. If the patient is lying on the pack, the amount of toweling needed may need to be more than doubled, in compensation for body weight compressing the toweling.

Direct contact with water at these temperatures can also burn the pack handler. Therefore, the pack should be removed from the container with tongs, grasping the pack tabs designed for this purpose. The pack should be held out of water until the excess has dripped off (about thirty seconds) to avoid soaking the insulating toweling. The layer of towel next to skin must be dry. Otherwise, a burn can result. If the patient complains at any time during the treatment that the sensation is more than comfortably warm, more toweling should be added. If the patient reports no sensation of warmth within two or three minutes after the pack has been applied, one or more layers of toweling should be removed.

In any case, it is the therapist's responsibility to inspect the skin in the area to be treated, before, during, and after treatment, regardless of patient statement of sensation. Any blemish on the skin before treatment should be described and recorded. The anticipated skin reaction from the standard treatment is that within five minutes the patient's skin will be warm to touch, with or without the appearance of hyperemia. If the hyperemia is an angry red, or if mottling has occurred, more toweling *must* be added, or the pack removed, to prevent a burn. Ideally, the first time the patient receives a hot pack treatment, the skin should be reinspected every five minutes throughout the treatment period. Once that patient's reaction to the treatment is established, on subsequent treatment, skin inspection prior to treatment and five minutes later may be adequate.

If the patient is emotionally disturbed, has a neurological deficit, or is on medication that could impair sensation, regular skin inspection during each treatment is mandatory. Any lesion resulting from the treatment is the therapist's responsibility, regardless of patient behavior during treatment.

Because of the large volume of bath towels and other linen needed if the clinic has much demand for use of hot packs, many departments have installed automatic washers and dryers. Over a period of several years, this cost will be more than returned by the savings in commercial laundry bills and lower investment in the actual numbers of towels needed by the department.

THE PARAFFIN BATH

The paraffin bath has been in clinical use longer than the hot pack. It is especially useful for pain relief in *chronic* orthopedic lesions, such as in rheumatoid, osteo-, or mixed arthritis, involving joints distal to the elbow or knee.

The contents of the paraffin bath are actually a mixture of paraffin and paraffin oil, mineral oil, or petroleum jelly. Perhaps the most widely used mixture for a standard-sized upper extremity bath is 25 Kg of solid paraffin to 1 liter of paraffin oil. The paraffin is a solid at room temperature and is supplied in slabs weighing 4 to 5 Kg. This paraffin liquifies when stored at temperatures above 40°C. Hence, it is placed in a thermostatically controlled stainless steel container of suitable dimensions to immerse an arm (up to and covering the elbow) or a leg (up to the knee). The other ingredient is added to the bath to make it easier to remove solidified paraffin from hairy skin. If the bath is intended for upper extremity use, most clinics set the temperature within the range of 52° to 58°C. If primarily for lower extremity use, the temperature is usually within the 45 to 52 degree range.

Physical Differences Between Paraffin and Water

One might immediately wonder how a patient can tolerate immersion of a body segment into paraffin at these temperatures when it was previously stated that heating of normal tissue to 45°C is likely to cause irreversible damage. There are several physical reasons why paraffin, but not water, can safely come into contact with skin at these higher temperatures. One difference is in the quantity of thermal energy released per degree drop in temperature by water as compared to paraffin. The amount of energy needed to raise the temperature of water one degree is nearly double that needed to raise the temperature of paraffin. The specific heat (S.H.) of water is arbitrarily set at 1.0. The S.H. of clinically used paraffin is approximately 0.65. The S.H. of paraffin oil, mineral oil, and petroleum jelly is about 0.45. When cooling, therefore, less energy is released by these liquids.

Secondly, when living tissue is immersed in the bath, the paraffin in contact with the skin cools to a solid almost instantaneously because of the low skin temperature. This one or two millimeter layer of solidified paraffin now acts as a thermal insulator so that the surrounding liquid paraffin, which is of higher temperature, can no longer transmit as much thermal energy to the skin. A small volume of air also frequently becomes trapped between the skin and the solidified paraffin, especially upon repeated movement of the segment into and out of the paraffin. The trapped air acts as additional insulation.

For both of the above reasons, and possibly more, the starting temperature of the liquid paraffin mixture can be higher than if the applied liquid were water.

Physiological Differences Between the Paraffin Bath and Water

The next question might well be, why not substitute use of water at a lower temperature. This is done with both the whirlpool and Hubbard tank. Why bother to have both whirlpool and paraffin available? It is the clinical experience of many therapists and physicians that the patient with a *chronic* orthopedic lesion will usually perceive a greater and longer-lasting pain relief when the paraffin bath can be used as the source for adding thermal energy, as compared to water.

The reasons for this are not known. There is a useful working hypothesis. The paraffin close to the skin is a solid and a very effective insulator, especially if the solid layer is built up by repeated immersion to a thickness of more than 5 mm. The net result is that the cutaneous receptors are cut off from all extrinsic stimuli except the thermal stimulus. This enables the local cutaneous sensory system to be maximally flooded with thermal input. If one accepts the gate control theory of pain and pain relief (Chapter 1), optimal conditions are set up for pain relief. Furthermore, the insulating capability of paraffin diminishes heat loss by evaporation (in the area where the paraffin is applied). The end result is a greater local TTR, a more pronounced hyperemia, and pain relief that lasts for an hour or more.

It is not practical, however, to apply paraffin to the more proximal body segments, nor is it recommended for use when local circulation is impaired. The whirlpool (or Hubbard tank) then becomes more practical and safer.[7]

Technics of Application of Paraffin

Two technics are in common use when applying paraffin. One is usually called the "dip and wrap" technic. The distal extremity is slowly dipped into the hot liquid and withdrawn. This is repeated until a glove of solidified paraffin of 5 to 10 mm has been built up. The number of dips required will depend largely on the temperature differential between the skin and the liquid paraffin. The hotter the paraffin, the more dips needed to make an effective glove. When the glove is adequate, the segment enclosed by the glove is inserted into a loosely fitting plastic bag and then into an insulating fabric several layers thick. Paper toweling may be substituted for the plastic bag and bath toweling for the fabric bag. Any cloth that must be laundered should not come into contact with paraffin. It is difficult to separate one from the other. After the part is adequately insulated, the patient is allowed to rest comfortably for about twenty minutes. The paraffin glove is then removed and saved for reuse after reheating; whatever additional treatment is needed is then done. The skin will invariably be moist, supple, and hyperemic.

If mottling is present to a significant extent, the number of dips used at the next treatment should be diminished. Mottling is more apt to appear with treatment by paraffin than with treatment by any other form of infrared. This is due to the initial liquid temperature and to the extreme insulating capacity of paraffin, even at room temperature.

The other widely used technic of paraffin application is called "dip and leave in." The dipping procedure is as was described for the "dip and wrap" technic. After a thick glove of solidified paraffin has been built up, the distal segment and its glove are reimmersed in the constant-temperature bath for a fifteen- to twenty-minute period. The patient should be seated comfortably during the "leave in" period. With this technic, the anticipated skin and subcutaneous TTR will be higher during and for a longer period of time after treatment. Therefore, it is recommended that bath temperature not exceed 52°C (hand) or 45°C (foot).

Precautions

The risk of burn is greater with paraffin application as compared to hot pack use, especially with the "dip and leave in" procedure. Therefore it is recommended that an easily readable thermometer be immersed in the liquid paraffin before each treatment. Until the thermometer stem warms up to a higher temperature than that at which paraffin solidifies, a coating will form on the stem and give a false low reading, by as much as 5°C. It is also recommended that the thermometer stem be placed deep in the bath and kept moving until the reading is stable. The heating units are in the bottom, and the paraffin is frequently hotter toward the bottom of the bath.

The thermostats on paraffin baths are usually reliable, but they can fail. There is an additional danger with paraffin, that of a flash fire if a malfunctioning thermostat raises the paraffin temperature above 85°C. The paraffin and other ingredients all have flash points below the temperature at which water boils. Therefore, a working fire extinguisher should always be near but not too close to the paraffin unit. It should be of the CO_2 type rather than one of those in which water is a major constituent.

Because of the strain placed on cutaneous and subcutaneous circulation by application of paraffin, many therapists are reluctant to use it on lower extremities. Circulation is always less efficient in the lower as compared to the upper limb, and a majority of arthritic patients are of an age where they will have an appreciable circulatory impairment affecting the blood flow in the calf and foot. Hence, it is recommended that a separate bath, set at a lower temperature (48° to 52°C), be used.

Cleaning the Paraffin Bath

In normal usage, perspiration, dirt, and other skin debris will accumulate because of the immersion in the liquid paraffin. Water and most of the debris will settle to the bottom, since paraffin is of low density. Most baths will have some kind of perforated cover between the tank bottom and the immersion area. The heating elements are never open, so they cannot be touched, but the liquid near the bottom is always hotter, and the bottom itself is very hot to touch. Since the top several millimeters of the paraffin is usually solid, because of prolonged exposure to room air, the debris and water at the bottom are not usually visible to the therapist or patient.

If the bath is in repeated daily use, it must be taken out of service and cleaned about every six months. This is a two- or three-day procedure. The liquid paraffin does not drain out easily because of instant solidification at exposure to room temperatures. If an attempt is to be made to salvage some of the paraffin, it is common to add several tablespoons of powdered boric acid to the liquid. This will tend to pool the accumulated water. If the draining paraffin is run through a cheesecloth seive, most of the debris can be collected and discarded. The last several centimeters of sludge at the bottom should always be discarded. Mechanical scraping of the sides and bottom, followed by scrubbing with a fat solvent, will complete the cleaning. Alcohol, toluene, benzene, carbon tetrachloride, and ether are all useful for the scrubbing. All except alcohol are also highly volatile and toxic to humans. Hence, the room where this is done must be well ventilated, and smoking should be prohibited.

Debris accumulation can be kept to a minimum by thorough

washing of the part to be treated, including rinsing and drying, before immersion.

Treatment by means of the paraffin bath is inevitably messy, even with careful technic. Some scraps of solidified paraffin will always reach the floor. This can be a major hazard because solidified paraffin is very slippery to walk on. The floor around the bath should be scraped at least at the end of each day and lightly scrubbed with alcohol or other fat solvent.

HOT MOIST AIR

Although not in widespread use because of equipment cost for safe and efficient utilization, if water is heated to form steam and the cooling vapor is transmitted to the trunk, hot moist air is a very effective way of inducing "reflex heating" to the extremities. The water temperature is thermostatically controlled so that the vapor reaching the patient's skin is readily adjusted within the range of 70° to 90°C. This will produce a strong hyperemia in all exposed skin and induce a distal extremity skin temperature rise of 5° to 10°C. Skin temperature does not return to pretreatment levels for up to six hours if ambient temperature is reasonably constant. Rise in body temperature is rare and not desirable. If it occurs, the patient's thermoregulatory mechanisms are not functioning adequately and treatment should be discontinued.

Practical and commercially available equipment consists of a stainless steel plinth of usual dimensions to which is attached a foldable platform extension large enough to hold the water heating unit. This hood-shaped unit is designed to roll freely into position over the supine or prone patient.

Technic of Application

The patient is placed on the padded plinth with all but essential clothing removed. The heating unit is then rolled into position over the trunk area. Plastic curtains attached to the inverted U-shaped hood are then tucked around the neck and shoulders, trunk, and hips. The heating unit is turned on. Within five minutes, an adequate quantity of hot water vapor fills the enclosed space. The heating unit is left running at the desired temperature for twenty to forty minutes. Pain due to orthopedic trauma (such as muscle spasm) is usually reduced with the shorter treatment time. Chronic arterial vasospasm usually responds better to a lower temperature and longer treatment time. If the room temperature is over 28°C, administration of salt tablets during or after treatment may be indicated, since sweating will be profuse. Most patients go to sleep during the treatment. After treatment, the patient must be thoroughly dried and kept in a draft-free area for at least one-half hour. As a precautionary measure, it is recommended that for the first several treatments the patient's oral temperature, blood pressure, and toetip skin temperature be recorded before and after treatment.

The authors are unaware of any definitive study comparing attempts at pain relief by hot moist air and with any other form of infrared energy. If there is a significant difference, it may be due to the fact that a greater number of cutaneous thermal receptors are receiving maximum stimulation, resulting in thorough muscle relaxation and reduction in vasomotor tone, with exposure of a large part of the trunk to hot moist air.

INFRARED LAMPS AND BAKERS

As with the application of hot packs or a paraffin bath, when one uses an infrared lamp (IRL), a 5° to 10°C skin temperature rise is anticipated in the area of application. Infrared lamps and bakers have the advantage of being able to cause a superficial TTR in an area where the patient cannot tolerate the weight of a hot pack or where a skin lesion precludes significant temporary skin hydration. Furthermore, it is easier to control intensity of energy absorption with an IRL or baker as compared to the paraffin bath. Finally, the quantity of linen necessary when radiant heat is used, as compared to conductive heating, is negligible.

Despite the above advantages, radiant heat is not in common use at this time. It does not give as effective pain relief as either hot packs or paraffin. The reasons for this have not been explored in detail.[7] However, speculation, on the basis of the gate control theory of pain relief (Chapter 1), could indicate that because the patient is not in direct contact with the source of thermal energy, the cutaneous receptors are not as isolated from other external stimuli, such as air currents. Numerous studies in the 1940s, and 1950s have shown that the depth of tissue temperature rise within a standard twenty-minute treatment is essentially equal for any clinical source used to add thermal energy. These data have been well presented in earlier literature.[5-7]

Bakers are rarely used today. Presumably, this is because they are relatively heavy, bulky, and hard to move on and off the patient. Also, they fall easily if jarred by the patient or therapist. The standard baker consists of four to eight incandescent bulbs with a wattage rating of 25 to 60 per bulb. These are evenly spaced within an inverted U-shaped reflector. They are wired so that four, six, or eight bulbs are radiating infrared energy simultaneously, thus giving easy control of intensity. It is practical to use a baker to induce a superficial TTR on the posterior trunk, hips, or on segments of the lower extremities. It is rarely possible to use a baker to supply heat to the upper extremities because of awkwardness of patient positioning.

The authors are not aware of any company that manufactures a nonluminous infrared lamp at this time. Several manufacturers do continue to make luminous lamps. It was shown late in the 1920s that, because of certain unique characteristics of human skin, infrared at a wavelength of about 12,000 Å will penetrate slightly more deeply than either longer (nonluminous and carbon filament incandescent bulbs) or shorter wavelengths. Tungsten filament bulbs and special "quartz" rod sources produce significant amounts of infrared at the 12,000 Å wavelength. Both types of luminous sources present a major problem with glare from the source or its reflector. When a luminous lamp is used at an angle or in an area in which glare can irritate the patient's eyes, the lamp should be shielded. This is done usually by fastening a sheet around the reflector. When this is done, care must be taken to avoid covering the reflector's ventilating holes. Otherwise, the draping material may catch fire, as the source reflector becomes quite hot.

When an infrared lamp is indicated, the authors prefer a luminous source with a ruby-red colored glass envelope. Essentially, no radiation as short as 12,000 Å is passed by the colored envelope. The standard 250 watt incandescent bulb generates adequate thermal energy for treatment of surfaces in one plane up to 50 cm diameter at a distance of 50 cm from the skin. The colored envelope filters all the glare-producing visible radiation. This eliminates the need for draping the source. Most patients find the resulting visible red radiation very soothing psychologically, while receiving the same benefits as from any other source of infrared energy.

Technique of Application

Most infrared lamps are mounted on casters so that with reasonable care the lamp is easily moved. The lamp is adjustable in height through a wide range and can be tilted vertically and/or horizontally. Frequently, there is provision for moving the reflector and its bulb laterally with respect to the upright. When this adjustment is provided, the base should be weighted.

There are two physical laws that the therapist should keep in mind when applying either an infrared or an ultraviolet lamp (Chapter 6) to a patient.

THE COSINE LAW. The cosine law states —

> The energy per square centimeter is proportional to a constant multiplied by the cosine of the angle made by a line connecting the source and the patient, and a line perpendicular to the patient's body. That constant is the light per square centimeter when the patient is perpendicular to the line joining the light and the patient.[8]

Clinically, this means that if energy is to be absorbed rather than reflected from the skin, the source should be approximately perpendicular to the surface being treated. In practice, deviation of 10° from the perpendicular is acceptable. Such an approximation of a right angle is easy to achieve without a measuring device.

THE INVERSE SQUARE LAW. The inverse square law states —

> The intensity of radiation from any source of light varies inversely with the square of the distance from the source.[8]

One might assume that when a light source is 40 cm from the surface to be treated, the amount of energy absorbed would be twice as great as compared to when the source is 80 cm away.

This is incorrect. If the lamp is twice the distance away, the radiation intensity is only one fourth as great, if all other factors are equal. For example, if one squares 40 (40 × 40 = 1600), squares 80 (6400), and then divides 6400 by 1600, it is seen that the square of 80 is four times greater than the square of 40.

Clinically, if a patient reports that a source of radiant heat is uncomfortable, or if mottling becomes visible during treatment, two things could be done. One could either increase the distance between the source and the patient or cover the patient surface with a towel. In either case, energy reaching the patient will be decreased. If the distance is increased, the inverse square law should be kept in mind, thus realizing that an increase of a few centimeters can result in a significant decrease in energy reaching the patient.

The distance between source and patient will necessarily be different if the IR source is 250 as compared to 1250 watts (w). A 250 w lamp with an 18 to 40 cm diameter reflector would usually be placed 40 to 50 cm distant. A 1250 w source would commonly be positioned 75 to 90 cm away from the skin. The larger source will usually have a larger reflector. Because less energy per unit area may reach the patient when a larger reflector is used, the therapist must select the appropriate distance with both wattage and reflector size in mind.

Adequate provision for locking the source in place at the desired distance is critical for patient safety. It is the therapist's responsibility to see to it that the reflector cannot drop onto the patient during a treatment period. A serious burn could occur. The lowest-temperature nonluminous source of infrared will have an operating temperature of about 400°C, and the common luminous source, a tungsten filament incandescent bulb, a temperature of about 3000°. In both cases, the reflector becomes too hot to touch.

Skin Inspection

Whenever treatment is given with the objective of causing a TTR, it is the therapist's responsibility to inspect the skin in the area to be treated *before* treatment and to descriptively record any skin lesion. Furthermore, the skin should be inspected after treatment to make sure no damage (burn) has occurred. Damage with application of any form of infrared is rare, *unless* the patient is emotionally disturbed or has diminished or absent cutaneous sensation. If either of the above circumstances are known to be a factor with an individual patient, the therapist should visually inspect the skin *at least* every five minutes during treatment and adjust intensity as necessary.

Movement of a Lamp or Baker After Treatment

For safety, as soon as the treatment is over, the lamp or baker should be removed from its position over the patient. Then the lamp should be lowered to its lowest adjustment in height and moved out of the treatment area. When the lamp is at its lowest height, its center of gravity is as low as possible and it is less apt to tip over on lateral movement. The baker reflector will be too hot to touch except at its handles. Care should be taken to lift it *up* and then off away from the patient; it should then be placed on the floor until it is cool.

FLUIDOTHERAPY*

In spite of its trade name, this treatment is the dryest of all forms of infrared in clinical use. Presumably the term Fluidotherapy was coined because the dry powder used to transmit the infrared is kept in motion while the patient is treated. The extremity segment(s) to be treated are inserted via an airtight port into a container that holds several cubic feet of a low density powder. The powder can be preheated through a clinically suitable range of temperatures. A comparative study by Borrell et al. (1980) showed the treatment is most effective in causing a TTR inside small joint capsules when the powder temperature is maintained at 48°C (118°F).[11] After the part to be treated is immersed into the powder, a variable speed blower is used to set the material into motion. Standard treatment time is twenty minutes. After treatment, the powder can be heated to sterilizing temperatures to minimize risk of contamination of other patients. If the patient has an open wound, it can be covered with an airtight dressing prior to treatment.

---

* Fluidotherapy is the trade name registered by Fluidotherapy Corporation Therapy Devices, Houston, Texas 77081.

Presumably this treatment provides mechanical as well as thermal stimulus to cutaneous receptors. Hence it would represent, as does aerated water, a more intense pain replacement stimulus as compared to application of a hot pack or paraffin. This treatment came into clinical use in the 1970s. Several reports have appeared demonstrating its rationale and effectiveness in the management of chronic musculoskeletal pain problems.[9-11]

WHIRLPOOLS AND HUBBARD TANKS

The whirlpool (WP) and Hubbard tank (HT) are convenient sources of infrared energy which can be used to cause either a mild tissue temperature rise (TTR) or a slight drop in superficial tissue temperature. If the water temperature is at or above the skin temperature of the area being treated, a superficial TTR will occur. If the water temperature is more than 1°C less than the skin temperature, the net effect produced within the standard ten- to twenty-minute treatment will be a drop in temperature of the exposed skin and superficial subcutaneous tissues. The WP is used to treat adult-size body segments, most commonly the distal segments of the upper or lower extremity. The HT is used when one or both lower extremities plus the trunk and upper extremities need a change in superficial temperature for relief of pain and/or increase in range of motion. The areas treated with WP or HT are usually larger than can be conveniently treated with other forms of infrared.

Water Temperatures for Causing a Tissue Temperature Rise

The surface and volume of tissues treated by hydrotherapy is larger than is the case with hot packs or other forms of infrared. Consequently, if the skin temperature of these large body segments is raised as high as it is with other forms of infrared, a rise in core temperature would be likely. This is rarely desirable. Hence, with rare exception, the water temperature should not exceed 40°C. When an HT is used, its water temperature should not exceed 38°. Also, when a larger body segment is exposed to heat, there is a greater demand on regional circulation. If the patient has a chronic arterial insufficiency in the segment being treated, the larger the area exposed, the less the capability of adequate dilation to supply the demand and the greater the chance of causing an increase rather than decrease of pain because of the vasospasm induced by rebound.

Water Temperatures for Causing a Tissue Temperature Drop

If the objective of the WP or HT treatment is to cause a drop in local tissue temperature, for both physiological and psychological reasons it is recommended that immersion should be started at or near a neutral temperature (33° to 36°C), followed by a gradual decrease in water temperature over the usual ten-minute treatment period. The extent of the gradual temperature drop should vary in proportion to the size of the body segment exposed to the cool water. Thus, if exposing one lower extremity, distal to the knee the drop in temperature could be greater than if both extremities were simultaneously exposed. If both lower extremities plus the trunk are to be exposed, the temperature decrease should be smaller still.

The major indications for use of a cold WP are for *acute* orthopedic trauma, *acute* edema, and *acute* muscle spasm. The HT is more likely to be needed when dealing with moderate to severe *chronic* spasticity due to a central nervous system lesion. However, when using cold (or heat) with such patients, it must be predetermined whether their vasomotor regulatory controls are intact. If they were damaged by the lesion, the patient can undergo a critical *core temperature* crisis when large body segments are exposed to either heat or cold. A reasonable rule of thumb for water temperature drop in a Hubbard tank would indicate *no more than* a 5°C drop from the neutral starting temperature during the first treatment while never exceeding a 10°C drop in water temperature on any subsequent treatment. Knowledgeable personnel should be on hand at all times whenever a patient who has damage to his thermoregulatory controls is in a Hubbard tank.

Operation of Whirlpools and Hubbard Tanks

The smallest whirlpool in clinical use will have the capacity to hold about 120 liters (30 gallons) of water. It is designed for immersion of an upper extremity from the elbow distally. Whirlpools of 200 to 300 liter capacity are used for immersion of one or both lower extremities distal to the knee. The largest size permits an adult to sit in it and is used for immersion of the body distal to the navel. All such units require an additional 10 to 20 percent of the initial volume of water to clean the WP after each treatment. A standard Hubbard tank requires 3200 to 4000 liters for each filling. All hydrotherapy units require a large volume fast-recovery source of hot water as well as provision for mixing hot and cold water to obtain the desired temperature.

Each unit will have one or more electrically driven water pumps (turbine), with a manually adjustable flow rate for varying the degree of water aeration and provision for adjusting the height of the turbine impeller in the water. The pump shaft bearings are water lubricated. Hence, the turbine should never be switched on unless the impeller is immersed in water. Since warm water plus the turbulence created by the pump are excellent for loosening adhesive dressings and cleaning debris from the skin, the therapist must be alert to dressings floating loose and being sucked into the impeller. If this occurs, the turbine should be shut off immediately to prevent clogging, with subsequent damage to the impeller, its drive shaft, or its bearings. Since the pumps are electrically driven, care must be taken to avoid splashing water onto the motor housing or its electrical connections.

Patient Safety and Comfort

It is the therapist's responsibility to see that the patient is positioned safely and comfortably. When an upper extremity is treated, the patient sits in an armless chair, resting his lateral trunk against the outside of the whirlpool. If the patient is short, the top edge of the whirlpool may press into his axilla. If this is the case, some kind of padding should be added to the tank edge to minimize the pressure, or the chair seat should be raised. The chair should have a back rest, and the patient's feet should be supported by the floor or a footstool so that he can be safe and relaxed while receiving treatment.

If one or both distal lower extremities are treated, the patient often is placed in a special swivel chair whose seat is several centimeters above the brim of the WP. The patient climbs into the chair when it is facing away from the WP and then swings around, with or without assistance, until he can immerse the lower extremities. If only one leg is treated, the other foot should be supported outside the tank by another chair or stool. If there is any question that the patient could fall from his high seat, he should be strapped in. Care must be taken that the seat is high enough so there is no pressure from the edge of the tank on the posterior thigh.

When the patient is to be seated in the whirlpool, he would first climb onto the high seat, immerse his legs, and then slowly slide into the water and onto the seat in the whirlpool. Normally, his arms would rest on the padded edges of the tank. Care must be taken that the water level in the WP is not so high that when the turbine is turned on water is spashed out of the whirlpool.

If the patient has any past history of suicidal tendencies, or of fainting, knowledgeable personnel should be in constant attendance and should keep the patient in sight at all times.

For entrance into a Hubbard tank, the patient is manually transferred from a wheelchair or stretcher onto an immersible litter. The litter is then connected to a motor-driven, ceiling-mounted hoist, manually transferred over the tank, and then lowered into the water. The head end of the litter is fastened to the head supports in the tank while the foot end of the litter continues its descent to the bottom of the tank. After the litter is in its final position, the connections to the hoist are removed from the litter and away from the tank area. If the patient's behavior is not under voluntary control, for either physical or psychological reasons, he may need to be strapped onto the litter for transfer and treatment.

It is recommended that anyone responsible for patient transfer into a Hubbard tank experience such a transfer as a patient, in order to fully appreciate the apprehension which the patient may feel.

Care must be taken to keep the patient's head out of water at all times. Adequate provision for rapid drying of the patient after removal from the tank is necessary to prevent chilling. Since HT (and WP) rooms will invariably be quite humid, provision should be made for good air circulation. Likewise, the floor of such rooms will be wet during treatment periods. Good non-skid floor surfaces and adequate floor drains will minimize the obvious hazards.

Physiological Advantages of Hydrotherapy

Whirlpools and Hubbard tanks are excellent for cleaning debris from skin and/or open wounds, for promoting muscle relaxation (heat) or reduction of muscle spasm or spasticity (cold), and for permitting a transient increase in passive or active range of motion.

Although the authors know of no comparative study, they prefer, as soon as the patient has some control over his joint motion, to let the patient rest and relax as completely as possible while in the WP or HT and then to guide the patient in performing any indicated exercise after transfer of the patient out of the water. Other therapists routinely supervise the indicated exercise while the patient is in the water, during the time the patient has the best chance to relax. The buoyancy effect of the water is not likely to be critical for the exercise, except in a few peripheral nerve lesion problems. The buoyancy makes it harder for the therapist to adequately stabilize the patient and to observe substitution of motion due to muscle imbalance. The buoyancy effect is important when a patient is relearning how to walk in a walking tank or therapeutic pool, but very few physical therapy departments have such expensive hydrotherapy sources available.

The Cleaning of Hydrotherapy Units

Bacteristatic or bacteriocidal agents are commonly added to the water when open lesions are to be immersed. Acute burn patients and all persons with open lesions will inevitably discharge pathogenic microorganisms into the WP or HT. Careful cleaning of the unit can be critical in preventing cross contamination. Most departments that treat open lesions with hydrotherapy rely on regular culture testing to prove or disprove the efficiency and thoroughness of their cleaning procedures. Discharge of urine or fecal material into the water can be as much or more of a problem than open lesions. Tank seams, water inlets and outlets, and the insides of turbine shafts are especially difficult to keep clean. Each department should establish its own cleaning procedures, usually on recommendation and monitoring from the institution's pathology or microbiology departments.

Costs of Hydrotherapy

The initial cost of whirlpools and Hubbard tanks are high. They are custom-made of heavy gauge stainless steel. If the area where they are placed was not designed for hydrotherapy, addition of floor drains can be a major item. The ceiling to hold the Hubbard tank hoist requires a special design. Floors may have to be reinforced.

A department with, for example, five whirlpools and two Hubbard tanks in regular use may consume water at a rate in excess of 400,000 liters (100,000 gallons) per day. Much of that water has to be heated. For these reasons, more and more large hydrotherapy departments are installing water purification and recirculation systems. Initial costs are high, but a properly installed system will recover its cost in about five years.

The point to remember is that hydrotherapy is one of the most expensive physical agents, especially in the form of the Hubbard tank, in initial cost plus installation plus water consumption. Hydrotherapy is also high in personnel and linen costs.

COLD PACKS

Cold packs are similar in construction to hot packs. However, they are supplied in sealed, waterproof plastic bags so that if stored at temperatures below the freezing point of water they are not unusably stiff. It is possible to store the water-soaked pouch below freezing because the sand-water slurry has a lower freezing point than that of water alone. If the plastic cover is torn or removed, in time the ratio of water to sand will change (through evaporation). Then the pack will become stiff when frozen. The commercially available storage unit is thermostatically equipped to maintain pack temperature at any desired temperature between 20° below and 20° above 0°C. Many clinics store their packs at 0° to 10°C.

The storage cabinet should not be filled with water. The thoroughly soaked pack should be placed in its plastic bag and the bag sealed and placed into the dry storage cabinet. When first used, the pack needs to have been stored at the desired temperature for about twenty-four hours. After initial use, replacement in the storage cabinet for one-half to one hour should return the pack to an effective temperature.

Treatment Procedures

The pack (in its plastic bag) should never be placed next to the skin. At least one layer of bath toweling should be used. Clinics will vary in election as to whether the toweling toward the patient should be wet or dry. Wet toweling will speed the process of withdrawal of thermal energy from the patient. Water plus moist air are better thermal conductors than dry toweling and dry air. Several layers of dry toweling are standardly placed on the side of the pack away from the skin, so that not as much of the cold effect is lost to room air.

The usual treatment time is ten to fifteen minutes. Depending upon the differential in temperature between the pack and the skin, after five minutes of application, one may expect to see hyperemia or a marked pallor of the skin. If hyperemia is present, it indicates that the normal vasomotor regulatory system has been able to bring in enough warm blood so that even though the skin temperature may have dropped 5° to 10°C, the cutaneous blood supply is adequate to prevent tissue damage. Damage will occur if the temperature of the skin approaches 13°C.[12, 13]

Pallor indicates that arterial dilation has been inadequate to maintain skin temperature within physiological limits, and so cutaneous vasoconstriction has occurred to conserve heat loss from underlying tissues. If the pack was applied to a distal extremity, by the time ten minutes has elasped, few patients will have hyperemia, and pallor should be anticipated. Since cutaneous temperature and circulation is normally better in the trunk areas, pallor rarely appears here. If the temperature differential between the pack and skin was initally great and was maintained by replacement with a fresh pack after five minutes, by ten minutes pallor is very likely to appear. If the skin becomes cyanotic in appearance, severe vasoconstriction has occurred and the treatment should be discontinued.

Physiological Effects of Cold Pack Application

The cold pack is widely used in *acute* orthopedic lesions in an attempt to control traumatically induced edema. It is better to use cold for ten to fifteen minutes out of each half hour rather than a single longer application. Injured tissues must receive some nutrition, even in the presence of massive swelling. It should also be realized that the pack will come to equilibrium with skin temperature within ten to fifteen minutes after application. If an intense cold application is indicated, the pack should be changed every five minutes. The temperature change in the patient will be confined to the skin and adjacent subcutaneous tissue rather than penetrating to muscle unless the pack is changed frequently and the cold differential is maintained for at least one-half hour.[12, 13]

A decrease in axon temperature will slow conduction velocity. If the temperature drop is great enough, no conduction will take place. The critical axon temperature has not yet been established, but in most patients a decrease in skin temperature of 5°C will be adequate to cause a reduction in *motor nerve* activity, with subsequent reduction of muscle spasm. It has been shown that in the presence of a CNS lesion, spasticity is dramatically reduced within one minute after exposure of the skin to cold.[14] The mechanisms involved are not understood.[12-16] It cannot be due to decrease in motor nerve or muscle temperature within such a short time period. However, if pain is due to acute muscle spasm or to spasticity, local application of cold can be very effective in temporarily decreasing muscle hyperactivity and hence reducing pain.[14-17]

Many patients with a CNS lesion will have diminished or absent sensation. This is especially true for patients with a spinal cord lesion. If this is the case, the spasticity will not be accompanied by pain, but even so the spasticity can be transiently reduced with appropriate application of cold. If the volume of muscle in spasticity is small, this can be done with cold packs. If the area to be treated is large, a cold whirlpool or Hubbard tank (as described earlier in the section on hydrotherapy) may be indicated.

Precautions for Cold Application

It is probably wise prior to first exposure to cold on any patient to check blood pressure before and after treatment. There have been occasional clinical notes of a sharp transient rise in systolic pressure. This could be hazardous if the patient has a history of high blood pressure. Presumably, the pressure change is due to a massive reflex vasoconstriction.

SUMMARY

Infrared sources of various kinds have been in use over the centuries to transmit thermal energy to or from a patient. In the last several decades, increasing use of various types of cold applications has evolved.

Both moist and dry heat, as well as moist and dry cold, are part of the electromagnetic spectrum. Their wavelengths are short, and hence their effect is chiefly on cutaneous circulation, cutaneous axons, and the skin itself. Pain relief is achieved through application of heat or cold of infrared wavelengths that act directly on the skin and structures in the skin and, through these structures, cause certain reactions in deeper lying tissues.

Rationale and technics for judicious use of the many forms of the infrared energies through conduction, convection, and radiation are discussed, with emphasis on technics in widespread use at this time. The relative safety and ease of use of infrared as compared to the hazards associated with conversive heating (Chapter 4) are discussed.

REFERENCES

1. Sodeman, W. A. and Sodeman, W. A., Jr.: *Pathological Physiology*, 5th ed. Philadelphia, Saunders, 1974, p. 473.
2. Eddy, H. C. and Taylor, H. P.: Experiences with the Dermatherm in relation to peripheral vascular disease. I. Normal studies. *Am Heart J*, 6:683-9, 1931.
3. Shepard, J. T.: *Physiology of the Circulation in Human Limbs in Health and Disease*. Philadelphia, Saunders, 1963.

4. Davson, H.: *A Textbook of General Physiology,* 4th ed., Volume I. Baltimore, Williams & Wilkins, 1970, Chapter 6.

5. Glasser, O. (Ed.): *Medical Physics,* Volume I. Chicago, Year Bk Med, 1945, p. 1158.

6. Hollaender, A. (Ed.): *Radiation Biology,* Volume I. New York, McGraw, 1954, p. 20.

7. Licht, S. (Ed.): *Therapeutic Heat and Cold,* 2nd ed. New Haven, Licht, 1965.

8. Krusen, Frank H.: *Physical Medicine.* Philadelphia, Saunders, 1942, p. 235.

9. Borrell, R. M. et al.: Fluidotherapy: Evaluation of a new heat modality. *Arch Phys Med Rehabil, 58:*69-71, 1977.

10. Sharborough, R. J. and Hargot, T. S.: Effects of air-fluidized systems on microbial growth. In *Air-Fluidized Beds: Clinical and Research Symposium.* Medical University of South Carolina, 1975, pp. 76-82.

11. Borrell, R. M. et al.: Comparison of in vivo temperatures produced by hydro-therapy, paraffin wax treatment, and Fluidotherapy. *Phys Ther, 60:*1273-76, 1980.

12. Wolf, S. L. and Basmajian, J. V.: Intramuscular temperatures deep to localized cold stimulation. *Phys Ther, 53:*1284-8, Dec., 1973.

13. Beirman, W.: Therapeutic use of cold. *JAMA, 157:*189-92, 1955.

14. Miglietta, O.: Electromyographic changes with application of cold. *Arch Phys Med Rehabil, 45:*508-12, 1964.

15. Mense, S.: Effects of temperature on discharges of muscle spindles and tendon organs. *Pfluger's Arch, 374:*159-66, 1978. (In English)

16. Negrin, R.: Hypothermia to the spinal cord for relief of spasticity and rigidity. *Arch Phys Med Rehabil, 47:*169-73, 1966.

17. Mecomber, S. and Herman, R.: Effects of local hypothermia on reflex and voluntary activity. *Phys Ther, 51:*271-81, 1971.

Chapter 6

ULTRAVIOLET LIGHT

INTRODUCTION

Unlike the diathermy and infrared portions of the electromagnetic spectrum, which are used to induce a temperature rise in absorbing tissues, ultraviolet wavelengths are used clinically to stimulate a variety of chemical reactions in microorganisms, epidermis, dermis, and mucous membranes. The wavelengths that we arbitrarily designate as ultraviolet (UV) run from approximately 420 to 185 nanometers (nm) or 4200 to 1850 Anstrom units (Å) and are the shortest used by physical therapists. For reasons discussed in Chapter 2, these wavelengths have the least penetration into any liquid or solid. In biological tissues, all the ultraviolet absorption takes place within 0.2 mm (200 microns) of the absorbing surface, and 90 percent of the absorption occurs within the first 0.1 mm.[1] This means that somewhere between 80 and 90 percent of the radiation is absorbed within the epidermis and not more than 20 percent reaches the dermis in normal skin.[2, 3] In locations where the epidermis is normally thicker than usual (palms, soles of feet), none of the radiation penetrates to the dermis.

Normal skin is dehydrated and thickened by even a single exposure to UV. Repeated exposure increases stratum corneum thickness (hyperplasia) by as much as fifty times.[4] The dehydration and thickening are effective in treatment of acne and related diseases.

When an intense skin reaction is desired, photosensitizing compounds may be administered prior to exposure to UV, either topically or systemically.[4, 5] This is standard practice in the management of vitiligo and psoriasis. More often, the therapist needs to be aware if the patient is receiving medication that enhances skin reaction to UV. A too intense reaction can exacer-

245

bate rather than alleviate the pathology. Appendix A at the end of this chapter lists generically those commonly used drugs which are known to increase the hazard of overdose with UV.[5] If an attempt were made to produce an exhaustive list, it would run to about five pages, as of 1980. This rapidly growing list of compounds that can cause an undesirably strong reaction to UV is a major reason why if UV is to be used in the treatment of skin disorders, a sleeve test should always be performed to help in deciding appropriate treatment time for the individual. Details of the sleeve test are given later in this chapter.

Photochemical conversion of provitamin D (7-dehydrocholesterol) into previtamin D_3 by exposure of human skin to UV is a well-established reaction.[2, 6-8] Provitamin D is a normal constituent of human epidermis. Vitamin D_3 deficiency is a major factor in the bone disease osteomalacia (rickets).[6] This disease is still a major problem throughout the world, including the United States. If the individual (infant, adult, or geriatric) has an adequate supply of vitamin D *and is able to metabolize it normally,* calcium absorption becomes normal and the disease disappears.[6] Control of diet and oral administration of vitamin D are standardly adequate procedures in the management of rickets. Whole-body irradiation with small doses of UV are indicated if the patient does not respond to routine treatment. During the 1970s some of the mechanisms by which UV absorption enchances the interaction between serum calcium and provitamin D have been elucidated. They are discussed later in the chapter. Knowledge of the predominant wavelength(s) radiated by the various clinical sources of UV is critical and is summarized in Appendices B and C at the end of the chapter.

Psoriasis is perhaps the most common skin disease after acne. It appears in 2 to 3 percent of the entire population.[9] Its etiology remains unknown. Very few physicians would ever speak of a cure, but it can be well controlled, frequently on an outpatient basis. The key to its management is exposure of the abnormal skin to topically applied medication (photosensitizers) followed one to two hours later with exposure to moderate doses of UV, or by oral administration of other compounds (furocoumarins), again followed by UV. Treatment is commonly on a daily basis during an acute episode followed by maintenance treatment several times a week or month. Bryant has written a clinically useful review of trends in management of psoriasis as of 1980.[9]

Some of the mechanisms by which UV helps the medication return psoriatic skin toward normal have been determined.[2, 3, 7-9] There is now strong evidence that the absorbing tissue reaction results in alteration of its deoxyribonucleic acid (DNA) composition, both for calcium-vitamin D interaction and for control of psoriasis.[2, 3, 7-13] Again, therapist knowledge of predominant wavelength(s) of the UV source is critical.

Less common skin problems such as vitiligo and pityriasis rosea usually benefit from the use of ultraviolet along with appropriate medication more than from medication alone.[1, 5, 14]

When the healing of an open wound such as a bedsore is delayed by the inevitable infection that results from loss of the body's first barrier against microorganisms (the skin), regular exposure of the wound to heavy doses of UV is superior to either local or systemic administration of antibiotics. Bailey states that antibiotics are useful in the healing of pressure sores only if a streptococcal cellulitis is present.[15] The general lack of usefulness of antibiotics for control of infection in this type of wound is due to the poor blood supply in the wound area. One function of UV in such wounds is to kill the invading microorganisms. A major mechanism by which this occurs is alteration of the organism's DNA. Another result of exposure of open wounds to UV is that granulation tissue formation is stimulated. The mechanism remains unknown. Formation of granulation tissue is essential for the healing of any open wound.

CLINICAL SOURCES OF ULTRAVIOLET LIGHT

There are two major types of ultraviolet sources in clinical use in this country. They are classically designated as "Hot Quartz" (HQ) and "Cold Quartz" (CQ) mercury vapor arc lamps. It is easy to tell whether a given lamp is HQ or CQ (Figs. 6-1 and 6-2). The transparent envelope that contains the arc will appear as a straight hollow cylinder, or it will be seen at a flat coil (grid). HQ envelopes are straight, rarely exceeding 20 cm in length or 2 cm

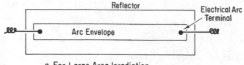

"Hot Quartz" Envelopes

a. For Large Area Irradiation

b. For Small Area Irradiation

Figure 6-1. (A) *The HQ Envelope for Large Area Irradiation.* The envelope will range from 10 to 20 cm in length and 1 to 2 cm diameter, depending upon the size of the reflector and intensity of the arc. The envelope is usually made of quartz in order to withstand extreme temperature changes. Commonly, the envelope is positioned 50 to 75 cm from the surface to be treated.

(B) *The HQ Envelope for Small Area Irradiation.* The envelope may be coiled into a single ring, as shown, or may be a single straight tube. In either case, the reflector diameter will be 3 to 5 cm. Modern lamps for high intensity area clinical use are air cooled by high speed fans. This permits their use as close as 10 cm from the surface to be treated with negligible risk of thermal tissue damage so long as the exposure does not last more than sixty seconds.

in diameter. CQ envelopes are coiled, usually in a circular fashion, with a uniform distance between turns of 0.5 to 1 cm. The number of turns will vary with the size of the lamp. Very large CQ sources may have rectangular coils more than a meter in length and be 10 to 15 cm in width. The envelope diameter in CQ sources rarely exceeds 1 cm.

All clinical UV sources contain small quantities of mercury, a semisolid at room temperature, and argon. Argon is an inert gas that is a very efficient conductor of electricity at ambient temperatures. When the metallic arc is energized, excitation of the argon, not the mercury, gives rise to the characteristic blue radiation. This visible radiation is *not* UV. UV is invisible to the human eye. As the temperature of the gas within the envelope begins to rise, the mercury starts to vaporize (at about 357°C).

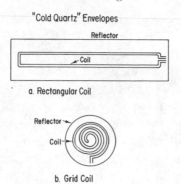

"Cold Quartz" Envelopes

Reflector

Coil

a. Rectangular Coil

Reflector

Coil

b. Grid Coil

Figure 6-2. (A) *The CQ Envelope for Large Area Irradiation.* The long dimension of the rectangularly coiled envelope may be as much as 90 cm, with a 5 to 10 cm distance between the sides of the rectangle. The reflector may be as much as 150 cm long and 30 cm wide. The diameter of the envelope is usually 0.5 to 1 cm. Distance from source to surface to be treated is usually 20 to 40 cm.

(B) *The CQ Envelope for Small Area Irradiation.* The reflector is usually circular in shape, with an envelope coiled into several turns wound in a grid fashion closely adjacent to the reflector. The diameter of the reflector often ranges from 10 to 20 cm. Diameter of the envelope is usually 0.5 to 1 cm. This type of lamp is commonly used at a distance of 1 to 2 cm from the surface to be treated.

When the average temperature of the mercury atoms reaches more than 8,000°C, an appreciable amount of UV, along with infrared and visible light, is emitted. The more intense the arc, the greater the thermal energy production, the more visible light production, and most importantly, the broader the UV spectrum.[16] No mercury vapor source will have more than 25 to 30 percent of its total radiation as UV.[3, 16] Those designed for use without medical supervision will radiate less than 5 percent as UV. The stronger the arc (wattage), the more intense the radiation. Clinical HQ sources require 5 to 20 amperes and a step-up transformer. Clinical CQ sources rarely require over 2 amperes. They do not need transformers. Ballast similar to that in residential fluorescent lights provides the short-duration high voltage needed to excite the CQ arc. Appendix B summarizes the physical differences between clinical HQ and CQ sources.

The arcs may be conveniently classified as high, medium, or

low pressure. These designations are relative to atmospheric pressure at sea level (760 mm Hg). High and medium pressure arcs are always HQ and always have a broad UV spectrum with strong peaks at 2537, 2800, and 2967 Å. The only high pressure arc in clinical use is the Kromayer type, which is used for application of intense radiation to a small area of diseased skin or infected subcutaneous tissue, as in bedsores. The total arc output is so great that the arc must be cooled to avoid thermal damage to the patient. Models built prior to 1940 were usually water cooled. Since the waterlines must be flexible in order to position the arc, leaks are inevitable in time. If any water should leak onto the high voltage transformer, the noise, damage to the lamp, and the risk to the therapist are very real. Development of small, high speed fans now permit safer cooling of these high pressure arcs. However, the closest distance permitted between source and absorbing tissue is 10 cm because of the tremendous infrared output.

For research (*not clinical*) use, extremely high pressure xenon arcs have been developed. The internal envelope pressure may be as high as 100 atmospheres. In addition to UV radiation at the previously mentioned wavelengths, they also have large output between 3200 and 4000 Å,[16] which is not needed in clinical UV treatment.

Most clinical UV sources are medium pressure (approximately 0.5 atm.) or low pressure (about 0.2 atm.) for safety reasons and for ease of control of the UV output. If a high pressure envelope is shattered, the contents are diffused with explosive force. Pieces of the envelope and the mercury vapor could badly burn the patient and the therapist. When the pressure inside the envelope is less than atmospheric (partial vacuum), if the envelope loses its seal for any reason, the envelope pieces and the mercury would not be driven towards the patient or therapist, but the laws of gravity would still be in effect. As manufacturing techniques and quality control have improved, explosion or implosion of envelopes has become rare, but if the lamp, and especially the envelope, receives a sharp blow, it will still shatter.

Even more important, as manufacturers have learned to achieve better vacuums while sealing the essential electrodes inside the envelope, they have been able to reduce arc intensity and the quantity of mercury needed to produce an adequate UV output. It has been known for many years that absorption of radiation at 2650 Å is the most lethal for all kinds of microorganisms.[16] To have a mercury arc produce adequate quantities of this wavelength and little other UV, the arc intensity must be low.[16] The clinical CQ sources have better than 90 percent of their UV output at a wavelength of 2537 Å, which is quite close to the 2650 Å wavelength insofar as its bactericidal effects are concerned. The total pressure within the envelope is low, the quantity of mercury is low, and the arc wattage is low. The net result is a CQ source whose envelope temperature rarely exceeds 60°C, even though the average mercury vapor temperature is more than 8000°C. In any gas, the interatomic and intermolecular distances are vast in comparison with the same distances for a solid. The higher the temperature of the gas, the more this is true. Hence, the confining solid that makes up the arc envelope will get hot but will not even remotely approach the temperature of the contained vapor because of the vastly greater number of molecules per unit area to absorb the thermal energy. The greater the vacuum (and therefore the fewer the number of gas molecules to transmit energy), the less the rise in envelope temperature. Hence, the low pressure (high vacuum) CQ sources are ideal for use close to any tissue. Because CQ arc intensities are low, these lamps are rarely used at distances greater than 25 cm from the area to be treated. However, one must bear in mind that they have no significant output at 2800 or 2967 Å.

Modern clinical HQ sources are in the medium pressure category. The quantity of mercury is larger than in the CQ envelope, the arc intensity is greater, and there is far more thermal energy radiated, along with a broad-spectrum UV output. The envelope temperature will be higher, usually reaching a temperature of 500° to 1000°C. Therefore, unless the HQ source is air cooled, it is rarely used at a distance closer than 50 cm. With an efficient HQ source of a size intended to cover one surface of the trunk or one surface of an extremity with one exposure, a distance of 75 cm from source to tissue is usual.

The envelope confining the mercury must be able to transmit UV, to stand repeated, severe temperature changes, and be sufficiently rigid to contain low or high pressure. HQ source envelopes are usually quartz cylinders. The melting point of the quartz used is about 1500°C. Quartz is expensive and hard to work with. Hence, it is rare to see an HQ source large enough to give whole-body irradiation in less than four exposures (two anterior, two posterior). CQ source envelopes usually use a UV transmitting glass such as *Vycor*®* which readily withstands the temperature of low pressure arcs. Both quartz and UV transmitting glasses block all radiation shorter than 1850 Å. Since most investigators agree that wavelengths longer than 3200 Å produce effects similar to visible light, clinical UV should be regarded as having a wavelength range of 1850 to 3200 Å.[3, 16, 17]

Hot quartz lamps require warmup time of at least two minutes before their UV output is stable. Where precise dosage is important, it is probably better to allow at least five minutes, especially after the first 100 hours of operation. Once shut off, HQ sources require at least a two-minute cooling period before they can be restarted. When mercury has been vaporized and is cooling toward room temperature, as long as its temperature is above approximately 100°C, the random motion of the cooling molecules is still so great that they will not conduct enough electrical energy to restart the arc. For both of the above reasons, if one is to give several HQ-UV treatments in a morning or an afternoon once the lamp is started for the first patient it is wise to leave it running until all treatments are finished for that day. However, it is important that care be taken that the radiation be confined by shutters or a fiberglass hood when a lamp is left running in a treatment area. Most HQ sources have adjustable shutters for this purpose. The shutters are manually opened only during actual intended patient exposure. If the lamp does not have shutters, the therapist must *not* use a pillowcase or other linen for this purpose. If the HQ source is of any appreciable size, the concomitant heat production may scorch or set fire to any linen attached to the reflector. A fiberglass cloth hood will easily

---

* *Vycor*® is the trade name for the 96% silica content UV-transmitting glass manufactured by Corning.

withstand these temperatures; it is easy to make and easy to put on or remove. Small HQ sources (Kromayer) will usually have a snap-on, clear plastic cover which blocks all UV radiation. More than a few times, the therapist has forgotten to remove the cover for treatment and has wondered why there was no apparent response to the exposure.

Because of the higher starting voltage, the smaller quantity of mercury, and the greater vacuum, CQ lamps do not need a warm-up period. Within a matter of a few seconds, their UV output is at maximum. Because of the smaller quantity of mercury and lower envelope temperature, the CQ lamp cools much more rapidly when shut off. Hence, a CQ lamp can be started and shut off many times a day with no worry about uniformity of output.

During the late 1960s and early 1970s impressive clinical evidence was presented indicating that long wavelength UV (4200-3200 Å) is superior to either middle (3200-2800 Å) or short wavelength (2800-1850 Å) UV in the management of patients with psoriasis.[18-23] Long wavelength radiation is called UVA. Middle and short wavelength UV is designated as UVB and UVC, respectively.

The UVA sources in clinical use have a predominant output at 3400-3600 Å.[24, 25] Although oral administration of 8-methoxypsoralen followed in two to three hours by exposure to UVA is clearly more effective than other methods in short- and long-term control of severe psoriasis, it has also become clear upon follow-up studies that the risk to the patient of developing skin cancer is significantly higher.[26-28] Hence it is now recommended that this treatment should *not* be used with children; it should be used in adults only when other treatment has not controlled their psoriasis, and then only if the patient has been informed of the increased hazard and consents to the risk of this treatment. The combination of oral ingestion of the psoralens (furocoumarins) followed by exposure to UVA is referred to as PUVA therapy.

Commercially available sources of UVA are not in standard use in physical therapy departments. Lamps designated as UVB (HQ) and UVC (CQ) are standardly available. It has been shown that *topical* administration of 8-MOP, or of crude coal tar, or of anthralin, followed by exposure to *UVB*, can be as effective as PUVA therapy.[9, 21, 24, 40]

TECHNIQUES OF ULTRAVIOLET TREATMENT

Cleaning the Lamp

Any dust or oil or water film on the envelope or reflector will diminish the UV energy reaching the patient. If not removed before starting the lamp, the contaminants can become baked onto the envelope or reflector. Output will be permanently impaired and nonuniform. Therefore, wiping off the envelope and reflector daily, if used daily, or before each treatment if usage is sporadic, is advised. Ether, toluene, carbon tetrachloride, or 95% ethyl alcohol are all good. Most other readily available and inexpensive alcohols contain a high percentage of water. Repeated use of water can cause rusting of areas of the reflector. All of these cleaning agents are volatile and flammable. Hence, they should be used in a well-ventilated room when the envelope and reflector are at or near room temperature. Nap- or lint-free toweling is preferred to cotton balls or terry cloth because of the likelihook of leaving fibers behind with the latter materials.

Output of the Lamp

All clinical sources of UV deteriorate with use. This is more of a problem with HQ lamps as compared to CQ sources and less of a problem with lamps built within the last several decades. When the electrical arc is energized and the mercury is vaporized, some of the mercury is inevitably baked onto the inside of the envelope. Therefore, there is always a decrease in intensity of output by about 20 percent during the first 100 running hours and by about 5 percent per year thereafter if the lamp is in daily use. Also, even with the best sealing techniques, over a period of years, the vacuum will decrease so that there will be more air molecules within the envelope to absorb more energy from the arc, causing more nonuseful collision of mercury and argon molecules with the increased air molecules. For these reasons, it is wise to regularly check on lamp intensity. The accepted clinical test is to do a sleeve test on the most lightly complected staff member, recording the number of seconds required to produce a standard visible response at a standard distance. In lamps used once daily, such a test should be done at least every six months. When the time required to produce an equivalent response has approximately doubled, it is time to consider repair or replacement of the lamp. This should be done for each UV source in the department, as each lamp will deteriorate at a different rate. The standard response time should be plainly visible and permanently attached to the lamp. There are a lot of variables to such a clinical test, especially medication the subject may be on and whether the test area is more or less pigmented than at the time of previous tests. Currently available UV meters are expensive and must be recalibrated at least twice a year. Since no one meter is valid for both HQ and CQ sources, few departments can justify this expense.

Eye Protection

The eyeball and adjacent structures are extremely sensitive to UV of any wavelength because of their relative avascularity. Since blood supply is poor, absorbed energy is not diffused rapidly. In addition, UV penetration is poor, leading to concentration of the energy in a small volume of tissue. Exposure to small quantities can lead to a painful conjunctivitis lasting several days. Exposure to larger quantities can lead to temporary blindness. Hence, eye protection is mandatory for patient and therapist alike. Glass commonly used in eyeglasses is effective as a UV filter, as are *Uvinyl*®* and *Mylar*®.† Unless tinted, they do not diminish the quantity of glare (from the reflector) or visible light, which can reach the eyeball. Because it is possible for UV to be reflected from skin to eyeglass lens and be redirected toward the eyeball, the glasses should fit snugly. Since the therapist should be able to see during treatment in order to time the treatment, he cannot wear heavily tinted glasses and may prefer

---

* *Uvinyl*® is the trade name for benzophenone compounds manufactured by the Antara Chemical Co., a division of General Aniline and Film.

† *Mylar*® is the trade name for polyester plastics manufactured by DuPont. Both are excellent filters for all UV wavelengths shorter than 4200 Å.

a clear or lightly tinted full-face shield. These are inexpensive and lightweight. Many therapists recommend the patient keep the eyes closed even when wearing goggles as a further precaution.

Protection by contact lenses is highly variable, depending on the material used. While most contact lenses would protect the human lens, iris, and retina, they are not large enough to offer any protection to the periphery of the eyeball. Therefore patients and/or therapists who are near an energized source of UV should wear ultraviolet-filtering goggles.

The Sleeve Test

Because each lamp will have its own output characteristics, and since human skin is very sensitive to UV, it is always wise to perform a sleeve test on an individual who is to receive clinical UV if skin is to be the absorbing tissue. This can be done in a number of ways. It is probably wise to select an area of skin that has not been appreciably exposed to sunlight for at least six months. Such areas are becoming increasingly difficult to find, especially in the younger population, but the skin of the abdomen inferior to the navel or the skin on the inside of the upper arms is usually less exposed. A series of holes at least 2 cm in diameter are cut into UV-filtering cloth or paper. As few as four and as many as fifteen holes have been recommended by various authors. This author prefers five or six holes unless the dosage must be extremely precise. The paper is attached snugly to the skin, with all holes exposed for a period of time (usually seconds) which, on the basis of past experience, should produce no visible response. Then, one hole at a time is covered at specified intervals until all holes are covered. The times used should be marked adjacent to each exposed area. The therapist should observe the exposed skin approximately twenty-four hours after the test exposures. Although there is a difference in opinion, a majority of therapists regard that exposure time needed to produce a faintly visible reddening of the skin present twenty-four hours after exposure as the minimal erythermal dose (MED). Test skin that has no erythema present twenty-four hours after exposure has received a suberythermal dose (SED). Test skin that retains reddish coloration for up to forty-eight hours after exposure will have been exposed to UV approximately two and one-half times as long as the skin that showed an MED.

The visible reaction lasting up to forty-eight hours is usually called a first degree erythemal response (1st D). If the response lasts from forty-eight to seventy-two hours, it is usually considered a second degree erythemal dose (2nd D). The 2nd D response skin will have been exposed approximately five times as long as the MED skin. Thus if the MED was established with a thirty-second exposure, a 2nd D response would result upon exposure to 5 × 30 (150) seconds. With exposures causing erythema to last more than seventy-two hours, blistering will usually occur in less than one hour after exposure, indicating destruction of epidermis and sometimes the dermis (3rd D). This is clearly a pathological dose and has no place in modern use of ultraviolet in treatment of diseased skin. However, one should remember that mucous membrane and subcutaneous tissues are far less responsive to UV than is skin. Therefore, in treatment of urine scalds, Vincent's angina ("trench mouth"), and other mucosal infections, such a dose may be used beneficially. These pathologies usually respond routinely to antibiotic therapy, and UV is needed only in stubborn cases. When 2nd or 3rd degree doses are used intentionally, care must be taken to prevent exposure of adjacent skin. Otherwise, a painful burn is likely to follow. When UV is used to control infection in a pressure sore, 2nd or 3rd degree doses are routine. Protection of surrounding skin with adequate draping is necessary.

The use of a sleeve test on a patient prior to treatment is becoming more important as medical therapy is becoming more complex. The dose that may yield an MED on a person not under medication may yield a 3rd D response when they are taking any photosensitive drug. Therefore, it is prudent to perform a sleeve test on each patient, especially if the skin is lightly pigmented.

The visible reddening of the skin (erythema) is brought about by a series of events to be discussed later. Erythema due to exposure to UV is always a delayed reaction, rarely appearing before two hours after exposure. Exposure at intensities that can later be classified as MED usually are visible by seven to eight hours after exposure and reach maximum intensity at eleven to twelve hours.[3] Stronger intensities may cause earlier appearance. It is well to remember that erythema from a CQ source will usually appear earlier and disappear sooner than will erythema from an HQ source.[2, 3, 16]

Doses of MED or greater intensity are followed by epidermal exfoliation, hyperplasia, and pigmentation. The hyperplasia and pigmentation appear to make the skin more resistant to UV. Hence, if it is desired to maintain a given level of reaction over a period of several weeks, repeated exposures must be of slightly greater intensity. For example, if the MED was established as thirty seconds at 75 cm and the treatment is to be given daily, progression of exposure might well be thirty, thirty-five, forty, forty-five, and fifty seconds. UV is not commonly given more than five days in a row. For each day of "rest," using the above scale, one should cut back five seconds. If on a Friday a fifty-second exposure was used, on Monday, the treatment would be resumed at forty seconds. If treatment is scheduled three times weekly, a more nearly constant dose would be used to maintain equivalent reaction.

The Inverse Square Law

This law states that as distance between source of radiant energy and absorbing tissue is altered, intensity is decreased (or increased) geometrically rather than arithmetically. Formal statement and significance are discussed in Chapter 5. At one time, therapists had to be able to calculate alteration in intensity with change in distance to maintain the prescribed dose level. With modern equipment this is rarely necessary, since it is unusual that a single exposure will require over sixty seconds. It is essential, however, when the sleeve test is done and when treatment is given, that the distance used be accurately recorded, to minimize the possibility for error in dosage. Equally important is accurate timing and recording of each actual exposure in seconds. This used to require a stopwatch, but wristwatches with sweep second hands are entirely adequate, readily available, and usually more convenient. If the department has more than one

UV source, it is wise to record which lamp was used on which patient.

The Cosine Law

This law states that for maximum absorption of radiant energy, the source should be perpendicular to the absorbing surface. Deviation of $\pm 10°$ from the right angle does not create a major energy loss problem. For this reason, visual positioning of the source is usually adequate, although when large areas, i.e. posterior trunk, are subject to a single exposure, the erythema production will be noticeably less where surface contour is curved rather than flat.

Reflection of UV

It is the therapist's responsibility to drape areas of the patient that should not be exposed to UV. A single layer of an ordinary sheet, bath or linen towel, or a pillowcase is adequate to block UV unless the linen is threadbare or torn. It is equally important that the therapist realize that white cloth is a very good reflector of UV. Many a therapist has received an inadvertent exposure to the arms and face by standing near the patient draping while the patient is being treated. Such reflection from cubicle curtains is a good reason for remembering to tell the patient to keep his/her eyes closed when being treated, even though the face is remote from the source and the area of exposure.

Therapists vary in opinion as to the merits of drape versus no drape. If a patient is to receive a series of treatments to a small area, it will be difficult to place the draping precisely the same way for each treatment. Yet if a first or second degree dose is indicated, and if nearby previously unexposed skin is exposed at a third or fourth treatment intensity, a serious burn can result. Some therapists advocate the use of fabric or paper templates, with cutouts to be placed over the lesion. If the lesion is becoming worse, or if it is responding to treatment, the cutout has to be revised on a regular basis. It would seem simpler to leave adjacent areas exposed at each treatment so that no margin receives a sudden intense exposure. Where draping might be called for on the grounds of modesty, it would seem simpler to have female therapists treat female patients rather than to drape for modesty alone. Nipples and external genitalia tolerate exposure to UV considerably better than less pigmented skin. Also, many a skin lesion has been inadequately treated because the therapist did not expose adipose or pendulous skin folds.

Patient Positioning

Thoughtful attention must be paid to patient positioning, expecially if whole-body irradiation is to be used. One half of the face and either the anterior or posterior surfaces of the upper extremities and the lateral aspect of the lower extremities are very likely to receive a painfully uneven dosage. To illustrate, suppose a patient is prone. For comfort, his neck will be fully rotated to the right or left and his forearms will be in full pronation so that the volar surface is exposed. When he is turned over and lies supine for the next exposure, unless the neck is rotated so that the other half of the face is exposed, one side will have received a double exposure. When lying supine, the forearms are commonly pronated, which is fine because the dorsal surface of the forearm and the anterior surface of the upperarm will be exposed. But if the patient happens to lie supine with forearms in full supination, the volar surface will receive a double exposure. In both the prone and supine position, many patients lie with their lower extremities in moderate external rotation. This is more readily visible when the patient is supine. If the therapist instructs the patient to keep the extremities neutral while supine but does not do so when the patient is prone, the lateral surfaces can receive excessive exposure. It is the therapist's responsibility to see to it that no surface is under- or overexposed.

Preparation of the Surface to be Treated

It is necessary to remember that ultraviolet light is not a penetrating form of energy. All investigators agree that more than 50 percent is absorbed within the first 0.1 mm (100 microns) and all is absorbed within the second 0.1 mm. Therefore, the treatment surface must be cleansed, rinsed, and dried before each exposure for best results. If a photosensitizing liquid or ointment has been applied to the diseased skin, only a very thin residue is needed or desirable upon exposure. This can be effectively achieved by gently rubbing the area with soft, dry toweling. If the medication stains fabric, use soft, disposable toweling. If an open wound is to be treated, it should be debrided before each exposure. Institutions will vary as to whether the task of debridement is assigned to physicians, nurses, or therapists. Hand-held electric dryers are very effective and efficient in temporary drying of both skin and open wounds.

PHYSIOLOGICAL EFFECTS OF CLINICAL ULTRAVIOLET LIGHT

Cold quartz (CQ) lamps produce more than 90 percent of their UV output at the 2537 Å wavelength. Hot quartz (HQ) lamps produce a substantial peak at that wavelength, as well as a strong peak at 2800 Å, and radiate very strongly throughout the range of 2900 to 3200 with a peak at 2967 Å.[2, 3, 16] Early studies indicated that less than 1 percent of any UV penetrated to the dermis. The conclusion was that all response to absorption of UV started in the epidermis and diffused to the dermis. Recent data[2, 3] indicate that 10 to 20 percent of UV reaches the dermis of lightly pigmented skin, especially when the epidermis is of normal thickness. Where the epidermis is thick (palms, soles of feet), none of the radiation penetrates to the dermis.

Human skin is classically described as having two major divisions — the epidermis (outermost) and the dermis. The epidermis has five layers. From the outside in, they are as follows: the stratum corneum (horney or keratinized layer) and stratum lucidium (clear layer), followed by the granular, prickle cell, and basal layers. Pigment cells (melanocytes) are within the basal (Malphigian) layer. No part of the epidermis has a direct nerve or blood supply.[4, 5]

Extensive study by Kligman (1964) has indicated that in most areas of the body, the epidermis is much thinner than was previously thought.[29] Except in atypical areas (callus), the epidermis is 60 to 100 microns in depth. Normal stratum corneum had a maximum depth of 15 microns and an average of 11 microns, regardless of degree of pigmentation. Both the stratum corneum and the entire epidermis are much thicker on the sole of the foot and, to a lesser extent, on the palm of the hand. Observable reaction to UV by the epidermis of the sole or palm is rare, irrespective of degree of pigmentation prior to treatment or of the dose administered.

Production of Erythema

The best known and most studied reaction of human skin is production of erythema. UV-induced erythema is a *delayed reddening* of the skin. It first appears several hours after exposure and lasts in direct proportion to intensity of exposure. The intensity of the erythema also varies depending upon which region was exposed. The chest is usually the most sensitive, followed by the abdomen and then the posterior trunk. The skin of the extremities ordinarily requires a significantly higher dose to produce an equivalent erythema.

There are differences in erythema production that depend on whether the skin was exposed to CQ (2537 Å = 254 nm) or to a HQ source (2967 Å = 297 nm).[2, 3, 16] Both the intensity and duration of response are significantly less when exposed to CQ, but the onset of erythema is earlier, in normal skin.

In all cases where erythema appears, there is active vasodilation of the cutaneous capillaries. Arteriolar dilation occurs only with an intense exposure.[3, 30, 31] Neither the mechanism nor the site of the reaction causing either type of dilation is known. For many years, it was thought that absorption of UV caused a photochemical decarboxylation of histadine, which is the usual precursor of histamine (Fig. 6-3). This reaction does occur when skin is exposed to a strong dose of infrared (*see* Chapter 5). Such a reaction has yet to be demonstrated *in vitro* using UV sources with major output in the 290 to 320 nm range. However, one well-known deamination product of histadine is urocanic acid (Fig. 6-4). Urocanic acid is normally present in human skin and is a major factor in protection of the skin from damage due to exposure to either natural or artificial sources of UV.[2] When urocanic acid absorbs at 290 nm, it undergoes a *cis-trans* isomerization.

If urocanic acid is applied to the skin prior to exposure to UV,

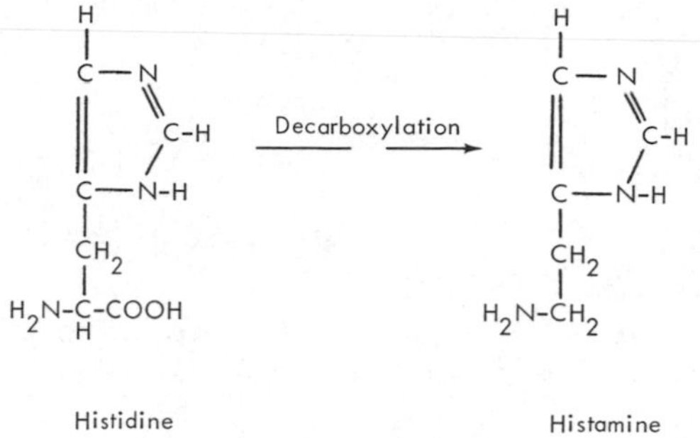

Figure 6-3. *Conversion of Histidine into Histamine.* For many years it was *assumed* that this reaction took place in human skin upon absorption of UV and that this reaction was the basis for erythema production. To date this reaction has never been demonstrated *in vitro*, even at intensities far above those clinically feasible.[7]

erythema production is suppressed. There is some evidence that decarboxylation of 5-hydroxytryptophan to 5-hydroxy-typtamine may be a factor in UV-induced capillary dilation (Fig. 6-5). The present theory is that all mercury arc sources have a direct action on the dermis and that the longer wavelengths (290 to 310 nm) also act directly on the epidermis.[32, 33] Apparently, some vasodilator substance is produced or activated within the stratum corneum by any UV wavelength.

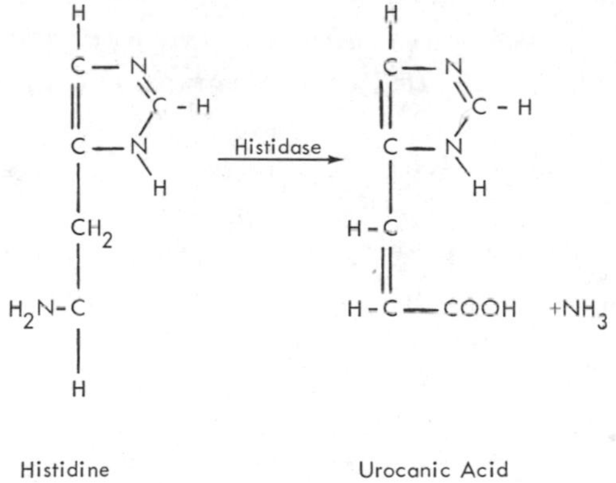

Figure 6-4. *Conversion of Histidine into Urocanic Acid.* Urocanic acid is a well-documented deamination product of histidine. This reaction is known to take place when human skin absorbs UV. Urocanic acid is a vasodilator.[2]

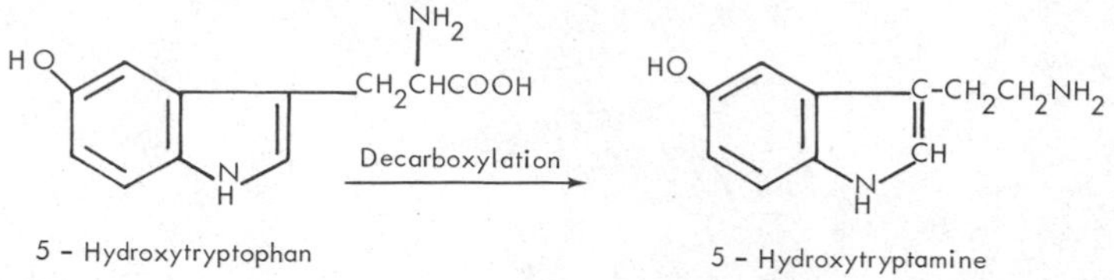

5 - Hydroxytryptophan   5 - Hydroxytryptamine

Figure 6-5. *Conversion of 5-Hydroxytryptophan into 5-Hydroxytryptamine.* This reaction is well established as taking place in human skin upon absorption of UV. It is a vasodilator. It *may be* a significant factor in erythema production.[2]

It has been known since 1950 that erythema production is *not necessary* for bactericidal or other effects of UV.[34] The major usefulness of erythema production is as a clinical dose scale.

Pigmentation Augmentation

Melanin is the pigment that protects skin against damage from overexposure to any source of UV. Although human skin, irrespective of racial genetics, contains the same number of melanocytes, darker-complected individuals produce more melanin.[35] Melanin is synthesized from the amino acid tyrosine, through a series of reactions, and combines with a protein.[36] Figure 6-6 illustrates the known steps in the reaction.

Pigmentation occurs when these pigment granules are transferred from the melanocytes to the keratinocytes. Both types of cells are found in the basal layer of the epidermis. The pigment granule remains colorless until it is oxidized. Exposure of the epidermis to either natural or man-made UV brings about the oxidation. Smaller quantities of HQ radiation cause more pigmentation than occurs with CQ sources. This makes sense if one recalls that natural sunlight at sea level has no wavelengths shorter than 290 nm. HQ sources have a large output between 290 and 320 nm. CQ sources have an insignificant output within that range.

In lightly pigmented skin, the level of activity of *tyrosinase* always increases when the skin is exposed to UV. Tyrosinase is

Figure 6-6. *Conversion of Tyrosine into Melanin.* One way in which melanin is formed is by absorption of UV by the amino acid tyrosine, which is normally present in human skin. The steps outlined in this series of reactions are known to take place in human skin.[37]

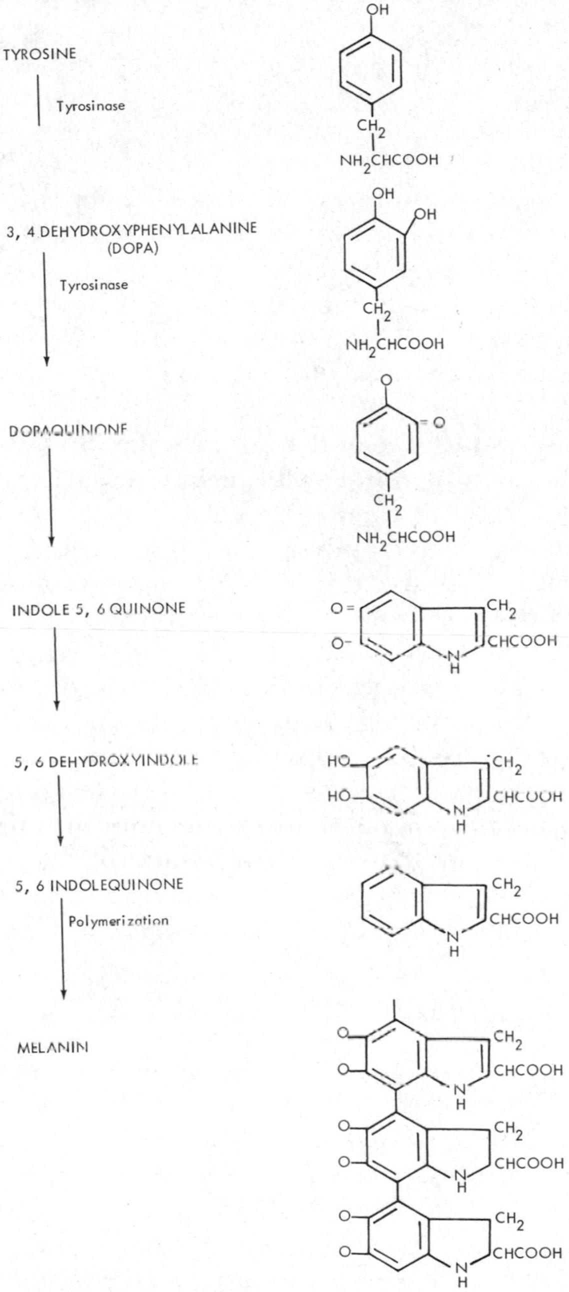

TYROSINE

Tyrosinase

3, 4 DEHYDROXYPHENYLALANINE
(DOPA)

Tyrosinase

DOPAQUINONE

INDOLE 5, 6 QUINONE

5, 6 DEHYDROXYINDOLE

5, 6 INDOLEQUINONE

Polymerization

MELANIN

the enzyme that catalyzes oxidation of tyrosine into dihydroxy-phenylalanine. If the level of tyrosinase is increased, more tyrosine will be metabolized. One of the results will be augmented pigmentation. There is some evidence that genetically darker skin contains more of a tyrosinase *inhibitor*.[2] The net effect of the inhibitor is to prevent already pigmented skin from darkening further upon exposure to wavelengths longer than 290 nm.

Certainly it can be shown in patients with vitiligo, a depigmenting disease, that vitiliginous areas will sunburn far more easily than the surrounding darker skin. A standard treatment for this disease is oral administration of 8-methoxypsoralen (a photosensitizing chemical) followed by suberythemal doses of HQ-UV.[4, 5]

Most redheads and blondes are far more apt to suffer from overexposure to the sun. Few brunettes or blacks need fear the sun. However, there are notable exceptions among both lightly and heavily pigmented individuals. These exceptions, plus individual treatment source differences in output, plus differences in recent over-the-counter or prescription medication make performance of a sleeve test almost mandatory if large areas of the skin are to be treated with clinical UV. Details of this test procedure are given in the technique section of this chapter. It is the therapist's responsibility to see that the same lamp that was used for testing is used for treatment. The sleeve test is not as critical when mucous membranes (inside of the mouth) or open wounds (pressure sores) are treated. These tissues will tolerate and benefit from far heavier doses. Doses standardly used on open wounds would cause a third-degree burn if applied to healthy skin.

The Bactericidal Effect

It is now well established that when any microorganism absorbs UV of a wavelength at or near 254 nm, the pyrimidine base fraction of deoxyribonucleic acid (DNA) known as thymine is the most strongly affected part of the molecule.[2, 3, 36] When DNA absorbs UV in the 250 to 270 nm range, thymine dimerization occurs. Only 1 to 2 percent of the thymine in a given molecule needs to be affected to suppress the ability of the cell to

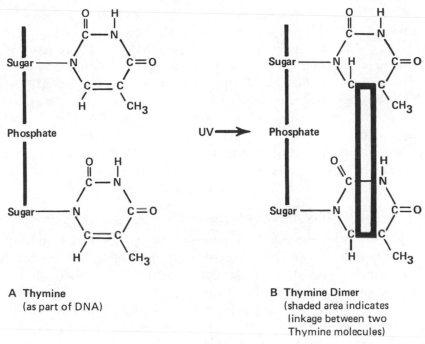

A **Thymine**
   (as part of DNA)

B **Thymine Dimer**
   (shaded area indicates
   linkage between two
   Thymine molecules)

Figure 6-7. *Conversion of Thymine into Thymine Dimers.* Thymine is a pyrimidine base fraction of human DNA and RNA. Absorption of UV by human DNA or RNA causes some of the thymine to dimerize. This prevents normal metabolism of the DNA. If enough thymine is converted, the cell dies.[2]

synthesize new DNA. Normally, no thymine fraction of DNA is ever directly linked to another thymine fraction. With dimerization, two thymine fractions break their normal linkages and join together. Figure 6-7 schematically portrays the theoretical appearance of a thymine dimer.

A UV dose several times *weaker* than that needed to produce an MED is completely lethal to the absorbing microorganism. Appendix C gives in tabular form the known physiological mechanisms excited by various UV wavelengths and intensities needed.

When human epidermis absorbs wavelengths in the 250 to 270 nm range in sufficient quantity, DNA synthesis is suppressed for twenty-four to forty-eight hours. This is followed by a period of increased synthesis, and hyperplasia.

The CQ-UV lamp major output is at 254 nm. Because its infrared output is low, there is little risk of concomitant thermal damage when massive doses of UV are needed. There is some evidence that the presence of histidine in the skin at the time of exposure will tend to block absorption of longer wavelengths of UV by the pyrimidine bases of DNA.[38] The molecular mechanism of this attenuation is unknown. Whether this has clinical significance is unknown. It is well known that HQ-UV, which produces significant quantities of UV in both the 250 to 270 nm and 290 to 320 nm ranges, is also highly effective as a bactericidal agent.

Photosensitization and Photoreactivation

The term *photosensitization* refers to the process by which an object becomes abnormally sensitive to light. The furocoumarins (psoralens) constitute a class of compound that, when administered either orally or topically to humans, enhances the effects of UV.[4, 5] It has been recently shown that the psoralens bind to the pyrimidine bases in both DNA and RNA, forming a new cyclobutane ring. This reaction is strongly enhanced when the skin is exposed to HQ-UV (290 to 310 nm) but is attenuated when exposed to CQ-UV (254 nm).[19] Thus, if one wishes to increase the effectiveness of UV by use of a psoralen, one should remember to use a hot quartz rather than a cold quartz lamp.

The authors are not aware of any similar study on the effects of crude coal tar preparations on DNA or RNA. Crude coal tar has been used for years as a topical ointment to enhance the effects of UV in the treatment of acute generalized psoriasis.

One coal tar preparation in common use in the latter part of the twentieth century is liquid carbonis detergens.[21, 44] Use of topical coal tar preparations followed by exposure to UVB was first reported by Goeckermann in 1925.[40] There are many modifications of the Goeckermann regimen in current use. They all consist of topical application of some form of coal tar as a paste, ointment, gel, or liquid to the psoriatic skin several times each twenty-four hour period. The patient is exposed to UVB one to two hours after application of the medication, once a day. Immediately prior to exposure to UV, the medication is removed mechanically with a soft dry towel. This leaves a *thin* residue of medication on the abnormal skin. No solvents are used.

The therapist's objective is to achieve the desired degree of erythema within the exposed skin. Opinions vary as to whether maintainence of an SED, MED, or 1st D erythema is most effective.[9, 21, 40, 42] It is generally accepted that neither the UV nor the coal tar alone is as effective as their combined use. The disadvantages of this treatment are that most of the crude tar preparations have a distinct odor and also tend to permanently stain many fabrics. The Ingram technique is similar to the Goeckermann regimen except that anthralin rather than coal tar is the topical medication.[9, 44]

In less severe psoriasis, i.e. only scattered small areas of skin involved, topical or intradermal application of various steroids (such as hydrocortisone) may be used. These applications are *not* followed by exposure to UV.[9]

Photoreactivation is the name given to the process that decreases the effects of UV. The process was discovered by Kelner in 1949.[41] He observed that bacteria that had been exposed to 100 percent lethal doses of 254 nm UV would survive if later exposed to daylight that had reached the bacteria through window glass. In time, it was shown that wavelengths from 320 to 400 nm were essential for photoreactivation, with exposure to radiation at 340 nm being the most effective. In the mid-1970s, conclusive evidence was reported demonstrating that human epidermal reaction to UV is attenuated by later exposure to similar longer wavelengths.[37]

This becomes important clinically if a patient is inadvertently given a massive overdose of UV. When this is known to have happened, the overexposed skin should be treated with a luminous infrared lamp (*see* Chapter 5) or to a residential-type fluorescent light within one hour after the overexposure to UV. The attenuating radiation should be applied for at least ten minutes. This will usually diminish the injurious effects of overexposure to UV.

INDICATIONS FOR ULTRAVIOLET THERAPY

There are three major categories of indication for the clinical use of UV. These are infections, noninfectious skin diseases in which transient exfoliation and hyperplasia are adjunctive in the return of the epidermis to its normal state, and in excitation of calcium metabolism.

The mechanism by which UV disrupts microbial infection is the dimerization of the thymine fraction of DNA.[2, 3, 37, 41] DNA and/or RNA is present in the nucleus of all microorganisms as well as in all human cells. Theoretically, CQ-UV should be more effective for this disruption because absorption of 250 to 270 nm wavelengths without the presence and absorption of additional longer wavelengths does not stimulate histidine inhibition of the thymine dimerization.[39] The presence of histidine in the intra- or extracellular fluid blocks or suppresses DNA disruption.

It has been the authors' clinical experience that HQ-UV is equally or more effective in combatting infection as compared to CQ-UV. The reasons for this are not known. It may be that the mixture of both long and short wave UV brings about additional chemical reactions which have not yet been isolated but which are synergistic to DNA alteration, or it may be simply that the total UV output per unit area is significantly greater with any clinical HQ-UV source.

With the evolution of antibiotic therapy since the 1940s, the need for UV to combat infection has markedly declined, except in the treatment of pressure sores. These open wounds do not respond well to antibiotics, presumably because of their poor blood supply.[15] It will be interesting to see whether development of new antibiotics will keep pace with the evolution of antibiotic-resistant strains of microorganisms.[43]

The authors would like to see the results of a carefully designed comparative study on patients whose clinical diagnosis indicates the likelihood of onset of pressure sores, with half the patients receiving regular suberythemal doses of UV to skin over bony prominences long before there is any sign of incipient breakdown and the other half not receiving UV until the ulceration is evident. It would be interesting to determine whether the difference in number and severity of the pressure sores would be statistically significant in a series of 100 patients.

The use of UV in the management of infections has a major drawback — its lack of depth of penetration. The absorbing microorganisms must be within a few microns of the surface being exposed in order to absorb the radiation. This requires cleansing and drying of the skin or debridement of the open wound prior to each exposure in order to achieve maximum effect.

The skin lesions which respond to UV but which are not caused by contagious pathogens are acne, seborrheic dermatitis, psoriasis, and pityriasis rosea.[5, 14] The role of dehydration, hyperplasia, exfoliation, and pigment augmentation in the treatment of these lesions is not known. It *is* known that these lesions respond better to exposure to UVB than to UVC.[5, 14] Use of UVA in noninfectious dermatoses has not been reported.

As of the 1980s, the mechanisms of interaction between UV and photosensitizing medications are not completely established. It now seems clear that when exposure to UVB follows either topical or oral administration of the psoralens, or topical application of anthralin or of the various crude coal tars, there is interference with the normal metabolism of DNA.[2, 3, 6, 17, 37-39, 41]

Likewise, the mechanisms for interaction of UV with provitamin D, serum calcium, and calcium absorption and excretion are not fully understood.[6-8, 10, 11, 18] However, it is clear that where urinary excretion has increased to levels indicative of significant osteoporosis, whole-body exposure to small doses of UVB on a regular basis can be highly effective in controlling the demineralization.[6-8, 11]

Psoriasis continues to be a major problem.[9, 44] Its cause remains unknown, and there is no cure, only remission. The wide variety of treatments recommended by various authors indicate that a number of approaches to management can play a role in remission. There is now some evidence that when the psoralens are used in conjunction with UVB or UVA, there is interference with normal DNA metabolism. There has been no report as to whether the same occurs with photosensitizers other than the furocoumarins.

CONTRAINDICATIONS FOR ULTRAVIOLET THERAPY

There are a few clear-cut contraindications for the clinical use of UV. These are mostly in rare metabolic disorders, such as in the porphyrias and pellegra,[6] or in the presence of either systemic or discoid lupus erythematosus, sarcoidosis, or xeroderma pigmentosum.[4, 5, 44] Because of extreme individual differences in skin reaction to exposure to UV, it is strongly recommended that a sleeve test be performed prior to treatment to enable the therapist to achieve the desired level of response. For this same reason, a detailed record should be kept of the source used, distance, and duration of each exposure. This should minimize the chances for error resulting in either over- or underdosage. Whenever skin absorbs UV, enough energy is absorbed per unit volume to bring about a massive stimulus-response reaction. Therefore, whole-body irradiation should also be avoided in patients who have severe cardiac, pulmonary, renal, or hepatic pathology.

SUMMARY

The physical and physiological differences between broad- and narrow-spectrum clinical ultraviolet sources are discussed, including advantages and disadvantages of each type of source. Differences in utilization on skin as compared to other tissue is stressed. Standard clinical treatment techniques, along with indications and contraindications, are reviewed. The importance of performing a sleeve test, especially when large areas of skin are to be exposed, is emphasized. Presently known mechanisms in erythema and pigmentation production, bactericidal effects, and excitation of calcium metabolism are discussed. The possible significance of photoreactivation in all of the above mechanisms is presented.

APPENDIX A

PHOTOSENSITIZING DRUGS*

I. Sulfonamides

II. Sulfonylurea Hypoglycemics
Tolbutamide
Chlorpromamide
Acetohexamide

III. Antibiotics
Demethyltetracycline
Griseofulvin
Tetracycline

IV. Chlorthyazide Diurctics
Chlorothiazide
Hydrochlorothiazide
Cyclothiazide
Methylchlorothiazide

V. Phenothiazines
Chlorpromazine
Promazine
Perchlorperizine
Promethazine
Neprazine

VI. Psoralens (Furocoumarins)
8-Methoxypsoralen

---

* From G. Sauer, *manual of Skin Diseases*, 3rd Ed., 1973. Courtesy of J. B. Lippincott Company, Philadelphia.

APPENDIX B

PHYSICAL DIFFERENCES BETWEEN HOT AND COLD QUARTZ ULTRAVIOLET LAMPS

	Spectral Output (UV)	Electron Temp.	Average Mercury Temp.	Envelope Temp.	Starting Voltage	Running Voltage	Starting Amperes	Running Amperes	Arc Warmup	Restart Characteristics
COLD QUARTZ	Narrow — more than 90% at 2537 Å	Higher than for Hg vapor	7000° to 9000°C	60°C	High — 1800 to 2000	Low — 110 to 120	Low — Less than one	Low — Less than one	Instant	Instant
HOT QUARTZ	Broad — Strong at 2537, 2800 & 2967 Å	Equal to that for Hg vapor	7000° to 9000°C	500 to 1000°C	Moderate — 800 to 1000	Moderate — 400 to 500	High — 5 to 20	High — 5 to 10	2 to 5 minute *minimum*	2 minute minimum after lamp is shut off

APPENDIX C

ESTABLISHED *PHYSIOLOGICAL* EFFECT DIFFERENCES BETWEEN HOT AND COLD QUARTZ ULTRAVIOLET LAMPS

	Bactericidal Effects	Conversion of Provitamin D Into the Active Compound	Excitation of Calcium and Phosphorus	Erythema Production	Pigmentation Augmentation
COLD QUARTZ	Excellent	None	None	Moderate — early onset, short duration	Usually poor, short duration
HOT QUARTZ	Good	Excellent	Excellent	Strong — delayed onset, long duration	Variable, usually strong

Under optimal circumstances, it requires about 20 microwatts/cm^2/second for ionization of Ca and P.[6]

Under optimal circumstances, it requires about 100 microwatts/cm^2/second for thymine dimerization when DNA is exposed to UV at 2537 Å.[38]

Under optimal circumstances, for lightly pigmented Caucasian skin, it requires about 700 to 800 microwatts/cm^2/second for production of a minimal erythemal dose when skin is exposed to UV at 2967 Å.[4,45]

REFERENCES

1. Licht, S. (Ed.): *Therapeutic Electricity and Ultraviolet Radiation*, 2nd ed. New Haven, Licht, 1967, p. 271.
2. Giese, A. (Ed.): *Photophysiology*, Volume IV. New York, Acad Pr, 1968, Chapter II.
3. Urbach, F. (Ed.): *Biological Effects of Ultraviolet Radiation*. New York, Pergamon, 1969.
4. Sulzberger, W., Wolf, J., and Witten, V.: *Dermatology: Diagnosis and Treatment*, 2nd ed. Chicago, Year Bk Med, 1961, pp. 85-96.
5. Sauer, G. (Ed.): *Manual of Skin Diseases*, 3rd ed. Philadelphia, Lippincott, 1973.
6. Thompson, R., and Wooten, I.: *Biochemical Disorders in Human Diseases*, 3rd ed. New York, Acad Pr, 1970, pp. 774-82.
7. Holick, M. F., and Clark, M. B.: The photogenesis and metabolism of vitamin D. *Fed Proc, 37#12*:2567-74, Oct., 1978.
8. Macleod, M. A., and Blacklock, N. J.: UVL induced changes in calcium absorption and excretion and in serum vitamin D_3 levels measured in black skinned and caucasian males. *J R Nav Med Serv 65*:75-78, Summer, 1979.
9. Bryant, B. G.: Treatment of psoriasis. *Am J Hosp Pharm, 37*:814-20, June 1980.
10. Ohayashi, T., Yoshimoto, S., and Yasamura, M.: Effect of wavelength on the photochemical reaction of ergocalciferol (vitamin D_2) irradiated by monochromatic ultraviolet light. *J Nutr Sci Vitaminol, 23*:281-90, 1977. (In English).
11. Corless, D., and Gupta, S. P.: Response of plasma 25-hydroxyvitamin D to ultraviolet irradiation in long stay geriatric patients. *Lancet, 23*:649-51, Sept., 1978.
12. Rogers, S. et al.: Effect of PUVA on serum 25-OH vitamin D in psoriatics. *Brit Med J*, 833-34, 6 Oct., 1979.
13. Giese, A. (Ed.): *Photophysiology*, Volume V. New York, Acad Pr, 1970, Chapters VI and VII.
14. Taylor, R. L.: Clinical study of ultraviolet in various skin conditions. *Phys Ther, 52*:279-82, 1972.
15. Bailey, B. N.: *Bedsores*. Baltimore, Williams & Wilkins, 1967.
16. Hollaender, A. (Ed.): *Radiation Biology*, Volume II. New York, McGraw, 1955.
17. Giese, A. (Ed.): *Photophysiology*, Volume IV. New York, Acad Pr, 1968, Chapter II.
18. Pathak, M. A., Harber, J. C., Seiji, M. et al. (Eds.): *Sunlight and Man*. Tokyo, U of Tokyo Pr, 1974, pp. 335-368.
19. Weber, G.: Combined 8-methoxypsoralen and black light therapy of psoriasis: Technique and results. *Br J Dermatol, 90*:317-23, 1974.
20. Parrish, J. A. et al.: Photochemotherapy of psoriasis with oral methoxsalen and longwave ultraviolet light. *N Engl J Med, 291*:1207-22, 1974.

21. Fischer, T.: Comparative treatment of psoriasis with UV-light, trioxsalen plus UV-light and coal tar plus UV-light. *Acta Derm Venereol, 57:*345-50, 1977.

22. Lynch, W. S. et al.: Clinical results of photochemotherapy. *Cutis, 20:*477-80, 1977.

23. Morison, W. L. et al: Controlled study of PUVA and adjunctive therapy in the management of psoriasis. *Br J Dermatol 98:*125-32, 1978.

24. Challoner, A. V. J. and Duffey, B. L.: Problems associated with ultraviolet dosimetry in the photochemotherapy of psoriasis. *Br J Dermatol, 97:*643-48, 1977.

25. Roenig, H. H.: Comparison of phototherapy systems for photochemotherapy. *Cutis, 20:*485-89, 1977.

26. Segal, S. A.: PUVA: A caution. *Pediatrics, 62:*253, 2 Aug., 1978.

27. Hardie, R. A. and Hunter, J. A. A.: Psoriasis. *Br J Hosp Med, 20:*13-23, 1978.

28. Stern, R. S. et al.: Risk of cutaneous carcinoma in patients treated with oral methoxsalen photochemotherapy for psoriasis. *N Engl J Med, 300:*809-813, 1979.

29. Montagna, W. and Labitz, W. (Eds.): *The Epidermis.* New York, Acad Pr, 1964, p. 408.

30. Holti, G.: Measurements of the vascular responses in skin at various time intervals after damage with histamine and ultraviolet radiation. *Clin Sci, 14:*143-55, 1955.

31. Sams, W., and Winkleman, R.: The effect of ultraviolet light on isolated cutaneous blood vessels. *J Invest Dermatol, 53:*79-83, 1969.

32. Van Der Leun, J. C.: Theory of ultraviolet erythema. *Photochem Photobiol, 1:*153-58, 1965.

33. Tronnier, H.: Zur Bedeutung der Hornschicht für die Lichttreaktionen der menschlichen Haut. *Strahlentherapie, 132:*128-33, 1967.

34. Grynbaum, B. et al.: Prevention of ultraviolet induced erythema. *Arch Phys Med Rehabil, 31:*507-92, 1950.

35. Gordon, M. (Ed.): *Pigment Cell Biology.* New York, Acad Pr, 1959, pp. 107-09, 127-37.

36. Giese, A. (Ed.): *Photophysiology,* Volume V, New York, Acad Pr, 1970, Chapters VI and VII.

37. Giese, A. (Ed.): *Photophysiology,* Volume VII. New York, Acad Pr, 1972, Chapters V and IX.

38. Giese, A. (Ed.): *Photophysiology,* Volume VI, New York, Acad Pr, 1971, Chapter III.

39. Peak, M. et al.: Inactivation of transforming DNA by ultraviolet light. II. Protection by histadine. *Mutat Res, 20:*137-41, 1973.

40. Marisco, A. R. et al.: Ultraviolet light and tar in the Goeckermann treatment of psoriasis. *Arch Dermatol, 112:*1249-50, 1976.

41. Kelner, A.: Photoreactivation of ultraviolet irradiated eschericoli, with special reference to the dose reduction principal and to ultraviolet induced mutation. *J Bacteriol, 58:*11-22, 1949.

42. Cram, D. L.: Psoriasis: Treatment with a tar gel. *Cutis, 17:*1197-1203, 1976.
43. Dulaney, E. L. and Laskin, A. I. (Eds.): The problems of drug resistant pathogenic bacteria. *Ann NY Acad Sci, 182,* June 11, 1971.
44. Maddin, S. (Ed.): *Current Dermatologic Management,* 2nd ed. St. Louis, Mosby, 1975.
45. Pringsheim, P.: *Fluorescence and Phosphorescence.* New York, Interscience, 1949.

Chapter 7

ULTRASONIC ENERGY

INTRODUCTION

U TILIZATION of ultrasonic energy for relief of pain and/or soft tissue relaxation was introduced into this country in the early 1950s. Prior to that time, extensive basic research, with subsequent clinical application, had been carried out in Europe, especially in Germany. Basic and clinical research has continued there and has developed in this country. Clinical application of ultrasonic energy for pain relief is now widespread and is perhaps second only to the use of hot packs.

Ultrasonic energy is a component of the acoustic spectrum of energy rather than a segment of the electromagnetic spectrum. Acoustic energy production, transmission, and absorption differ in major ways from that of electromagnetic energy. Acoustic energy of any wavelength cannot penetrate a vacuum. It must be conducted by molecules or larger units of matter. Electromagnetic energy travels best through a vacuum and does so at the speed of light (approximately 300,000,000 meters per second). Acoustic energy travels very inefficiently through any gas or mixture of gases. Electromagnetic energy travels well through gases. At sea level, its velocity is about 296,700,000 m/s. At sea level pressures, acoustic energy travels at a rate of about 330 m/s. Acoustic energy is transmitted well through degassed or gas-free liquids and travels best through high density solids. Since velocity equals wavelength times frequency, and wavelength equals velocity divided by frequency, any acoustic frequency will have a far shorter wavelength than electromagnetic energy of the same frequency.

Ultrasonic energy by definition is any vibrational energy of a frequency too high for stimulation of the sensory receptors of the human ear. Obviously the cutoff point between audible and

279

ultrasonic sound will vary, particularly with age, but in no case will audible sound have a frequency over 20,000 Hertz (Hz). Ultrasonic energy is almost entirely absorbed by the nitrogen, oxygen, and carbon dioxide in the atmosphere. Hence, in order to transmit ultrasonic energy to a patient, a liquid or a semisolid (ointment) must be used to insure significant transfer of energy from the source to the patient. Human skin is not a smooth surface, even when the transmitting applicator is applied with pressure. When the radiating surface is in contact with skin, air is always trapped within the pores of the skin. This leads to non-uniform energy transmission from the patient surface of the applicator into absorbing tissues. If the applicator (sound head or transducer) and the skin are immersed in a liquid or semi-solid, the amount of interfering air is markedly reduced. Both the efficiency and uniformity of energy transmission are greatly enhanced. Use of a coupling agent is standard clinical procedure.

Since human soft tissues consist of 70 to 90 percent water, plus proteins and other solids, the velocity of sound in water is standardly considered to be equivalent to that of sonic and ultrasonic energy in soft tissues. At ambient temperatures, that velocity is about 1500 m/s. Ultrasonic velocity in cortical bone, the body's most dense solid, is approximately 3500 m/s. For various reasons, to be discussed later in this chapter, the standard clinical ultrasonic frequency is 1 megacycle (1 Mc = 1000 Kc = 1000 KHz), although there are commercially available clinical generators with an operating frequency as low as 90 Kc and as high as 2 Mc. The relationship of operating frequency to depth of penetration is well documented.[1] With a frequency of 1 Mc, approximately 50 percent of the ultrasonic energy will penetrate to a depth of 5 cm within soft tissue. At 90 Kc, 50 percent will reach a depth of 10 cm. At 4 Mc, 50 percent will penetrate to a depth of 1 cm. It is then obvious that clinical ultrasound is indicated when good depth of penetration is needed. Ultrasonic energy has another important clinical advantage over any electromagnetic energy that physical therapists utilize, namely the more homogenous the tissue, the less the absorption. Subcutaneous fat is the most nearly homogenous human tissue and presents many problems when electromagnetic energy is being added for the purpose of causing a deep tissue temperature rise (TTR). Excessive fat temperature rise is no problem when ultrasonic energy is used. This fact, coupled with the depth of penetration, makes ultrasound the most effective physical agent when a TTR is required in a deeply seated joint.

A further advantage is that ultrasound may be safely used even though metallic implants are well within the depth of penetration of 50 percent of the energy.[2, 3] The metal does not absorb or concentrate the energy as would be the case if short wave or microwave energy were used, although there will be reflection, especially if the radiating surface of the application is not at a right angle to the implant's largest dimension. Hence, the presence of metallic implants does not give rise to tissue "hot-spots" with subsequent risk of damage to adjacent tissue. Actually, it has been shown that the metals used in the various wires, screws, plates, and joint replacements do not get as hot as surrounding tissues. Presumably, this is because the metal is more homogenous than living tissues and therefore transmits rather than absorbs the ultrasonic energy.

In the past, there has been major controversy as to whether the pain-relieving effects subsequent to exposure to ultrasonic energy are entirely due to the TTR, which always occurs under clinical conditions, or to a combination of thermal and nonthermal (mechanical or chemical) effects, or to the nonthermal effects alone. The leaders in basic and clinical research in this country agree that there are clinically significant nonthermal effects. Possibly Gersten and coworkers[4-6] were the first to demonstrate nonthermal effects of ultrasonic energy on peripheral nerve. In publications appearing as late as 1965, Schwann classified ultrasonic energy as a form of diathermy.[7] In 1969, he stated that he wished he could tear up that section of his chapter and give equal emphasis to the thermal and nonthermal effects of ultrasound.[8] Lehmann was well aware of the existence of nonthermal effects of ultrasound in the 1950s but did not regard them as clinically significant until much later.[9] Griffin and Touchstone demonstrated in 1962 that it is possible to drive topically applied hydrocortisone through skin and into underlying lumbosacral plexus with clinical ultrasonic energy.[10]

The reluctance of many investigators to conclude that nonthermal effects of ultrasound on intact tissues might have clinical significance is understandable if one reviews the intensive efforts made in the 1930s and 1940s to demonstrate nonthermal effects from exposure to short wave and microwave diathermies. It is now well accepted that the only effects of these latter forms of energy are due solely to the TTR that results from absorption of these electromagnetic frequencies.

Thus, treatment with ultrasonic energy can lead to pain relief where the lesion is beyond the reach of an infrared- or diather-my-induced TTR because of its superior penetration. It can be used safely in the presence of metallic implants whereas the diathermies cannot (*see* Chapter 4), and it can give pain relief by mechanisms not related to tissue temperature rise.

GENERATION OF CLINICAL ULTRASONIC ENERGY

Any unit of matter exposed to a pulsating stimulus will be set into vibration by the absorption of energy. Vibration is standard-ly defined as periodic motion in alternately opposite directions from a position of equilibrium. The rate of vibration will be in direct proportion to the rate of alternate periods of stimulus — no stimulus — stimulus, etc. In the case of a solid of finite dimension, there will be a certain rate of stimulus that will produce the maximum excursion of vibration for a given quanti-ty of energy absorbed. That particular rate is called the resonant frequency. What that rate will be depends largely on the dimen-sions of the solid and, of course, upon its composition. When the vibrating object is of homogenous composition, i.e. a crystalline material, its resonant frequency is controlled largely by the ratio of thickness to width or diameter. In general, the higher the ratio, the higher the resonant frequency.

One convenient way to set crystals into vibration is to attach two wires at some distance apart on the face of the crystal. If a direct current (DC) voltage of adequate amplitude is applied, the mass of the crystal will tend to deform as long as the voltage is applied, but in one direction only. This would not result in vibration in the usual sense, and if the energy applied were great enough, the crystal would eventually shatter. If an alternating current (AC) is applied, with each half cycle the crystal would bend first in one direction and then in the other, with maximum excursion if the AC frequency matched the ratio of thickness to diameter. If a liquid or solid is in contact with a face of the vibrating crystal, much of the energy applied to the crystal would be transferred to that other material in a periodic fashion.

When ultrasonic energy began to come into clinical use, most ultrasonic generators produced the mechanical energy by applying AC of appropriate frequency to natural quartz crystals. Quartz is expensive and hard to work with. Furthermore, quartz is a very poor conductor of electricity. Hence, high voltage is required to set quartz crystals into vibration. Fortunately, the technology for precise, controlled growth of synthetic crystals developed rapidly immediately after World War II, and some synthetic crystals are admirably suited for being driven by low voltage, high frequency AC. Now, almost all clinical ultrasonic generators utilize either barium titanate, lead zirconate, or a grown mixture of the two kinds of crystals to convert high frequency, low voltage AC into high frequency sound energy. For protection of the patient and of the crystal, the crystal is bonded to a metal plate (usually nickel-plated brass) or to a thin layer of glass. This surface is applied to the patient. The dimensions of the plate or glass are carefully selected so that their resonant frequency exactly matches that of the driven crystal. These synthetic crystals are cheaper to prepare for clinical use and require far less voltage to set into useful vibration as compared to quartz, so the cost of the necessary transformer for modifying house current is far less.

A crystal that has an operating frequency of 1 Mc will have a thickness of 3 to 4 mm. Clinically useful crystals will have a diameter of anywhere from 0.5 to 10 cm. Most of the transducers in use have an effective patient surface of from 2 to 10 cm^2. Different manufacturers vary widely as to how much of the apparent patient surface is actually producing a significant quantity of ultrasonic vibration.[11, 12] One should bear in mind that an operating frequency of 1 Mc means that the crystal is deforming one million times per second in each of two directions — toward and away from the patient. When the operating frequency is lower, the crystal is thicker. When the frequency is higher, the crystal is thinner. For any given diameter or thickness, the synthetic crystals will have a more nearly uniform energy output from the entire radiating surface as compared to natural quartz crystals. The latter are very apt to have a high intensity output at the center of the radiating surface and much less toward the periphery. Thus, if the radiating surface had an area of 5 cm^2 the center square centimeter might be producing two to five times more ultrasonic energy than that surface as little as 0.5 cm distant. Such a "hot-spot" effect is much less evident with barium titanate or lead zirconate crystals. The synthetic crystals respond to an applied AC voltage with a more nearly true piston action rather than a deforming or bowing effect.

To drive either kind of crystal, house current (60 cycle 110 v AC) is converted into whatever is the resonant frequency of the crystal to be driven. This frequency conversion is done by some form of oscillating circuit (*see* Chapter 8). The high frequency current is then led into a step-up transformer to supply a high voltage (quartz crystal, 2000 to 3000 v) or an intermediate voltage (synthetic crystal, 200 to 300 v). The modified electromagnetic energy is then coupled to the crystal, usually through a coaxial cable. Use of a coaxial cable is an effective way to minimize frequency alteration when high frequency current is to be transmitted from the electrical oscillating circuit to the crystal.

Early ultrasonic generators had problems with bonding the metal or glass face to the crystal and to the metal covering housing the disc edge. One could tell that the bond was becoming defective when it was audible as well as producing ultrasonic energy. Apparatus manufactured since about 1965 rarely becomes defective in this manner.

The crystals are driven with either continuous or pulse modulation AC. The former is in more common use. In apparatus designed to deliver pulsing ultrasound (US), there frequently is a manually controlled variation in ratio of power on to power off. Some arrangements for this duty factor control are very precise. Others leave much to be desired insofar as accuracy in timing and uniformity of intensity is concerned, especially when a given piece of apparatus has been in regular use for more than six months.[11] With pulsed ultrasonic energy, it is possible to use higher peak intensities with less risk of tissue damage.

CLINICAL ULTRASONIC FREQUENCIES

Perhaps more than 90 percent of all the clinical ultrasonic generators in use in this country are intended for operation at a frequency of 1 Mc. This frequency was deliberately chosen as a compromise frequency between those which produce predominantly thermal effects (2 Mc and higher) and those which produce nonthermal (mechanical and/or chemical) as well as thermal effects (500 Kc or lower) in human soft tissues. Theoretically, if the ratio of crystal thickness to diameter is kept constant, frequencies below 300 Kc should *not* produce a significant TTR.[12] This is true for at least two reasons. At lower ultrasonic frequencies, the energy spreads laterally to a much greater extent than is true for frequencies at or above 1 Mc, so that there is less energy available for absorption per unit volume of tissue. Also at low frequencies, the time between significant radiation pressure changes becomes great enough so that there is no net TTR. In practice, since it is not feasible to keep the ratio constant in a clinically useful transducer because of size of the patient surface, the lower frequencies also produce a strong TTR, in large part due to the thermal *(not acoustic)* energy production and transmission as well as US (ultrasonic) energy production.[13] A barium titanate crystal with a resonant frequency of 250 Kc will be about 2 cm thick. If its total patient surface area is 5 cm, its diameter will also be about 2 cm. Thus, the crystal would be very nearly symmetrical in its critical dimensions. Such a crystal will become quite hot when an AC voltage is applied with an intensity great enough to produce more than a few tenths of a watt per cm^2 of ultrasonic energy. Because of the liquid or semisolid coupling between the transducer and the patient, much of the thermal energy, along with the ultrasonic energy, is transmitted to the patient. The Acoustics Branch of the Bureau of Radiological Health is in the process of establishing regulations that will include requiring the manufacturer to state the expected crystal face temperature rise under standard operating conditions for any ultrasonic generator intended for clinical use.

Clinical Low Frequency Ultrasound

Summer and Patrick have stated that theoretically, US at frequencies lower than 300 Kc should not produce a significant tissue temperature rise.[12] This is true only if the *ratio* of crystal diameter to crystal thickness is kept the same as that for 1 Mc units. Since that is not practical for clinical use, low frequency generators will always generate significant thermal as well as acoustic energy. There is no known reason why this thermal energy should cause reactions different from those discussed in Chapter 5.

When Griffin and colleagues first began to experiment with clinically practical low frequency ultrasound, it was with the objective of increasing depth of penetration of acoustic energy.[10, 13, 65] These reports were *in vivo* studies on pigs and humans. They showed significant improvement in pain relief for the osteoarthritic patient where the affected joint was deeper than 5 cm below the skin, as compared similar patients treated with 1 Mc ultrasound. It was further shown that *in vivo* exposure of pig lumbosacral plexus to 90 Kc alone increases hydrocortisone content of the gross axonal complex.[10] The significance of this finding is not yet understood.

Griffin has routinely used 90 Kc ultrasound on osteoarthritic patients who did not respond to 1 Mc US, for twenty years, with excellent results. The only established difference as of 1981 is the fact that 90 Kc ultrasound does penetrate soft tissue approximately twice as deeply as does 1 Mc ultrasound, namely 50 percent to 10 cm versus 5 cm, respectively.

It seems likely that 90 Kc ultrasound generators will be commercially available as of 1981. Several major *in vitro* studies should appear during the 1980s.

Reasons why absorption of intermediate intensities of ultrasonic energy results in decrease of nerve conduction are not known at this time. It has been shown that the change in conduction velocity takes place when provision is made to prevent TTR as well as when a TTR is allowed to occur. The latter is the normal clinical circumstance.[6]

Physiological Effects of Clinical Ultrasonic Energy

This discussion will be limited to effects that have been demonstrated when the operating frequency is between 750 and 2000 Kc at intensities not exceeding 3 watts per cm^2 (w/cm^2). Under FDA regulations that became effective in 1979,[14] all clinical U.S. generators manufactured after February of that year must indicate through permanent labeling on the transducer or state clearly in the provided literature:

1. Output frequency of the transducer
2. Whether the output beam is focused or divergent
3. The *effective* area of the patient surface of the transducer, in cm^2
4. The recommended procedure for periodic recalibration of the meter. The meter must be accurate to within ±20 percent.
5. If the unit is designed to deliver pulsed ultrasound to the patient, the meter must be capable of indicating the temporal maximum effective intensity with a ±20 percent accuracy for all output greater than 10 percent of total possible output. There must also be some means of indicating the magnitude of each pulse duration and the pulse repetition rate.

There must also be a visual indicator, i.e. a pilot light, which is automatically turned on whenever the transducer crystal is actually excited by an alternating current of appropriate frequency.

Effects of Ultrasonic Energy on Peripheral Nerve

It has been known at least since 1950 that peripheral nerve *in situ* is more responsive to exposure to ultrasonic energy than is any other soft tissue.[15] It has been shown that there is more cortisol present in normal untreated peripheral nerve than in any human soft tissue except the adrenal cortex.[16] It has also been demonstrated that when the peripheral nerve (lumbosacral plexus) of swine is sonated *in situ,* its cortisol content increases significantly. Farmer established that there is significant change in conduction velocity when human subjects are exposed to ultrasound.[17] When ultrasonic intensity is between 0.5 and 1.5 w/cm^2, conduction velocity decreases. At intensities below 0.5 or above 2 w/cm^2, conduction velocity increases. When electromagnetic energy is absorbed in sufficient quantity to cause a TTR, conduction velocity invariably increases.

It is easy to demonstrate the decrease in motor nerve conduction velocity of human median nerve upon exposure to intermediate intensities of ultrasound with the direct contact moving sound head technique. Measure NCV by standard techniques at elbow and wrist. Expose the volar forearm, at whatever intensity generates a gentle sensation of warmth, for five minutes. Remeasure the conduction velocity. There will be a decrease in velocity of 5 to 10 meters per second in 80 to 90 percent of the subjects. Most other subjects will show no change. In a group of ten normal subjects one can anticipate a rise in NCV in one subject. Young normals of average build will usually tolerate an intensity of 0.5 to 1.0 w/cm^2 with the moving sound technique. The effect on velocity is transient and will return toward normal within thirty minutes.

Currier has shown that decline in NCV does *not* occur among cutaneous axons when treated in a similar manner.[18] He further showed that sensory velocity increases as skin temperature increases, just as is the case when either sensory or motor axons have their temperature raised by any form of electromagnetic energy.

Molecular Effects

Piersol and coworkers established that about 80 percent of ultrasonic energy is absorbed by proteins, in comparison with carbohydrates and lipids, and that absorption is equal in protein in plasma and in membranes.[19] Lota and Darling demonstrated that clinical intensities alter the diffusion of potassium and sodium across the red blood cell membrane.[20] When ultrasonic energy is applied with an intensity of about 1 w/cm^2, radiation pressure changes on the order of ± 1.5 atmospheres will take place within the absorbing tissues. This has been calculated to represent a change of about ± 4 milligrams per cell and is not regarded as destructive.[12] Both the pressure change and the normally occurring TTR could be factors in the well-established alteration of cell permeability. The pressure changes are usually considered to have a micromassage effect on the absorbing tissues.

Tissue Temperature Rise

Schwann,[21] Lota,[22] Lehmann,[23-25] and Abramson[26, 27] have shown that with clinical intensities applied with a continuously moving sound head, muscle temperature rises on the order of 1° to 2°C are common. Subcutaneous fat temperatures are about half that of the underlying muscle. If cortical bone lies within the limit of penetration of 50 percent of the energy being added, the bone temperature rise will be 5° to 6°C. All temperature changes due to exposure to ultrasonic energy occur much more rapidly than is the case when electromagnetic energy is the cause of the TTR. With ultrasound, the temperature rise occurs within twenty to thirty seconds. Presumably, this difference in rate in rise is due to the fact that a large percentage of ultrasonic energy applied to the skin is transmitted through the skin and subcutaneous fat, which in turn permits primary absorption in underlying muscle and connective tissue much more efficiently than can occur when electromagnetic energy is added. Subcutaneous fat acts as an insulator against penetration of electromagnetic energy at frequencies in clinical use. Hence, deeper tissue temperature rise is predominantly due to reaction by cutaneous nerve and/or secondary conduction. Demonstrable increase in local blood flow may persist up to an hour after a five-minute exposure to ultrasound. When electromagnetic energy is used, a treatment time of nearly ten times as long is necessary to produce equivalent change in deep blood flow.[26, 27]

One must remember there is considerable reflection of ultrasound at any tissue interface, i.e. skin-fat or tendon-bone. The reflection results in the more superficial tissue being exposed to greater intensities than would be the case if significant reflection did not occur. Reflection is greatest from tissues of high density. Theoretically, reflection from cortical bone should be on the order of 70 percent.[12] Actual *in vitro* measurements indicate it is more likely to be about half that amount.[23-25] The reflection of energy can give rise to sharply localized pathological temperature increases within the periosteum and to tendon at or near bone-tendon junctions. Both tendon and periosteum have a poor blood supply and a low water content. Hence, these tissues are poorly equipped to disseminate the reflected energy. The periosteum is richly supplied with sensory receptors, including thermal sensors. Therefore, if the patient has a normally functioning sensory nervous system, he will become aware of a characteristic noxious stimulus if the periosteal temperature approaches the critical level (45°C) and will move away from the source of energy before damage is done. The clinical response to periosteal overheating is commonly described as a deep, dull ache of very sudden onset. The sensation may occur at any time within the treatment and may recur several times during a single treatment. Whenever this sensation is reported, the intensity of the ultrasonic energy being applied must be decreased rapidly or long-lasting thermal damage can occur.

Alteration of Connective Tissue

There are numerous clinical reports that indicate that exposure to ultrasonic energy is effective in permanently diminishing pain due to the presence of neuromas and adhesive scars.[28-30] Also, it has been the authors' clinical impression that when patients with Dupuytren's contracture receive appropriate local sonation, there is long-lasting relaxation of the tight palmar fascia. On the basis of *in vitro* study, where pain is due to excess proliferation of connective tissue, relief of pain may be due to relaxation of polypeptide bonds after the absorption of ultrasonic energy.[4, 19-21] Joseph has reported that experimentally induced wounds heal faster upon exposure to ultrasonic energy. He presented evidence that indicates that improvement in tissue regeneration parallels systemic increase in the "male sex hormone" and that this increase occurs with local sonation at intensities that do not cause a significant TTR.[31]

Dyson, Webster, and colleagues have established some of the mechanisms by which wound healing is aided by exposure to ultrasound.[32, 33] Apparently the key to growth of replacement tissue at sites of injury is stimulation of protein synthesis in fibroblasts. Exposure of injured tissue to ultrasound at clinically practical doses seems to provide this stimulation.

Exposure to ultrasonic energy is also an effective way of increasing range of motion where limitation is due to massive hypertrophic scar tissue formation, as occurs in burns that have destroyed the dermis. Distinction must be made between hypertrophic and true keloid scars.[34-37] Exposure to ultrasound is not effective in regaining range of motion lost because of formation of true keloid.[35-37] The histological distinction between hypertrophic and keloid connective tissue proliferation is that in the former, proliferation comes entirely from the epidermal margin. In keloid proliferation, collagen production is predominantly from dermal rather than epidermal tissue, and there is massive hyalinization. Furthermore, hypertrophic scarring occurs with no predilection for race or age, whereas keloid scarring is considerably more common in Negroes, Malaysians, and Hindus and is more common between ages ten and thirty than at any other time of life. Keloids occur most commonly after trauma that has lacerated the dermis. The biochemical error, if any, that results in the formation of a keloid is not yet known. Recurrence after surgical excision occurs in more than 50 percent of the true keloids as compared to 15 to 20 percent in the more common hypertrophic scar. There is no known surgical, physical, or chemical technique which is consistently reliable in permanently removing the true keloid. Careful radiation therapy is the most reliable treatment to date.[37]

Regeneration and repair of connective tissue after injury is characterized by (1) watery edema, followed by (2) mucinous edema, containing at first hyaluronate and later chondroitin sulfate, and then (3) collagen cicatrization, and in the skin still later by epithelialization.[34] Fibroblasts synthesize the collagen precursors. Mast cells synthesize the acid mucopolysaccharides, i.e. heparin and hyaluronic acid, as well as histamine and serotonin. Repair of damage seems directly proportional to the amount of histamine produced. *In vitro* exposure of hyaluronic and chondroitin sulfuric acids to ultrasonic energy of intensities and duration of exposure close to those used clinically results in a sharp decrease in their viscosities.[38] With prolonged exposure (20 to 30 minutes), their viscosity approaches that of water. It is presumed that the viscosity change is due in large part to disruption of glucoside bonds. It has also been established that there is significant increase in tendon extensibility[39] and relaxation of skeletal muscle[40] upon absorption of ultrasonic energy. Hence, the therapist should anticipate being able to bring about the regaining of range of motion where the limitation is due to contracted fascia, muscle, tendon, and most scar tissue.

Mineral Deposition in Soft Tissues

A small percentage of patients with a clinical diagnosis of some form of periarticular pathology, i.e. tendonitis, bursitis, or fibrositis, have apparent calcium salt deposition upon or within the irritated tissue, as evidenced by x-ray visualization. Ultrasound has proven useful in relieving pain in many of these cases both with and without hard evidence that there has been mineral deposition within soft tissues.[41-44] Pain relief in such periarticular pathologies could be due to relaxation of skeletal muscle[40] and/or the apparent net result of resorption of abnormal calcium deposition on bone (spur formation), tendon (calcified tendonitis), or in muscle (myofibrositis). It is curious that with the widespread use of ultrasonic energy for relief of pain, no definitive study has been reported wherein pre- and post-treatment x-ray evaluation was used consistently. The author conducted an intensive search of American, British, and Canadian literature up through 1979 for clinical reports where abnormal calcium deposition was a likely cause of pain and was unable to find any study where x-ray evaluation of results was used through the reported series.

As of 1975, there was adequate documentation to state that absorption of ultrasonic energy as it is applied clinically will cause a physiological tissue temperature rise in underlying muscle, nerve, tendon, and bone. Furthermore, because it penetrates more deeply than any electromagnetic energy that physical therapists use, ultrasonic energy is more effective than other physical agents when stimulation of cutaneous nerve and vascular supply does not play a significant role in relief of pain. The significance, if any, of the fact that peripheral nerve is more sensitive to stimulation by ultrasonic energy than any other soft tissue is not yet understood. The fact that exposure to ultrasonic energy relaxes connective tissue in a more nearly lasting fashion than does any form of electromagnetic energy may be due to effects on plasticity, as opposed to elasticity, or to polypeptide bond disruption, or to reaction to radiation pressure changes. Much more laboratory study utilizing clinical parameters of ultrasonic energy needs to be done before the possible significance of nonthermal changes induced by absorption of this form of energy can be clearly stated.

TECHNIQUES OF APPLICATION OF
ULTRASONIC ENERGY

Heating of the Skin Prior to the
Application of Ultrasonic Energy

Some clinicians prefer to induce a rise in skin and sub-cutaneous tissue temperature prior to the use of ultrasonic energy (US). This is usually done with some form of infrared or diathermy. When it is done, the "preheat" treatment is usually given for about ten minutes. Clinicians who use this procedure feel that more of the US energy penetrates more deeply if immediately preceded by a local rise in superficial temperature. Other clinicians feel this procedure is unnecessary. One study was reported in 1979 indicating that pretreatment with hot packs does improve efficacy of transmission of ultrasound into deeper tissues.[45]

Until such time as a well-designed comparative study is reported, it would seem logical to try ultrasound alone for three or four treatments. If there is no lasting pain relief and/or gain in range of motion, preheating might then be tried for an equal number of treatments.

"Direct Contact"

This is the standard technique when the area to be treated is of reasonably regular contour. Some form of coupling material, liquid or semisolid (lotion, cream, or ointment) must be applied to the skin to minimize trapping of air in the skin pores when the transducer is applied to the skin and to minimize friction between the moving sound head and the skin. Degassed (boiled) water is the most efficient couplant for transfer of acoustic energy from the patient surface of the transducer into the patient because its acoustic impedance is reasonably close to that of the patient's soft tissues. However, its viscosity is too low to be practical when the direct contact technique is indicated. The sound head is likely to push all the water away so that the pores refill with air. Also, it is difficult for a clinic to maintain an adequate supply of degassed water, since as the boiled water returns to room temperature, the nitrogen, oxygen, and carbon dioxide that had been removed by boiling rapidly reenter the water. Hence, many commercially available coupling agents intended for use with the direct contact technique will have water mixed with some kind of thixotropic gel. Since their viscosities are greater than that of water, they will have less of a tendency to be pushed away by the weight or the movement of the sound head. Reid and Cummings measured the transmission of US through several readily available coupling agents, using near field measurement technics.[46] They found that a thixotropic gel transmitted better than 70 percent of the radiated energy, glycerol about 68 percent, water about 60 percent, and mineral oil about 20 percent. Mineral oil is perhaps the most widely used couplant because it is cheap and gets the job done.

In a later study, Warren and colleagues measured transmissivity through various couplants, using far field measurement technics through a thin layer of couplant and then a large volume of degassed water. Using water as a reference standard for transmissivity, Warren found that glycerol was 75 to 100 percent as efficient as water and that mineral oil was as efficient or more efficient compared to water, under several experimental conditions.[47] It is then reasonable to conclude that when the direct contact technic is used, it does not matter which coupling agent is applied, insofar as transmissivity is concerned. Griffin has shown that when large volumes of liquid are used as coupling agent, as would be the case for immersion technics, tap water is more efficient than either glycerin or mineral oil.[48]

Various emulsions of water and animal or vegetable fats are also in clinical use. One must remember the transducer will always become warm during a direct contact treatment, so the gels and emulsions will tend to liquify during treatment. One should then compromise between couplants that will remain as a semi-solid with a relatively high viscosity and hence require more effort on the part of the therapist to keep the sound head moving and the couplants that are liquids or become liquid during the treatment. A couplant that is adequate in body segments where the skin temperature is relatively low may be inadequate in segments that are more proximal. Furthermore, an agent that is adequate for use with a moving sound head may not be adequate with a stationary technic.

The coupling agent should be applied to the skin and the

sound head should be in place on the skin before the transducer is energized. Otherwise, if the crystal is set into vibration and there is no provision for unloading the vibrational energy, the crystal will develop standing waves which can interfere with resonant vibration within the crystal. In extreme cases, the standing wave load can cause structural damage to the crystal. When this has occurred, the sound head must be replaced and the oscillating circuit must be recalibrated.

In the most common clinical usage, once energized, the sound head is kept in continuous motion on the skin over the area being treated. Since the patient surface of the applicator is hard and rigid, care should be taken to avoid running into a bony prominence such as a vertebral spinous process or a greater trochanter. Such contact can be painful if the subcutaneous fat layer is thin. The authors feel strongly that movement of the sound head should be slow and steady — on the order of 60 cm per minute — for best relaxation for the patient. Other clinicians feel that by moving the sound head faster, they can use a higher intensity without causing periosteal overheating. In either case, two types of motion are in general use — a slow circle within a circle with concomitant translatory motion, or a pure stroking movement. There is more risk of hot-spot development if the pure stroke is used, since inevitably there will be deceleration of motion as the direction of the stroke is reversed. Possibly, the circle-within-a-circle technic results in a slightly more uniform pattern of energy absorption within the area being treated, especially if the radiating surface of the sound head has an area of 5 cm^2 or less. If the effective radiating surface is 10 cm^2 or greater, it is simple to achieve adequate overlap with either technic and hence more nearly uniform application of energy.

Intensity to be used should vary depending upon whether the objective of treatment is to cause a maximum tolerable TTR or whether nonthermal effects are also desired. Connective tissue relaxation and relief of perarticular pain do not require intensities in excess of 2 watts/cm^2.[4-6, 10, 18, 25] In general, the greater the volume of soft tissue, the higher the intensity. One needs to remember that the intensity indicated on the generator meter is not reliable, especially apparatus that has not been calibrated

within the last six months.[11] At least until such time as the federal
government standardizes and enforces acoustic rather than the
present electric power output measurement, it is better to use an
intensity that produces a gentle sensation of warmth as the
sound head is kept in slow motion rather than blindly picking a
meter reading and adhering to it regardless of the patient sensation of warmth. Obviously, there can be dosage problems when
ultrasonic energy is applied to patients who have a deficit in their
sensory nervous system and/or an emotional disturbance. Significant damage to the patient is unlikely to occur if the intensity
used on the trunk or proximal extremity does not exceed 1.5
w/cm^2 and on the distal extremity does not exceed 0.5 w/cm^2,
assuming an area of about 150 cm^2 is being treated over a
five-minute period with a steadily moving sound head.

Stationary Technique

There are occasions when a direct contact stationary technic is
preferrable to a direct contact moving sound head technic. If
there is a small, sharply localized area of pain and/or muscle
spasm and/or organized hematoma, the stationary technic may
be more effective. Specially designed transducers are more apt
to be used for this procedure. Those in widespread use have a
patient surface area of 50 to 100 cm^2. Very few pain-producing
orthopedic lesions will be so sharply localized that the more
common 5 to 10 cm^2 radiating surface will be adequate.

There are two important procedure differences when the
stationary technic is used. The intensity must be far lower, and
the coupling agent should have a greater viscosity as compared
to when the moving technic is used. Although intensities up to 2
w/cm^2 are common with the moving direct contact technic, very
few individuals can safely tolerate 0.2 w/cm^2 for more than two
or three minutes with the stationary treatment, regardless of the
volume of underlying soft tissue. Intensity on the order of 0.02
to 0.1 w/cm^2 is usually comfortable when the stationary sound
head is in place for five minutes or more. The usual treatment
time is ten to fifteen minutes, with the therapist always remaining close by to lower intensity as needed. Thus, if one is treating a
small, sharply delineated organized hematoma within an adult-

sized anterior thigh, the starting intensity might be 0.2 w/cm^2. Within three minutes, it is likely that the intensity will need to be reduced to 0.1 and by ten minutes to 0.01 w/cm^2 because of patient sensation of discomfort.

Periosteal overheating (to 45°C or higher), with concomitant sudden onset of a deep, dull ache, is much more apt to occur with the stationary procedure. Also, since the transducer is not in motion, the *thermal* energy that is inevitably generated within the crystal is going to be transmitted to a much smaller area and volume of tissue for a longer period of time. Of course, the same holds true for the transmitted and absorbed acoustic energy. Both types of energy will cause a TTR, and since the sound head is not moving, there is less chance for the absorbing tissue to cool down during the treatment period in comparison with the moving technic. Hence, one should select a coupling agent whose viscosity will not decrease significantly until the couplant temperature is over 40°C. If the previously viscous couplant liquifies and drains off the area being treated, energy transmission to the patient can become very nonuniform. Lotions, creams, or ointments with no more than a 50 percent water content and with a high glycerol content would seem very useful when the stationary technic is indicated.

Immersion Technic

Immersion of the part to be treated in a relatively large volume of coupling fluid is needed in treatment of elbows and distal upper extremity joints, as well as for the ankle and more distal lower extremity joints. Since there is much bone close to the surface in these areas, it is difficult if not impossible to maintain uniform contact between the skin and the radiating surface of the sound head. The net result if direct contact is tried is that where there is a bony protuberance, the quantity of absorption may be painfully great, but immediately adjacent tissue may absorb an ineffective quantity of energy. There is also the factor of the rigid patient surface of the transducer being pushed against a protuberance and causing a painful pressure point. Both these problems are minimized if the part to be treated is immersed in a liquid and the sound head is kept moving close to the skin (0.5 to 1 cm) over the area where the greatest absorption is desired.

Theoretically and practically, tap water is the best couplant when the immersion technic is indicated because it transmits ultrasonic energy efficiently even in the presence of massive bubble formation.[48] Large volumes of glycerol or mineral oil do not exhibit any significant bubble formation on prolonged exposure to clinical ultrasound.[48] Glycerin is superior to mineral oil in the near field transmission[46, 48] and approximately equal to mineral oil in the far field.[47, 48] The nonaqueous couplants do have a significant rise in temperature when the intensity is at 1 w/cm^2 or more for five minutes. The temperature increase is on the order of 3° to 6°C. Increase in water temperature is less than 1° under similar conditions. Therefore, it is a reasonable working hypothesis that if the therapist desires to obtain maximum thermal and nonthermal effects with the immersion treatment, the couplant should be preheated water (not exceeding about 42°C) or mineral oil or glycerin starting at room temperature. The temperature rise in glycerin is significantly greater than the rise in mineral oil. The cost of glycerin is about four times greater than that of mineral oil. However, both can be reused many times with insignificant loss in volume and can be heat sterilized much more safely than paraffin if contamination is a problem.

The Fluid-filled Bag

There are certain body areas where it is not practical to use either direct contact or an immersion technic for sonation. If, for example, it is desired to treat the anterior aspect of the knee, including the patella, or the lateral hip, including tissues attached to the greater trochanter, or the perianal area, via immersion, the volume of couplant needed would be so great that little energy would actually reach the target tissues. Most of the radiated energy would be absorbed by the large volume of couplant. If the direct contact procedure is used, because of irregular contour, with or without bony protuberances in the examples given, it would be difficult to get uniform energy distribution from the transducer to the absorbing tissues, and since the radiating surface is rigid, it can cause pain when sliding into a protuberance.

Under such circumstances, it is feasible to fill a finger cot (condom) with degassed water or glycerol or mineral oil and attach the lateral margins of the transducer to the open end of the finger cot with heavy rubber bands or adhesive tape. Care *must* be taken that no air is trapped between the surface of the transducer and the coupling liquid, or essentially no energy will reach the patient. The same coupling fluid is also applied to the outside of the finger cot and to the skin over the target area. The fluid-filled bag is than applied to the skin, using either the moving sound head or stationary direct contact technic. The elasticity of the bag permits a more nearly uniform energy transmission to areas of irregular contour. If there is abrupt contact with a bony prominence, it will not be painful, as could be the case if the radiating surface were in direct contact with the skin. The same fluid-filled bag can be reused many times.

Phonophoresis

Phonophoresis is the movement of a substance away from the patient surface of the transducer by virtue of having been exposed to ultrasonic energy. The movement is due to radiation pressure changes caused by the transmission of the high frequency sound waves through the couplant and into tissues.[12] In clinical physical therapy, a liquid or an ointment containing the desired ingredient is applied to the skin over the area to be treated. Medication strengths on the order of 0.5 to 10% (5 to 100 milligrams per gram of vehicle) have been reported.[49, 50] The vehicle functions as the coupling agent. The radiating surface of the transducer is placed into the couplant and energized in the usual manner, using either the moving or stationary technic. Laboratory data indicate that large, complex whole molecules such as hydrocortisone and lidocaine are easily driven through skin *in situ* and can be recovered from deeply underlying muscle and nerve using standard treatment parameters.[10, 13, 50, 51] Significant amounts of the medication can be recovered 10 cm deep to the skin after a five-minute exposure with the stationary procedure. Early in the 1950s,

Aldes and Jadeson[52] and Fellinger and Schmid[53] reported that chronic periarticular and osteoarthritic symptomatology responded better when intramuscular or intra-articular injection of hydrocortisone was immediately followed by exposure of the injected area to ultrasonic energy than do these pathologies when treated with either ultrasound or injected hydrocortisone alone. Presumably, the well-established ability of US energy to transiently increase membrane permeability is responsible for the improvement in pain relief, since diffusion of an analgesic, anesthetic, or anti-inflammatory agent is increased by external application of ultrasound. The technic of phonophoresis minimizes the possibility of a pain increase immediately following intramuscular or intra-articular injection where the pain increase was caused by the quantity of liquid injected.

Clinical studies using phonophoretic administration of several drugs compared to other treatment have been reported. Griffin et al. and Kleinkort and Wood demonstrated advantages of treatment with hydrocortisone administered by phonophoresis.[50, 56] Wanet and Dehon reported using phenylbutazone and Alphakadol®.[66] Aspirin has also been widely administered by phonophoresis (Myoflex® Creme), but no formal report has appeared. Burgudzhieva and Chuchkov reported phonophoretic administration of hydrocortisone as very effective as treatment in chronic vulvar dystrophies.[67]

Phonophoresis seems to be superior to iontophoresis (*see* Chapter 3) as a method of driving topically applied medication deep into underlying soft tissue. There is no hazard of skin damage when ultrasound is used. There is a very real hazard of an electrical burn when DC with continuous modulation is used as a driving agent. Very few individuals can tolerate iontophoresis at an intensity of more than 30 milliwatts/cm^2.[54, 55] Ultrasound is standardly used at intensities of 1 to 2 w/cm^2 with a moving sound head and at 0.1 to 0.2 w/cm^2 with a stationary transducer, with no risk of injury to the skin and only a remote possibility of periosteal overheating.[49] If the latter should occur, the patient is far more apt to become aware of it and report it than he is apt to be aware of warning signals for skin damage from absorption of too much continuous modulation DC.

With phonophoresis, there is no dissociation of the driven compound into ionized fragments. Hence, one does not need to know whether the ionized fragment that is physiologically active is driven in from the positive or negative pole. When iontophoresis is used, one must know this factor. Neither does one need to know about the ideal pH of the solution or ointment used when ultrasonic energy is the driving agent. At best, penetration of the driven compound will be to a depth of 1 cm with iontophoresis.[55] When US is the driving agent, there can be significant penetration to 5 cm with the standard clinical frequency (1 Mc) and to at least twice that depth in soft tissues when lower frequencies are used.[1, 12, 13] Lastly, if the area to be treated is no greater than 150 cm^2, a five-minute treatment appears adequate to drive in enough medication to provide substantial pain relief.[56] Iontophoresis requires at least a ten-minute treatment. Treatment for twenty to thirty minutes at a time is more common.[54, 55]

Selection of Intensity to be Used

Clinical opinion as to appropriate intensity to use when treating with ultrasound has undergone major change in the thirty or more years that this physical agent has been employed in this country. There are at least two major reasons for the steady *decrease* in intensity selected for most patient problems. First, more and more therapists have become aware that benefits from ultrasound are due to thermal as well as nonthermal effects.[4-6, 9, 10 17, 32, 33, 40, 49, 51] It is well established that a patient sensation of intense heat while undergoing treatment is quite likely to lead to a dull ache of delayed onset which may last for several hours after treatment. This slow-onset ache should not be confused with the sudden-onset ache which may occur during treatment and which is due to periosteal overheating. The delayed-onset ache is not necessary as a prelude to pain relief and/or gain in range of motion. The original logical procedure of the physician prescibing an intensity (in w/cm^2) for a specified length of time (in minutes) for a given patient was dealt a severe blow by the report of Stewart et al. (1974) on the wide disparity of actual acoustic output among clinical ultrasound apparatus depending upon how long since the instrument was last calibrated and how badly it had been abused.[11] Up until 1979, all clinical ultrasound generator meters measured electrical energy applied to the crystal rather than even roughly approximating the actual acoustic output directed toward the patient.[14] As of 1979 it became possible to build a clinical generator whose meter monitors actual acoustic output rather than electrical input to the crystal.

Secondly, as the capabilities for synthetic piezoelectric crystal growth improved, along with key developments in electronic oscillating circuits, the efficiency of the crystals has improved from the usual 8 to 10 percent (through the 1970s) to as high as 60 percent (in the 1980s). The net result is that clinical generators are now commercially available whose maximum acoustic output is 1 w/cm^2. These units are highly effective in all the standard treatment techniques.

Consequently, it is now unwise to apply ultrasound at a fixed intensity for a given patient and/or diagnosis. It is, in the opinion of the authors, wiser to select an intensity on the basis of what gives the patient a sensation of gentle warmth during treatment of that area with that generator, regardless of whether that intensity be 0.001 or 1.0 w/cm^2. If the patient does not have normal sensation, it is wiser to decrease the intensity, from the start, over what previous experience with that generator has indicated would be adequate under otherwise similar circumstances.

INDICATIONS AND CONTRAINDICATIONS FOR ULTRASONIC THERAPY

Chronic Arthritis

Ultrasonic energy is in widespread use for relief of pain due to osteoarthritis, chronic rheumatoid arthritis, and the nonarticular pathologies that are usually grouped together as periarticular arthritis. Chronic bursitis, myositis, fibrositis, and tendonitis are classical examples of periarticular pathology which responds well to exposure to US. Assuming that pain relief is due to a rapid rise in muscle temperature, with subsequent vasodilation and reduction in skeletal muscle tension, ultrasonic energy is the treatment of choice if vasodilation and muscle relaxation are needed in tissues that are 2 cm or more deep to the skin. It is well documented that ultrasonic energy penetrates more deeply and that there is a faster deep temperature rise when tissues are exposed to US as compared to tissues exposed to hydrotherapy or other forms of infrared or to the short wave or microwave segments of the electromagnetic spectrum.[1, 5, 19, 20, 22, 23, 43]

In addition to being useful in pain relief in the more common arthritic and/or collagen disorders, ultrasonic therapy appears to be at least as effective as x-ray therapy for pain relief in ankylosing spondylitis (Marie-Strumpell arthritis) and does not present the hazards, which are well documented, that occur when x-ray therapy is used in the management of this problem.[57, 58] Since the distance from skin to the bodies of the vertebrae in adults is more than 2 cm, the superior penetration of US over other forms of energy whose absorption causes a physiological tissue temperature rise, the transient increase in temperature could be a factor in pain relief. However, the authors have observed that patients suffering from the residual effects of gouty arthritis sustain excellent lasting pain relief and rapidly regain pain-free range of motion of the metatarsophalangeal joint upon one or two exposures to US, using the glycerol immersion technic. The patients were treated after their blood uric acid levels had returned to normal. The reasons for the apparent superiority of US in aiding return of damaged joints to normal function are not known. X-rays taken before and after treatment might provide part of the answer. Depth of penetration should not be a factor in treatment of such superficial joints.

Neuromas

Exposure of posttraumatic neuromas to ultrasound seems highly effective in relieving the pain. Such neuromas may be seen in patients who have had an amputation.[2, 29] It is usually not difficult to pinpoint the location of neuroma, so the stationary technic can be used with good results. The pain relief could be due to a deep TTR or to relaxation or dissolution of the excessively proliferated connective tissue. Since most neuromas cause more pain when subjected to externally applied pressure, as occurs when a prosthesis is worn, it would seem more likely that absorption of ultrasonic energy has caused a permanent relaxation or dissolution of the neuroma rather than just intermittently warming it up.

Adhesive Scars

Adhesive scars resulting from natural repair of lacerated tissues or from surgical intervention also show excess connective tissue proliferation. The range-limiting effects of adhesion formation are effectively and permanently relieved by exposure to ultrasonic energy.[28, 30] Exposure to US is also an effective means of increasing range of motion where limitation is due to massive hypertrophic scar tissue formation, as in the residual phase of a burn that has destroyed the dermis. Distinction must be made between the hypertrophic scar and the true keloid.[30, 35, 37] The histologic distinction is that, in the hypertrophic scar, the proliferation comes entirely from the epidermal margin. In the keloid, the collagen proliferation is predominantly dermal rather than epidermal in origin, and there is massive hyalinization. Ultrasound does not seem effective in releasing tissues bound by a true keloid scar.[35] The reasons for this difference are not known.

Plantar Warts

There is sharply divided clinical opinion as to the benefit of treating plantar warts with ultrasonic energy. Some have reported excellent results.[59, 60] Others have indicated that ultrasound is of no benefit.[61] There has been wide variation in treatment parameters. There has also been debate as to what are the proper criteria for arrival at the clinical diagnosis of a plantar wart as compared to other causes of indurated skin. The most careful diagnosticians require demonstration of the virus verruca plantaris.

Laboratory investigation of deactivation of viruses by exposure to ultrasound indicate that far higher intensities are required for such deactivation *in vitro* than are feasible clinically.[38] Study of verruca plantaris was not included in that report. If exposure to ultrasonic energy were going to remove the wart, it would seem necessary that absorption of the energy lead to the dissolution of the connective tissue binding between the normal and abnormal tissue or that the wart itself be softened. Detailed pathology reports of removed tissue have yet to be published. When treatment has been reported as successful, both direct contact and immersion technics have been used. Direct contact with exposure at about fifteen minutes per treatment and for a series of ten to fifteen treatments seems most likely to obtain removal of the wart. There have been no reports of harm to adjacent normal tissue with the use of ultrasound; the treatment is less painful than when chemical technics are used, and the patient does not suffer through a postsurgical severe pain period. Hence, at this point, it would seem that ultrasound should be given a reasonable trial before more drastic methods are used.

Pressure Sores

Exposure of pressure sores to ultrasonic energy appears to significantly increase the rate of healing.[62] At each treatment, the cavity is filled with mineral oil. The sound head is then energized in the liquid. Obviously, eschar and other debris would be removed prior to each treatment, and there should be no evidence that a sinus runs from the wound to deeper tissue. If the wound is pale in color prior to treatment, a visible hyperemia is likely to appear within a five-minute treatment, and a better local blood supply will be maintained until external pressure again diminishes local blood flow. Sonation of adjacent intact tissues immediately before sonation of the ulcer itself would probably enhance duration of the improved circulation. To the authors' knowledge, no comparative study has been reported using infrared energy in any form as compared to ultrasonic energy for transient improvement of local circulation. Certainly infrared in the form of radiant energy, as well as hydrotherapy, had been used for this purpose long before US was available. Infrared is not often regarded as effective in helping to maintain the blood supply to a pressure sore area.

Chronic Systemic Peripheral Arterial Diseases

In the early and moderately far advanced stages of arteriosclerosis and atherosclerosis, arterial vessels react to the salt and lipid deposition with persistent vasospasm in varying degree. Vasospasm can be transiently relieved by local exposure of the affected vessels to ultrasonic energy and by paravertebral sonation of the sympathetic nervous system. It is not known at this time whether the local sonation has any effect on the rate of deposition or dissolution of the material that is decreasing lumen diameter. It would seem reasonable as part of the overall management of such chronic arterial insufficiency problems to try three or four treatments, using paravertebral sonation to the lumbar and sacral areas, followed immediately by local sonation as indicated. Skin temperature testing, before and after treatment, and/or oscillometric index testing, would indicate whether that particular patient obtains enough transient reduction in vasospasm to make continued treatment worthwhile. If posttreatment temperatures show a rise on the order of 2° to 5°C at the toetips, and a lesser rise more proximally, lasting for an hour or more, ultrasonic therapy would seem beneficial for that particular patient. Lota has shown that in normal individuals, paravertebral sonation will increase distal remote skin temperature by 1° to 2°C.[22] This rise in skin temperature is assumed to be due to the effect of ultrasonic energy on the sympathetic nervous system, leading to a transient reduction in vasomotor tension. Local sonation would be contraindicated when there is clinical evidence of thrombophlebitis or phlebothrombosis because of the possibility of fragmenting an attached thrombus, thus converting it into an embolus, with the risk of causing a life-threatening intrathoracic infarct.

The Organized Hematoma

Anytime soft tissue is subject to trauma, small blood vessels are likely to be crushed and/or ruptured. Edema always occurs as a result of the marked increase in interstitial fluid. The outpouring of blood from the circulatory tree lasts only a few seconds if the injury is minor. It can last much longer, and can be fatal, in major trauma. In the case of small arteries, not more than a millimeter or two in outside diameter, instantaneous vasoconstriction takes place. This reduces the blood flow to the area, and escaping platelets start to adhere to the rupture margins. The damaged mural cells release chemicals, which, in conjunction with platelet activity, rapidly leads to clot formation in three major stages.[63] For the purposes of this volume, the important point is that ionizable calcium must be present in the extracellular fluid for each of the stages to take place. The reaction of serum and/or interstitial fluid calcium with the proteins released by the injured cells leads to the formation of a hard lump. The complete process leading to this lump formation may take several days to a week, depending upon extent of injury and whether the patient's clotting mechanisms are functioning normally. After natural or surgical repair of the leak(s) in the vascular tree, further intrinsic chemical activity dissolves the indurated mass.

If the clot is large, occupying many cubic centimeters, natural dissolution may take weeks to months for complete resorption. If a slowly dissolving clot is pressing upon nerve, muscle, or periosteum, it can be quite painful, restricting muscle contraction and/or joint motion. When this occurs, exposure of the clot to ultrasonic energy is one way to speed resorption. If the clot is deep, this is the treatment of choice because of the penetrating power of ultrasound. The US-induced TTR causes local vasodilation and transiently increases cell permeability. There is no hard evidence to date that US also decreases the binding of calcium ions to fibrin or other proteins that are essential to clot formation. However, it has been established that when whole blood is exposed to US *in vitro,* clotting time is significantly increased.[38] This is not known to happen with any form of electromagnetic energy in use by physical therapists.

It follows that once there is clinical evidence that continuing vascular leakage has stopped, exposure of the injury site to ultrasonic energy is an effective way of minimizing the pain and other problems that can result from a large and fully organized hematoma. In the situation where there is evidence of a mural thrombosis in venous circulation, there is a very real hazard that exposure to US could fragment the thrombosis and lead to an intrathoracic infarct. If there is any possibility of a venous thrombus in the area to be treated, the intensity of the ultrasound should be exceptionally low in order to minimize the possibility of embolus formation. To the best of the authors' knowledge, no report has appeared indicating that conversion of a thrombus into an embolus was due to exposure to ultrasound.

Contraindications

There are very few contraindications for the use of ultrasonic energy. It should be contraindicated whenever a TTR would hinder return to normal function.It should probably not be used in the thoracic area if the patient is using a cardiac pacemaker of any kind. Absorption of ultrasonic energy by the pacemaker or by adjacent tissues could lead to error in pacemaker response to instant cardiac status. Since US energy absorption is far more localized than is the case for most other forms of energy that physical therapists use, there is no reason why it cannot be used on other body areas in the presence of a pacemaker. This is not true for the application of nerve and muscle stimulating currents (Chapter 3) or the diathermies (Chapter 4).

The use of ultrasonic energy is contraindicated in an area of the body where a malignancy is known to be present. This is because of the established ability of ultrasonic energy to increase local arterial blood supply, which would tend to increase the rate of growth of the neoplasm. If the malignancy has reached the stage where it is untreatable by surgery or medication, and the patient is not obtaining satisfactory pain relief from narcotics, exposure of the local area to US is occasionally helpful in giving transient pain relief. This is probably due to transient relaxation of muscle spasm, where the cause of the muscle irritation is pressure from an expanding lesion.

Ultrasonic energy should not be used on a regular basis over or near growth centers of bone until bone growth is essentially complete. Absorption of this form of energy by cells making up the growth center tends to disrupt normal growth. Damage to growth centers has been clearly demonstrated in experimental animals when the exposure has been a long series at clinical intensities or a short series at high intensities.[64] However, since a big factor in selection of ultrasound for pain relief is its superior depth of penetration, it is rarely needed in treatment of children. If the ultrasonic energy is being used to promote lasting extensibility of tendon, the series of treatments would be small; hence the risk of damage to a child's epiphyseal centers would be small, but it could happen.

It should follow that a healing fracture should not be exposed to US, since this might delay or prevent completion of callus formation. When the radiologist is satisfied that bone repair is complete, and there is need of exposure to US for pain relief, then there should be no harm in such treatment.

SUMMARY

Physical and physiological differences between electromagnetic and acoustic energy absorption are discussed. Critical factors in equipment choice are given in broad outline. Factors that need to be considered in application of ultrasonic energy to patients are presented. Physiological effects that are known to occur at clinical intensities and with clinical frequencies are documented. On the basis of these known effects, indications and contraindications for the use of ultrasonic energy are given.

Much of the value of ultrasonic energy in providing pain relief is due to its superior depth of penetration and to its ability to induce permanent relaxation of connective tissues, especially when there has been excess proliferation of such tissue as a result of trauma or where a neurological deficit has lead to muscle or tendon shortening.

REFERENCES

1. Goldman, D. E., and Heuter, T. F.: Tabular data on velocity and absorption of high frequency sound in mammalian tissues. *J Acoust Soc Am., 28*:35-37, 1956.
2. Brunner, G. D. et al.: Can ultrasound be used in the presence of surgical metal implants? *Phys Ther, 38*:823-24, 1958.
3. Gersten, J. W.: Effect of metallic objects on temperature rises produced by ultrasound. *Am J Phys Med, 37*:75-82, 1958.
4. Gersten, J. W.: Thermal and non-thermal changes in isometric tension, contractile protein, and injury potential produced in frog muscle by ultrasonic energy. *Arch Phys Med Rehabil, 34*:675, 1953.
5. Gersten, J. W.: Non-thermal effects of ultrasound. *Am J Phys Med, 37*:235, 1958.
6. Madsen, P. W., and Gersten, J. W.: The effect of ultrasound on peripheral nerve. *Arch Phys Med Rehabil, 42*:645, 1961.

7. Licht, S. (Ed.): *Therapeutic Heat and Cold,* 2nd ed. New Haven, Licht, 1965, Chapter 3.

8. Schwann, H. P.: Personal communication, 1969.

9. Lehmann, J. F., and Guy, A. W.: *Ultrasonic Therapy.* In Reid, J. M. and Sikov, M. R. (Eds.): *Proc Workshop on Interaction of Ultrasound and Biological Tissues.* Washington, D.C., HEW (FDA 73:8008), Sept. 1972, pp. 141-152.

10. Griffin, J. E. et al.: Ultrasonic movement of cortisol into pig tissues. II. Peripheral nerve. *Am J Phys Med, 41:*20, 1965.

11. Stewart, H. F. et al.: Survey of use and performance of ultrasonic equipment in Pinellas County, Florida. *Phys Ther, 54:*707, 1974.

12. Summer, W., and Patrick, M.: *Ultrasonic Therapy.* New York, Elsevier, 1964.

13. Griffin, J. E., and Touchstone, J. C.: Effects of ultrasonic frequency on phonophoresis of cortisol into swine tissues. *Am J Phys Med, 51:*62, 1972.

14. *Ultrasonic Therapy Products: Radiation Safety Performance Standard.* Washington, D.C., *Federal Register, 43(34):*7166-72, February 17, 1978.

15. Rosenberger, H.: Über den Wirkungsmechanismus der ultraschall Behandlung ins besondere Ischias und Neuralgien. *Chirurg, 21:*404, 1950.

16. Touchstone, J. C. et al.: Cortisol in human nerve. *Science, 142:*1275, 1963.

17. Farmer, W. C.: Effect of intensity of ultrasound on conduction velocity of motor axons. *Phys Ther, 48:*1233, 1968.

18. Currier, D. P. et al.: Sensory nerve conduction: Effect of ultrasound. *Arch Phys Med Rehabil, 59:*181-185, 1978.

19. Piersol, G. M. et al.: Mechanism of absorption of ultrasonic energy in blood. *Arch Phys Med Rehabil, 33:*327, 1952.

20. Lota, M. J., and Darling, R. C.: Changes in permeability of the red blood cell membrane in an homogenous ultrasonic field. *Arch Phys Med Rehabil, 36:*282, 1955.

21. Schwann, H. P.: Absorption of ultrasound by tissues and biological matter. *Proc IRE, 47:*1959, 1959.

22. Lota, M. J.: Electronic plethysmographic and tissue temperature studies of the effects of ultrasound on blood flow. *Arch Phys Med Rehabil, 46:*315, 1965.

23. Lehmann, J. F. et al.: Temperature distributions upon exposure to ultrasonic energy. *Arch Phys Med Rehabil, 48:*662, 1967.

24. Lehmann, J. F. et al.: Comparative study of the efficiency of shortwave, microwave, and ultrasonic diathermy in heating the hip joint. *Arch Phys Med Rehabil, 40:*510, 1959.

25. Lehmann, J. F. et al: Heating of joint structures by ultrasonic energy. *Arch Phys Med Rehabil, 49:*28, 1968.

26. Abramson, D. E. et al.: Oxygen uptake and tissue temperatures produced by therapeutic physical agents. II. Effects of shortwave diathermy. *Am J Phys Med, 39:*87, 1960.

27. Abramson, D. I. et al.: Oxygen uptake and tissue temperatures produced by therapeutic physical agents. I. Effects of ultrasound. *Am J Phys Med, 39:*51, 1960.

28. Rubin, D. and Kuitert, J.: Use of ultrasound vibration energy in treatment of pain arising from phantom limbs, scars, and neuromas. *Arch Phys Med Rehabil, 36:*445, 1955.

29. Rubin, D. et al.: Application of ultrasound to experimentally induced neuromas in dogs. *Arch Phys Med Rehabil, 38:*377, 1957.

30. Bierman, W.: Ultrasound in the treatment of scars. *Arch Phys Med Rehabil, 34:*209, 1954.

31. Joseph, J.: Healing with ultrasound. *Medical Chronicle, 18:* May, 1970.

32. Dyson, M., and Suckling, J.: Stimulation of tissue repair by ultrasound: A survey of mechanisms involved. *Physiotherapy, 64:*105-8, 1978.

33. Webster, D. F. et al.: The role of ultrasound induced cavitation in the "in vitro" stimulation of collagen synthesis in human fibroblasts. *Ultrasonics, 18(1):*33-37, 1980.

34. Asboe-Hansen, G.: Regeneration and repair of connective tissue. In Valette, D. G. (Ed.): *La Cicatrization.* Paris, Editions du Centre Nationale de la Recherche Scientifique #145, 1965. (In English).

35. Wright, E. T., and Haase, K. H.: Treatment of keloids with ultrasound. *Arch Phys Med Rehabil, 52:*280, 1971.

36. Lewis, J. R.: *The Surgery of Scars.* New York, McGraw, 1963.

37. Inalsingh, C. H.: An experience in treating five hundred and one patients with keloids. *Johns Hopkins Med J, 134:*284, 1974.

38. El'Piner, I. E.: *Ultrasound: Its Physical, Chemical, and Biological Effects.* New York, Consultants Bureau, 1964, pp. 154-56.

39. Lehmann, J. F. et al.: Effects of therapeutic temperatures on tendon extensibility. *Arch Phys Med Rehabil, 51:*481, 1970.

40. Brust, M. et al.: Some effects of ultrasonic energy and temperature on the contraction of isolated mammalian skeletal muscle. *Arch Phys Med Rehabil, 50:*677, 1969.

41. Bearzy, H.: Clinical application of ultrasonic energy in treatment of acute and chronic sub-acromial bursitis, *Arch Phys Med Rehabil, 34:*228, 1953.

42. Echternach, J.: Ultrasound: An adjunct treatment for shoulder disabilities. *Phys Ther, 45:*865, 1965.

43. Lehmann, J. F. et al.: Comparison of ultrasonic and microwave diathermy in the physical treatment of periarthritis of the shoulder. *Arch Phys Med Rehabil, 35:*627, 1954.

44. Goodman, C.: Ultrasonic therapy for chronic acromio-clavicular separation with calcific deposits. *NY State J Med, 72:*2884, 1972.

45. Miller, L. E. et al.: Sequential use of hot packs and ultrasound. *Phys Ther, 59:*559-60, 1979. (Abstract of unpublished B.S. thesis presented at the 1979 APTA Conference).

46. Reid, D. C., and Cummings, G. E.: Efficiency of ultrasound coupling agents. *Physiotherapy, 63:*255-57, 1977.

47. Warren, C. G. et al.: Ultrasound coupling media: their relative transmissivity. *Arch Phys Med Rehabil, 57:*218-22, 1976.
48. Griffin, J. E.: Transmissiveness of ultrasound through tap water, glycerin, and mineral oil. *Phys Ther, 60:*1010-1016, 1980.
49. Griffin, J. E., and Touchstone, J. C.: Low intensity phonophoresis of cortisol in swine. *Phys Ther, 48:*1336-44, 1968.
50. Kleinkort, J. A., and Wood, F.: Phonophoresis with one percent versus ten percent hydrocortisone. *Phys Ther, 55:*1320-26, 1975.
51. Nowak, E. J.: Experimental transmission of lidocaine through intact skin by ultrasound. *Arch Phys Med Rehabil, 45:*231, 1964.
52. Aldes, J. H., and Jadeson, W. J.: Ultrasonic therapy in treatment of hypertrophic arthritis in elderly patients. *Ann West Med Surg, 6:*545, 1952.
53. Fellinger, K., and Schmid, J.: *Klinik und Therapie des Chronischen Gelenrheumatismus.* Vienna, 1954, p. 549.
54. Abramowitch, D., and Neousskine, B.: *Treatment by Ion Transfer.* New York, Grune, 1946.
55. Murray, W. et al.: The Iontophoresis of C_{21} esterified glucocorticoids: Preliminary report. *Phys Ther, 43:*579, 1963.
56. Griffin, J. E. et al.: Patients treated with ultrasonic driven hydrocortisone and with ultrasound alone. *Phys Ther, 47:*595, 1967.
57. Tschannen, F.: Effects of ultrasonic therapy on rheumatic diseases and circulatory disorders. *Br J Phys Med, 15:*7, 1952.
58. Aldes, J. H.: Ultrasound in arthritis. *J Arkansas Med Soc, 54:*39, 1957.
59. Cherup, N. et al.: Treatment of plantar warts with ultrasound. *Arch Phys Med Rehabil, 44:*602, 1963.
60. Vaughn, D. T.: Direct method versus underwater method in treatment of plantar warts with ultrasound. *Phys Ther, 53:*396, 1973.
61. Braatz, J. H. et al.: Ultrasound and plantar warts: A double blind study. *Milit Med, 139:*199, 1974.
62. Paul, B. J. et al.: Use of ultrasound in the treatment of pressure sores in patients with spinal cord injury. *Arch Phys Med Rehabil, 41:*38, 1960.
63. Sodeman, W. A., and Sodeman, W. A., Jr.: *Pathologic Physiology,* 5th ed. Philadelphia, Saunders, 1974.
64. DeForest, R. E. et al.: Effects of ultrasound on growing bone: Experimental study. *Arch Phys Med Rehabil, 34:*21, 1953.
65. Griffin, J. E. et al.: Results of frequency differences in ultrasonic therapy. *Phys Ther, 50:*481-86, 1970.
66. Wanet, G., and Dehon, N.: Clinical study of ultrasonophoresis with a topical application of phenylbutazon and *Alphakadol. J Belge Rhum Med Phys, 31(2):*1976. (In French)
67. Burgudzhieva, T., and Chuchkov, Kh.: The influence of treatment with ultrasound or with phonophoresis by hydrocortisone ointment on uncapsulated skin receptors in the presence of chronic vulvar dystrophies (according to electron microscopic data). *Vopr Kurotol Fizioter Lech Fizi Kult, 4:*75-78 (July-Aug), 1978. (In Russian)

Chapter 8

PRINCIPLES OF INSTRUMENTATION

INTRODUCTION

BASIC ELECTRICITY AND ELECTRONICS

THE PROJECTED TOTAL MARKET for medical electronic equipment in 1974 was 673.9 million dollars, as compared to 524.6 million dollars in 1972. In the same two-year span of time, the market for just diathermy and ultrasonic therapeutic equipment went from 12.4 to 14.9 million. If these figures are any indication, today's physical therapists can expect to find themselves confronted with an increasing amount of therapeutic instrumentation in the near future. Not only will the number of devices increase but also the sophistication and complexity of those devices. In order to competently use such equipment, the therapist must have an understanding of the fundamental physical principles employed in its design.

It is the purpose of this section to provide the physical therapist with a working knowledge of electricity, electronics, and the basic theory of instrumentation as employed in physical therapy.

It is assumed that the reader has a background in physics and algebra. However, the material is presented in a descriptive manner in order to accommodate the widest reader population, including those therapists whose physics and math are a "few" years behind them.

Fundamental Circuit Theory

The basis upon which all electrical and electronic instrumentation is founded rests on three fundamental quantities and six types of electrical components. The conclusion to be drawn from this all-encompassing statement is that with a good grasp of these nine items, the reader should be able to understand any electrical or electronic device and how it functions, once given the appropriate instrument data.

The three fundamental quantities mentioned above are as follows:

1. Voltage
2. Current
3. Resistance

These quantities are related by the following equation, commonly referred to as Ohm's Law:

$$i = \frac{v}{r}$$

Simplified definitions of the above quantities will suffice to give the reader a working knowledge of electrical activity; therefore, no rigorous analysis will be attempted.

Voltage, Current, and Resistance

VOLTAGE. Voltage is defined as the difference in electron population between two points. This electrical "difference of potential" can be used to cause the orderly, directed movement of electrons through a conductor; hence, it is also termed *electromotive force* (e.m.f.).

CURRENT. Electrical current can be defined as the *directed* flow or movement of electrons through a conducting medium, as opposed to the *random* drift of electrons.

RESISTANCE. Resistance is a characteristic inherent in any substance. It is related to the number of "free" electrons in a substance and hence to the ease or difficulty with which a current can be passed through the substance. The greater the number of free electrons in a substance, i.e. metals, the easier it will pass a current; hence, its resistance is termed *low*. Materials with few free electrons, i.e. glass, mica, have correspondingly higher resistances.

A useful analogy often used to facilitate an understanding of electrical circuits is the "fluid system analogy"; however, the reader is warned not to be caught holding too firmly to the analogy, as it can become confusing.

Simply stated, the fluid system analogy compares voltage to pressure, current to fluid flow, and resistance to pipe diameter. Hence, where

$$\text{current} = \frac{\text{voltage}}{\text{resistance}}$$

this is equivalent to

$$\text{fluid flow} = \frac{\text{pressure}}{\text{pipe diameter}}$$

It is obvious that where an increase in pressure will cause more fluid to flow, also an increase in voltage will cause a greater current to flow. In turn, a decrease in pipe size will decrease the fluid flow at a given pressure, while an increase in resistance will decrease current flow.

This simple law holds true in all metallic conducting systems and electronic devices, and no matter how complex an electronic circuit is, it can, with the appropriate calculations, be simplified down to the fundamental relationship between voltage, current, and resistance given in Ohm's Law.

Components

As noted in the previous section, all electronic instrumentation is made up of various combinations of six types of electronic components:

1. Resistors
2. Capacitors (condensers)
3. Inductors (coils)
4. Vacuum tubes
5. Semiconductors
6. Integrated circuits (I.C.s)

These components may differ in size and appearance from each other; in fact, in some instances, there may be no resemblance whatever between two components of the same type. Nevertheless, each *type* of component can be described by way of a brief operational description as given below. A more detailed operational description is included in a later section.

RESISTORS. A resistor is a device used generally in one of three ways: (1) to limit current, (2) to provide current-to-voltage transformation, (3) to produce voltage division. Resistors may be fixed or variable; they may be made of carbon, wire, or metallic film. The specific form of a resistor is dictated by its application.

CAPACITORS (condensers). A capacitor is a device that (1) stores energy in an *electric field* and (2) tends to oppose *voltage* changes. Capacitors may be small or large, fixed or variable, with solid dielectric interiors, mica or even air filled. They are used most often to decrease or dampen power supply voltage variations as well as to filter out unwanted signals.

Capacitors are also found as the air spaced plate electrodes in the diathermies. The patient is the dielectric.

INDUCTORS (coils). An inductor is a device that (1) stores energy in an *electromagnetic field* and (2) tends to oppose changes in *current*. (The reader should note the general similarity to the action of a capacitor but also should beware not to confuse the two.) Inductors also play a role in controlling power supply output variations and in selective filters. In addition, specialized applications of the principles of electromagnetic induction are found in transformers, galvanometers, motors, meters, and generators not to mention diathermy applicator coils.

VACUUM TUBES. Vacuum tubes are principally monodirectional current devices; that is, they allow current to flow in only one direction. Depending upon the number of electrodes they have, they are used (1) to *rectify* alternating current into direct current and also (2) to *amplify* small signal voltages into larger ones.

SEMICONDUCTORS. This general class of components includes the ubiquitous "transistor." Semiconductors are all miniature solid-state crystalline devices having the same general capabilities as vacuum tubes and providing the additional advantages of smaller size, longer life, and less power consumption.

INTEGRATED CIRCUITS. These microminiature devices are today's state of the art in electronic technology. Where a single conventional semiconductor discrete component (for example, a transistor) is roughly the size of the head of a pin, an integrated circuit "chip" the same size may contain 200 transistors and numerous resistors — truly the ultimate in miniaturization. All electronic functions that are adaptable to vacuum tubes and transistors can be accomplished using I.C.s, with the additional ability of housing complete circuits, i.e. voltage regulators, multivibrators, etc., in a single I.C.

Current Sources

The majority of medical electronic instruments in use today contain circuitry that requires direct current voltages to operate. To obtain D.C. voltages, one has two choices: (1) to use battery supplies or (2) to use a power supply that converts wall power (117 VAC, 60 Hz) to the required D.C. values. The former method is used primarily in portable devices, while the latter method is the form of power source found in most instrumentation.

CELLS AND BATTERIES. The word *battery* is often used incorrectly by the layman to refer to a cell, as in the "battery" used in a flashlight (really a "dry cell"). Hence, a battery is a combination of two or more cells. In all cases, the terminal voltage produced by a cell or battery is generated by chemical means and thus can eventually be depleted.

Batteries are of two types, based on whether or not their cells can be recharged. A *primary cell battery* is nonrechargeable; a *secondary cell battery* is rechargeable. The common everyday flashlight cell is a primary cell; the automobile battery is an example of a secondary cell battery.

The three most common types of primary cells are (1) zinc-carbon cell (Leclanche cell), (2) zinc-mercuric oxide cell (mercury cell), (3) zinc-manganese dioxide cell (alkaline cell). These cells are predominantly of the low voltage variety, ranging from the 1.5 volt flashlight cell to the 9 volt transistor radio battery. A recent introduction into the primary cell market is the *lithium cell*. This type of cell generates as much as thirty times the energy per unit volume as a more conventional cell — 15 watt-hours as opposed to 0.5 watt-hours for a zinc-carbon cell. The cost of a lithium cell is also proportionally larger ($11.48 for a D cell).

POWER SUPPLIES. Most commercial electronic devices, in order to operate, are plugged into wall receptacles that deliver 117

VAC, 60 Hz. Consequently, there must be some circuit within the instrument that changes that AC into DC; such a circuit is called a power supply. Power supplies will be covered in more detail in a later section; however, a brief summary will be given here.

The essential components of a power supply are as follows (from AC in to DC out):

1. A *transformer* — to step up or down the input voltage and to provide one or more secondary voltages.
2. A *rectifier* — to convert the high voltage AC into a pulsating DC.
3. A *filter network* — to remove the "pulsations" from the DC leaving "pure" DC.

Additional items that may or may not be included in a power supply are (1) *voltage dividers* to provide multiple DC voltages from a single high DC voltage and (2) *voltage regulators* to provide a constant voltage supply even though the current demands change. The complexity of a power supply is dependent upon its application. The requirement for a perfectly steady DC output over a wide current range will necessitate more complexity than a low voltage, low current, unregulated DC output.

DC Series and Parallel Circuits

An electrical circuit simplified down to its constituent parts is made up of (1) a power source, (2) a closed (or complete) conduction path, and (3) some form of driven element (or load) which constitutes the circuit resistance (or resistances). The manner in which the loads are connected to the power source requires an understanding of series and parallel circuits.

Figure 8-1 shows a simple series circuit. In such a circuit, total current (I_t) flows through each component so that its measurement at any point in the circuit will yield the same value. ($I_t = I_1 = I_2 = I_3$, etc.) In turn, the total resistance (R_t) that must be overcome by the current is seen as the sum of the individual resistances. ($R_t = R_1 + R_2 + R_3$, etc.) The total applied voltage of the power source (V_t) is "dropped" proportionally by the resistances in the circuit such that the sum of their voltage drops equals the applied voltage. ($V_t = V_{R1} + V_{R2} + V_{R3}$, etc.)

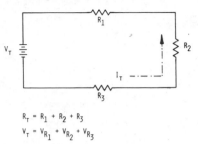

$$R_T = R_1 + R_2 + R_3$$
$$V_T = V_{R_1} + V_{R_2} + V_{R_3}$$

Figure 8-1. A simple series circuit.

The difference in potential (voltage) measured at the terminals of a load or resistance represents the energy lost (or voltage "drop") necessary to sustain a current through the resistance. Such lost energy is designated "power dissipation" and most often is given off as heat. Power is measured in watts, and the amount of power dissipated by a given load is found by the following formulae:

$$P = I^2R \quad P = IV \quad P = V^2/R$$

It is important to note that in all circuits there is only one path for current to get from one terminal of the power supply to the other.

When two or more paths exist for current to pass between two points, A and B, in an electrical circuit, it is a parallel circuit. As shown in Figure 8-2, two paths (R_1 and R_2) allow current to flow between points A and B, each path represented by a resistive element. From Ohm's Law it is known that the current through a given resistance is dictated by the quotient of voltage over resistance, and from this one can conclude that when a second resistance is placed in parallel with the existing resistance, circuit current increases as each resistance feels the same voltage at its terminals. This points out the sometimes confusing (to the layman) fact that when resistances are added to a parallel circuit, the *effective* total resistance decreases. Looking at the example from another point of view, suppose R_1 was the only resistance (and hence conduction path) between A and B. Any addition of a parallel conduction path, no matter how high its resistance, can only increase the ability of current to get from A to B. This effect can be observed in the home when too many electrical appliances have been plugged into a single outlet by use of a three-way plug, and a fuse has blown. Ohm's Law shows why. Resistances in parallel equals decreased effective R. Therefore,

$$I = \frac{V}{R}$$

decreasing R means an increasing I. When calculating effective resistance, the following formula is used:

$$R_{eff} = \frac{1}{1/R_1 + 1/R_2 + 1/R_3, \text{etc.}}$$

As a general rule of thumb, it should be remembered that the *effective resistace* of parallel resistors *is equal to or less than the smallest resistance.*

From the previous example, one can also conclude that total current (I_t) in a parallel circuit is found by adding the currents in the individual legs. ($I_t = 1R_1 + 1R_2, + 1/R_3$, etc.) In addition, since the potential felt at the terminals of parallel connected resistances is the same, then $V_t = V_{R1} = V_{R2} = V_{R3}$, etc.

Comparing and at the same time summarizing series and parallel circuits, the following may be observed:

In a *series* circuit,
—current is the same at all points
—voltage is the sum of the individual voltages
—additional resistances in series increases total resistance

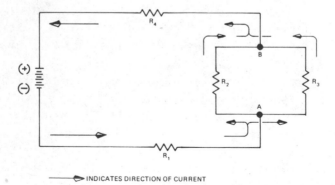

INDICATES DIRECTION OF CURRENT

Figure 8-2. A series-parallel circuit. From Terence Karselis, *Descriptive Medical Electronics and Instrumentation*, 1973. Courtesy of Charles B. Slack, Inc., Thorofare, New Jersey.

While in a *parallel* circuit,
   —voltage is the same across all legs
   —current is the sum of the individual leg currents
   —additional resistances in parallel decreases effective total
      resistance

Electromagnetism and AC Generation

Although the predominant form of voltage used to drive
instrument circuits is DC, the method of choice of transmitting
electrical energy is by way of alternating current (AC) voltage.
All electrical power generated in the United States is commonly
produced by a hydroelectric generating plant delivering 6600
volts at 60 cycles per second (referred to as 60 Hertz). This
voltage is stepped up by way of a transformer to 66,000 volts
before being applied to the high power transmission lines one
sees crisscrossing the countryside.

At distribution substations, the voltage is stepped down again
(via transformers) to 2200 volts (commercial power) and finally
stepped down again on the utility poles in individual neighbor-
hoods to 240 volts, two phase (two phases of 120 VAC each).
Hence, heavy appliances (range and dryer) can be driven by 240
VAC while wall power is 120 VAC, 60 Hz.

A closer look at the basic principle of AC generation will yield
some insight into its cyclic nature. When a current is passed
through a conductor, a magnetic field is generated around the
conductor; a steady current (DC) produces a steady magnetic
field, a fluctuating current and a fluctuating magnetic field. The
process is called *electromagnetism.*

A magnetic field produced in this way can be used to operate
electromagnetic devices such as relays, but it is the same process
acting in the reverse direction that is used to generate electrical
currents. If a conductor is passed perpendicularly through the
flux of a magnetic field, a current will be induced into that
conductor; this process is called *electromagnetic induction.* It
should be noted that the process will occur whether the field *or*
the conductor is the moving element, as long as there is relative
motion between the two. The direction of the conductor's motion determines the direction of the induced current such that a

conductor moving down through a given magnetic field would have an induced current in one direction, while if it were moved up through the same field, the current would flow in the opposite direction. It is this principle that provides the basis for electric *generators, transformers,* and even *tape recorder* heads.

An *electric generator* consists of a series of conductors, wound on a rotating element called an armature and caused, by mechanical effort, to rotate in a circular path through a magnetic field. Since the conductors cross the field in one direction for one half of a rotation and the opposite direction for the second half, the result is induction of an alternating current (Fig. 8-3). At two points in the circular path of the conductor, the motion is parallel to the magnetic flux; hence, no current is induced at these points, i.e. at 0° and 180° there is no voltage. If the conductor makes sixty rotations in a minute, sixty waves or cycles are generated.

A *transformer* (Fig. 8-4) consists of two coils wound on a common metallic core. When an alternating current is passed through one coil (called the primary), the magnetic field generated cuts the second coil (called the secondary), inducing a current into it. By manipulating the number of windings in the secondary, the induced voltage can be stepped up (more coils) or down (less coils). The metallic core is used only to concentrate the magnetic flux.

If a metal such as iron or aluminum is brought into the flux of

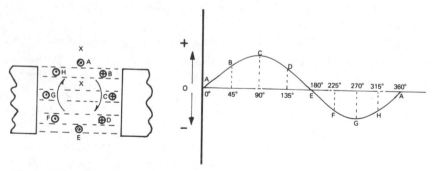

Figure 8-3. Electromagnetic induction. From Terence Karselis, *Descriptive Medical Electronics and Instrumentation,* 1973. Courtesy of Charles B. Slack, Inc., Thorofare, New Jersey.

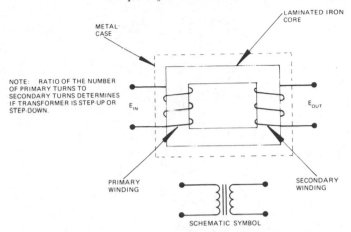

Figure 8-4. A simplified diagram of an iron core transformer. From Terence Karselis, *Descriptive Medical Electronics and Instrumentation*, 1973. Courtesy of Charles B. Slack, Inc., Thorofare, New Jersey.

an electromagnetic field, it will take on the property of a magnet, i.e. it becomes temporarily magnetized. This process, as mentioned earlier, is called *electromagnetism*, and it is the basis upon which such components as relays, solenoids, meters, and motors operate.

A *relay* is actually nothing more than an electromagnetically activated switch. It consists of a coil with a fixed iron core and a movable arm with contacts. When current energizes the coil, the magnetized core attracts the movable arm, closing (or opening) the switch contacts.

A *solenoid* is similar to a relay except its core is movable, providing mechanical action that can open or close valves or engage gears (as the starter solenoid does in an automobile).

One should note that relays and solenoids function employing only *one* magnetic field, that of the energized coil. *Meters* and *motors* on the other hand employ the use of *two* magnetic fields, one stationary or fixed, the other capable of rotation.

A simple *meter* (Fig. 8-5) consists of a permanent magnet with a sensing or detecting coil suspended between the magnetic poles. A pointer is attached to the sensing coil. When a detected current passes through the sensing coil, it takes on the properties of

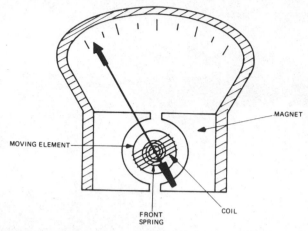

Figure 8-5. A typical meter movement. From Terence Karselis, *Descriptive Medical Electronics and Instrumentation,* 1973. Courtesy of Charles B. Slack, Inc., Thorofare, New Jersey.

a magnet and attempts to align its own field to the permanent field, thereby producing deflection of the pointer. Fine springs are used to return the movement back to its original (zero) position and the whole sensing assembly is mounted in jeweled bearings, providing minimal inertia.

The same "two magnetic field" principle applies also to elec-

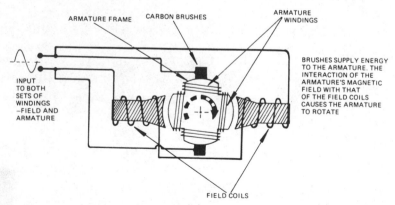

Figure 8-6. Pictorial diagram of a simple motor. From Terence Karselis, *Descriptive Medical Electronics and Instrumentation,* 1973. Courtesy of Charles B. Slack, Inc., Thorofare, New Jersey.

tric motors, with some slight changes. The stationary field is not provided by a permanent magnet but by two electromagnetic field coils. The moving element is called the armature, and it consists of many coils whose terminals (called the commutators) are sequentially energized by current tapped from graphite brushes. As one coil is energized and its magnetic field provides motion, the armature turns, the first commutator segments leave the brushes, and another set comes in contact, thereby generating another magnetic field. This process is repeated, continually providing constant motion of the armature (Fig. 8-6).

Inductance, Capacitance, and Reactance

It was stated previously under the section on components that capacitors and inductors are capable of storing energy in electrostatic and electromagnetic fields, respectively. A slightly more detailed discussion will be helpful in showing *how* these devices function.

When a magnetic field is generated around a coil and then the current that produced the field is interrupted, the field will collapse; but in doing so, the conditions for electromagnetic induction, i.e. a moving magnetic field and a stationary coil, are present. Hence, a current is induced back into the coil. This action is called self induction, and it is property of all inductors. Since the field collapses in the opposite direction (inward) to which it was generated (outward), it is reasonable to expect that the current it induces will also be in the opposite direction to the current that caused its generation. Such is not the case. Self-induced currents are *always in a direction opposite* to the *change* that caused them. (If a current increases, the self-induced current *opposes the increase*. If a current decreases, the self-induced current tends to increase the net current — it *opposes* the decrease.) It should be noted that if the current originally passed through the coil is an alternating current, constantly increasing, decreasing, and changing direction, a continual self-induced current is generated in the coil. This property of an inductor to oppose a change in current is called *inductive reactance*, and it is a frequency-dependent property in that it increases with an increase in the frequency of the applied current. Inductive reactance (X_L; X = reactance, L = inductance) is measured in units of resistance — ohms — and is found by the following formula:

$$X_L = 2\pi FL$$

Where

F = frequency in Hertz
L = inductance inductance in Henries
X_L = inductive reactance in ohms
2π = a constant

The effects of inductive reactance are such that a *phase difference* between voltage and current is produced in inductive circuits. The result is that voltage changes appear to lead (or occur) before current changes.

The inductive components found in electronic devices are used in specific applications based on the exploitation of one of the above three effects. For example, relays and solenoids exploit the magnetic effects, filter inductors and chokes exploit the reactive effect, and oscillators use the phase shift effects.

Between any two charged objects there exists an electrostatic field; this is the basis for the operation of *capacitors*. All capacitors consist of two metallic plates separated by a material called the dielectric. By choosing an appropriate material to place between the charged plates, the amount of electrostatic energy capable of being applied (or stored) can be increased. Increasing the area of the plates will also increase the amount of charge that can be stored. When a voltage is placed across the capacitor's plates, electrons flow into one plate and away from the other plate until such a time as the plates are at the same potential as the applied voltage. The charge is "stored" by way of the applied field distorting the electric field of the atoms in the dielectric. A simple analogy is the energy stored when stretching a rubber band. When stretched and held that way, it represents potential energy; when released, it gives up its energy. In a capacitor, the dielectric atoms are "stretched" when a charge is applied, and if no discharge path is available, it will hold the charge. When the charge is allowed to bleed off, the atoms return to their normal condition. Capacitors can be damaged by too large a charge in much the same way as a rubber band can be broken by over-stretching it. The overall effect of a capacitor's storage activity is a tendency to oppose changes in voltage. This effect leads to a primary application of capacitors as stabilizing devices in power supplies, where they are used to smooth out fluctuations in DC voltages.

The charging and discharging currents of a capacitor are at a maximum as the charging process begins, gradually slowing down to eventual zero as the charging or discharging process is complete (for example, capacitor not charged — charging current maximum, and vice versa). This brings about a phase difference opposite to that found in inductive circuits; current changes appear to lead voltage changes. A simple memory aid for the phase relationships occurring in inductive and capacitive circuits is "ELI the ICE man," where I equals current, E equals voltage (or electromotive force), C equals capacitance and L equals inductance. E before I in inductive circuits, I before E in capacitive circuits.

The capacitor's action in opposing voltage changes gives rise to reactance in a similar manner in which inductive reactance arises from opposition to current changes. Capacitive reactance (X_C) is also measured in ohms and can be found by the following formula:

$$X_C = \frac{1}{2\pi FC}$$

Where

$\quad$ F $\quad$ = $\quad$ frequency in Hertz
$\quad$ C $\quad$ = $\quad$ capacitance in farads
$\quad$ X_C $\quad$ = $\quad$ capacitive reactance in ohms
$\quad$ 2π $\quad$ = $\quad$ a constant

Note that for a given value of capacitance, capacitive reactance is proportional to $1/F$, indicating that it decreases exponentially as frequency increases. As with inductors, the reactive effects of a capacitor are employed in filter circuits. In addition, note that at zero frequency, i.e. DC, X_C is infinite, implying that capacitors can effectively block DC currents to which they exhibit an infinite opposition. This DC blocking effect is employed in filters as well as coupling circuits between amplifiers.

An important application of capacitors is in timing circuits. The time required for a capacitor to charge to 63.2 percent of the applied voltage is called a *time constant* (t) and can be found as follows: t = R × C, where t is in seconds, R is in ohms, C is in farads. For any given capacitor, since the charging process is nonlinear [it follows the equation $V_c = V_a (1 - e^{-t/RC})$], the time required to fully charge or discharge is five time constants. By altering the value of resistance through which the capacitor charges, the time constant is changed; hence, the frequency of the resulting signal is changed. For example, lowering R means a more rapid charge-discharge; therefore, more cycles per second equals higher frequency. This is a common method of making small changes in frequency. Also, if capacitance is changed, the frequency changes (since t = R × C). Switching in different values of capacitance is a method used to obtain large changes in frequency. This technique is used in some muscle stimulators as a method of varying pulse frequency.

Impedance, Selectivity, and Loading

The combined current-opposing effect of resistance, capacitive reactance, and inductive reactance is termed *impedance* (Z) and is most often used in referring to the "AC resistance" of a circuit. The effects of capacitive reactance and inductive reactance are opposite in two ways: (1) inductive reactance (X_L) causes voltage to lead current, while capacitive reactance (X_C) causes current to lead voltage, and (2) as L_L increases in magnitude with an increase in frequency, X_C decreases with a similar change in frequency. Combining both effects into a single circuit means that at some frequency X_L equals X_C, and hence, reactance becomes zero (their effects cancel). This point is called *resonance,* and the frequency is termed the resonant frequency of the circuit. The circuit is then said to be "tuned." The property of circuit resonance is employed in (1) filter circuits, where the resonant frequency signals are allowed to pass but signals at frequencies other than the resonant frequency are attenuated, and (2) oscillator circuits, where at resonance any opposition to current in an oscillator is due to the tuned circuit's residual resistance alone, since X_L and X_C are equal and therefore cancel, and the absence of reactance enables the oscillating elements to charge-discharge and recharge, etc., with little energy loss.

An important item to be considered in discussing tuned RLC circuits is the *selectivity* of the circuit. Selectivity refers to a filter circuit's ability to discriminate between signals that are close in frequency or to an RLC tank circuit's ability to oscillate. The term used to describe selectivity is "Q" (or quality), which is circuit coil reactance divided by coil resistance. This is because the coil is the weak link in any tuned circuit. It should be obvious that the higher the Q of a circuit, the better its selectivity. It also appears that the higher the frequency involved, the better the Q, since ($X_L = 2\pi FL$) inductive reactance is directly proportional to frequency. This is only true, however, up to about 20 MHz; above that, tuned circuits become inefficient (*see* section on microwave oscillators).

Impedance is also an important factor in considering circuit *loading.* When any two circuits are connected together in order to transfer a signal between them, each may draw current from the other; hence, each acts as a "load" for the other. In the case shown in Figure 8-7, all signal sources can be modeled as a voltage generator (V) and a series resistance (R_S; the impedance of the source). In the diagram shown, the objective is to measure accurately the source voltage. When a voltmeter with an internal

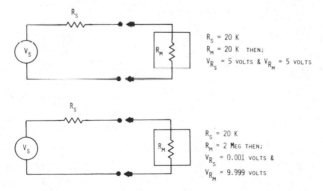

Figure 8-7. An example of circuit loading and the solution

impedance equal to the source impedance (20K or 2×10^4 ohms) is placed across the signal source, R_S and R_L are in series and the source voltage will be dropped across them according to Ohm's Law; hence, the meter will actually measure only 5 volts — an error of 50 percent! If, on the other hand, R_L were 2 megohms (2×10^6 ohms), virtually all the source voltage would be felt across R_L. The conclusion to be drawn from this is that when the circuit objective is signal transfer (voltage transfer), the load impedance must exceed the source impedance by at least 100. On the other hand, if the circuit objective is power transfer (current transfer), source and load impedances should be equal. This concept is employed in some diathermy units where the patient is part of the output circuit and the output circuit must be 'tuned" to obtain maximum efficiency.

Active Devices and Circuits

Basic Circuit Applications

Resistors, capacitors, and inductors are considered to be "passive" devices in that no excitation energy other than the signal voltage is required for them to perform their function. Vacuum tubes, semiconductors, and integrated circuits, on the other hand, are "active" devices in that they require excitation by a DC voltage in addition to the signal voltage.

All electronic instrument circuits, whether vacuum tube or semiconductor, are modifications of one or more of the following four basic circuits:

1. Rectifiers
2. Amplifiers
3. Wave generators
4. Logic circuits

RECTIFIERS. The purpose of rectifiers is to change AC voltages into DC voltages, primarily in power supplies. Rectifiers can be (1) metallic, (2) vacuum tubes, (3) gas filled, or (4) semiconductor in nature.

AMPLIFIERS. Basically, it is the function of an amplifier to take a small signal voltage and enlarge it to a useful magnitude. Amplifiers constitute the largest and most varied group of electronic circuits, and, as a consequence, special purpose amplifiers exist that will not only amplify but in addition will perform special functions such as integration, division, etc. Amplifiers can be of the (1) vacuum tube, (2) semiconductor, or (3) integrated circuit variety.

WAVE GENERATORS. Wave-generating circuits provide a wide variety of waveforms, from simple sine waves to complex, staircase-type square waves. The three most basic types of wave generators are (1) sine wave oscillators, (2) square wave generators, and (3) sawtooth generators. Some wave generators, including all oscillators, require no trigger signal in order to operate; they are termed self excited in that they spontaneously jump into operation as power is applied. Other generators require some form of external excitation pulse to cause their operation. As with amplifiers, wave generators can be of the vacuum tube, semiconductor, or integrated circuit variety. (As of 1974, one manufacturer has marketed a single I.C. chip that will provide sine, square, and sawtooth waveforms simultaneously.)

LOGIC CIRCUITS. Logic circuits constitute an area of electronics all their own — digital electronics. Although wave generators find wide application in digital electronics, the majority of digital circuits are of the "gate" variety, functioning in a go/no-go capacity. A typical example is the two-input *AND gate,* a circuit that will yield an output only when two input signals are present simultaneously. Although semiconductor logic circuits can be built from discrete compounds, today all digital circuitry is of the integrated circuit form.

Vacuum Tube and Semiconductor Theory

The overriding principle upon which all vacuum tubes and most semiconductors function is the principle of *monodirectional current flow* (current flow in one direction). This principle was first applied in the use of diodes as rectifiers.

DIODES. A vacuum tube diode consists of an electron-emitting cathode, an anode, and a filament which heats the cathode to facilitate electron emission. These components are encased in a "tube" of glass or metal from which the air has been removed; hence the name "vacuum tube." Since the cathode is the elec-

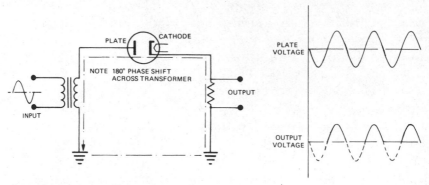

Figure 8-8A. A diode functioning as a half wave rectifier (broken line indicates current path). From Terence Karselis, *Descriptive Electronics and Instrumentation*, 1973. Courtesy of Charles B. Slack, Inc., Thorofare, New Jersey.

tron-emitting element, when a voltage is placed across the tube such that the anode is positive with respect to the cathode, electron current will flow from cathode to anode. If the polarity of the voltage is reversed, no current will flow, since the anode is not an electron emitter. Figure 8-8A shows how a diode is used as a rectifier. In the circuit shown, when an AC signal is applied, during the first half cycle the anode is positive, the tube con-

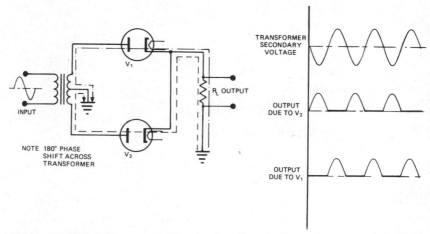

Figure 8-8B. A full wave rectifier (broken lines indicate current paths). From Terence Karselis, *Descriptive Medical Electronics and Instrumentation*, 1973. Courtesy of Charles B. Slack, Inc., Thorofare, New Jersey.

ducts, and the signal is reproduced across R. During the next half cycle the anode is negative with respect to the cathode, no conduction occurs, and no signal voltage is produced across R. The resulting voltage seen across the resistor is called a half wave rectified voltage and the circuit is a half wave rectifier.

Figure 8-8B shows a full wave rectifier. Both the positive and negative swing of the input signal are seen across R as positive-going voltages, since each diode conducts for one alteration — one for the positive half cycle, the other for the negative half cycle.

A semiconductor diode consists of two crystals of germanium or silicon chemically treated (doped) in such a way as to give one an excess of electrons (N-type semiconductor is a negative charge carrier) and the other a deficiency of electrons (P-type semiconductor is a positive charge carrier). The crystals are chemically bonded, and the bonding point is called the junction. When a voltage is placed across a semiconductor diode such that the P- and N-type material are connected to positive and negative potentials respectively (+ to P, − to N), the diode conducts. This is referred to as forward biasing the junction. When the polarity is reversed (+ to N, − to P), the junction is reverse biased and virtually no conduction occurs. Figure 8-9 shows a semiconductor full wave rectifier.

Two additional types of specialized semiconductor diodes are the *Zener diode*, which is used as a voltage regulator or voltage reference source, and the *silicon controlled rectifier* (SCR), a rectifier with three elements (anode, cathode, and gate) that must be triggered by an external excitation voltage at the gate electrode before it will conduct, even though it may be forward biased.

TUBES, TRIODES, AND TRANSISTORS. When a third element is

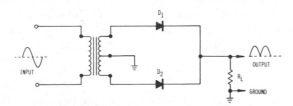

Figure 8-9. A semiconductor full wave rectifier.

placed between the anode and cathode of a diode tube, the result is a triode. The third element is called the control grid, and it is used to control the amount of current flowing from cathode to anode. When the grid potential is made more positive or more negative, the current through the tube will increase or decrease respectively. In this way, a normally high current through the tube can be controlled by a small voltage applied to the grid. It is the application of this process that allows amplification to take place.

The biopolar transistor is the three-element analog of the vacuum tube triode. Transistors are of two types, NPN or PNP. In either case, the device is simply a sandwich of two P- or N-type semiconductor crystals between which a very thin slice of oppositely doped crystal is bonded. As noted previously, P- and N-type semiconductor material refers to where the crystal is an electron charge carrier (N-type for negative) or a proton charge carrier (P-type for positive). The center element of the sandwich is called the *base,* and the other two elements are the *emitter* and *collector.* Comparing the transistor to the vacuum tube, the emitter is analogous to the cathode, the base to the grid, and the collector to the anode. In much the same way that the grid-to-cathode potential controls current through a triode, the base-emitter potential controls transistor current flow. When emitter-base forward bias is increased, transistor current increases. When it is decreased, transistor current decreases. As with triodes, this effect can be utilized in using small signals to control large currents, thereby amplifying the signal.

Figure 8-10 shows the schematic symbols for NPN and PNP transistors. Note that the emitter arrow always points toward the N-type material. When used as amplifiers, the fact that a transistor is PNP or NPN has little effect upon the simplification process. One amplifier is just like the other; the only circuit characteristic altered is the direction of the circuit current.

A second-generation transistor, called a Field Effect Transistor (FET), provides the same amplification capability as a bipolar transistor with the added advantage of exhibiting an extremely high input impedance. This makes it extremely useful in the input stages of amplifying instruments, since it prevents loading

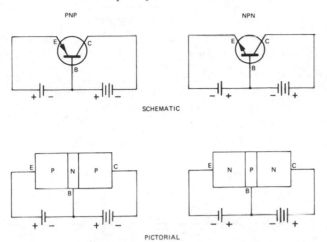

Figure 8-10. PNP and NPN transistor biasing. From Terence Karselis, *Descriptive Medical Electronics and Instrumentation*, 1973. Courtesy of Charles B. Slack, Inc., Thorofare, New Jersey.

of the signal source. These devices find application in pH meters, EKG and EMG devices, and virtually all instruments that are required to amplify very small signals.

Adding a second grid to a triode tube yields a *tetrode*. The second grid is called the screen grid, and its principle action is to reduce interelectrode capacitance between the other tube elements at high frequencies. Tetrodes are the evolutionary dinosaurs of the vacuum tube family; they were just the bridge from triodes to pentodes. *Pentodes* are tubes with three grids: (1) a control grid, (2) a screen grid, and (3) a suppressor grid. Pentodes overcome the frequency and power handling limitations of the triode, yielding greater amplification, a capability to operate at higher frequencies, and the ability to yield greater power outputs.

In the last few years, as industry has attempted to provide smaller and smaller instruments with more reliability, the move has been away from vacuum tube devices to predominantly solid-state instruments. Semiconductor technology has provided the capability with more advanced components such that today virtually any electronic function previously performed by vacuum tubes can be accomplished in a smaller, less power-consuming way with semiconductors. For instance, solid-state rectifiers capable of handling 740 amps are now available; transistors capable of amplifying signals at frequencies as high as 2 gigahertz (2×10^{12} Hertz) are everyday items; a tubeless, flat television screen capable of being hung on a wall like a picture frame is within economically feasible range.

INTEGRATED CIRCUITS. A conventional glass envelope amplifier tube is about the size of a big man's thumb. A transistor capable of the same amplification would be about the size of a small pencil eraser. In both cases, each device consists of a single amplifier stage. On a square crystal chip about the size of the tip

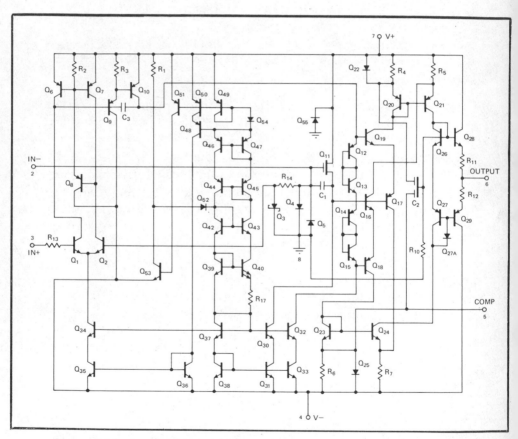

Figure 8-11. A typical integrated circuit-contains fifty-two transistors and diodes.

of a jeweler's screwdriver, an integrated circuit may contain as many as 200 stages of amplification, including all necessary transistors, resistors, and even capacitors! Figure 8-11 shows the equivalent circuit of a linear integrated circuit amplifier containing fifty-two transistors and diodes.

OTHER DISCRETE DEVICES. With vacuum tubes on the way out in electronics, bipolar transistors, FETs and I.C.s make up the bulk of active devices found in instrument circuits. There are, however, other devices that find use in special applications.

It was mentioned in a previous section that an SCR (silicon controlled rectifier) is a three-element device that will conduct in one direction, but only after it has been "gated" or triggered. A *triac* is much like an SCR except it will conduct in *either* direction after it has been triggered. The big problem inherent in both SCRs and triacs is that once triggered, they will not shut off until the anode-cathode voltage across them is virtually zero. This led to the development of the silicon controlled switch (SCS), which is basically an SCR with a second gate terminal added.This device can be turned off by shorting the anode gate to the anode momentarily. It is turned on by conventional gate triggering. SCRs, SCSs, and triacs all find application in areas involving turning on and controlling high current loads, such as motors, power supplies, etc.

Power Supplies and Amplifiers

The material previous to this point dealt with individual components and simple circuits and how they operate. This section will "put it all together" and look at how multiple-stage circuits function in examples of practical application.

The functional stages of a power supply were noted previously to consist essentially of three components: a transformer, a rectifier, and a filter network. Figure 8-12 shows a schematic diagram of a typical instrument power supply. Note that there are more components than previously indicated in the simplified discussion.

The AC input to a power supply is derived from commercial "wall" power, consisting of 115 VAC, 60 Hz. When an instrument is plugged into a wall receptacle and turned on, the 115

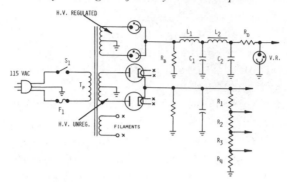

Figure 8-12. A typical power supply schematic.

VAC is fed by way of the line cord into the instrument, through the on-off switch (S_1) and line fuse (F_1) appearing at the primary of the transformer (T_p). The transformer has multiple secondary windings supplying three different circuits: (1) high voltage — regulated, (2) high and low voltage — unregulated, and (3) filaments. Each winding supplies a specified group of circuits.

The high voltage regulated supply is obtained by way of a full wave rectifier employing two gas-filled diodes. The AC voltage appearing at the transformer secondary is rectified by the diodes and appears across R_B, a bleeder resistor. Gas diodes are used in circuits requiring good regulation and high current loads.

The capacitors (C_1 and C_2) and inductive chokes (L_1 and L_2) filter the pulsating DC into a pure DC voltage. The capacitors function as follows: As the supply voltage pulse rapidly reaches its peak value, the capacitors charge up to that value. As the voltage rapidly drops off, the capacitors are unable to discharge rapidly due to R_B; hence, the voltage tends to remain high — the capacitors are "opposing a change in voltage." In a like manner, the inductive chokes "oppose current changes" that tend to appear due to the supply pulsations. The result is a relatively pure DC output voltage appearing across the voltage regulator tube (V_R) and its dropping resistor (R_D).

The voltage regulator, a gas-filled cold cathode diode, operates with the gas in the ionized state. In this way, a constant voltage is felt across the tube, even though current through the tube may vary because of the demands of the load. This is accomplished due to the fact that ionization requires that a specific potential be maintained (the V_R potential). Current changes, on the other hand, are absorbed by the degree of ionization. An increase in load current means a decrease in regulator current; hence, a lesser degree of gas atoms are ionized.

The high voltage unregulated section of the power supply utilizes indirectly heated high vacuum diodes and employs only RC filtering with no voltage regulation; however, an additional circuit is made up by resistors R_1, R_2, R_3, and R_4. This is a voltage divider used to provide more than one voltage from a single HVDC source. Since they are hooked in series, the full DC output is "divided up" by the resistances into voltage drops proportional to their resistance. Hooking a circuit from ground to any of the points marked will yield the indicated voltage. In this manner, multiple circuits having individual voltage requirements can be driven off a single rectifier.

Figures 8-13A and 8-13B show two other types of power supplies common to instrumentation. Figure 8-13A shows a metallic bridge rectifier with RC filtering and electronic voltage regulation as opposed to a V_R tube. The advantage of this type of supply is threefold: (1) no filaments are required; (2) higher DC output voltages are possible without correspondingly higher transformer voltages, since the full secondary voltage is used rather than one half, as with center tapped rectifiers; and (3) voltage regulation is obtained over a wider range of load currents. The electronic voltage regulator is a type of feedback-sensing network; the voltage divider (R_1, R_2, R_9) senses the output voltage of the circuit. Should load current demands change, V_O, the sensed voltage, would also tend to change. This voltage in turn controls conduction of Q_2, which controls conduction of Q_1, through which all circuit current (load and sensing) flows. For example, if load current decreases, divider current tends to increase, increasing sensed voltage (V_O) at Q_2 base. This in turn increases Q_2 conduction, thereby decreasing the potential at Q_1 base. Consequently, Q_1 conducts less and V_O remains stable. The Zener diode in Q_2 emitter circuit provides a constant reference potential for Q_2.

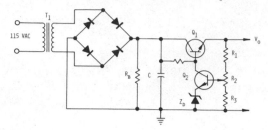

Figure 8-13A. A full wave bridge rectifier with electronic voltage regulation.

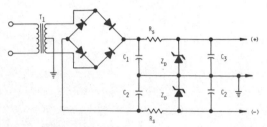

Figure 8-13B. A double-ended power supply with Zener regulation.

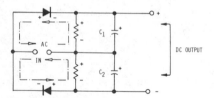

Figure 8-13C. A voltage doubler.

Figure 8-13B is a power supply finding increasing use in instrumentation today. It is a dual polarity (± 15 VDC) supply used to drive operational amplifier circuitry. The circuit is a bridge rectifier with a center tapped transformer and RC filtering and Zener regulation at each of the outputs.

A unique power supply often encountered in instrumentation is the full wave voltage doubler. It is unique in that it requires *no* transformer (although it can be used with one). The circuit as shown in Figure 8-13C operates as follows: On the negative alternation of the input, D_1 conducts and C_1 charges to the peak voltage (V_p). On the positive swing of the input, D_2 "sees" not only the peak input voltage but also the voltage of C_1, since C_2 is, in effect, in series with the input. As a result, C_2 charges to 2 V_p, or *double* the peak input voltage.

The application of diodes as rectifiers relies principally upon conduction or nonconduction of the device. On the other hand, the process of amplification depends upon (1) a variation in conduction that is proportional to the input signal and (2) the process of voltage division.

An amplifier, in the simplest sense, is a signal-sensitive voltage divider. In order to understand amplification, a simple analogy is often used: a voltage divider with one fixed resistance and one variable resistance in series (Fig. 8-14A). The law for voltages in a series circuit states that the applied voltage will be dropped proportionally across the resistances R_1 and R_2. If R_1 and R_2 are initially equal, the potential at point A will be 5 volts. However, if R_2 increases in value, the potential at A increases. If R_2 decreases, the voltage at A decreases. In an amplifier circuit, R_2 is represented by a triode or bipolar transistor, which in turn changes conduction in response to an input signal at grid or base, respectively. The change in conduction represents a relative change in the resistance of the device. For example, in Figure 8-14B, as the signal at the base of the transistor goes positive (+ 100 mv), the conduction of the device increases (increase forward bias means an increase in conduction) such that the voltage drop across the transistor decreases to 3 volts. As the input signal goes negative (− 100 mv), the conduction of the transistor decreases (decreasing forward bias means a decrease in conduction) and the voltage across the transistor increases to 7 volts. Thus, a signal voltage variation of 200 mv has produced an output voltage variation of 4 volts, a gain or amplification of 4/.2 = 20. It should be noted also that in addition to amplification, a phrase reversal has occurred. As V_{in} goes positive, V_O goes negative, etc. This circuit is called a common emitter amplifier. If the input signal were injected at a emitter, no phase reversal would occur and the circuit would be a common base amplifier.

A vacuum tube amplifier functions in much the same way as the previously discussed transistor common emitter amplifier. The signal is injected at the grid and taken off the anode or plate,

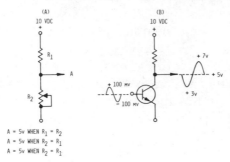

Figure 8-14A&B. Amplification.

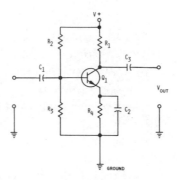

Figure 8-14C. A correctly biased transistor amplifier.

and a 180-degree phase reversal takes place. The major difference is in the high voltages used in tube circuits; as a result, more power dissipation occurs.

Having seen how an individual transistor (or tube) amplifies, it is now possible to examine a typical transistor amplifier circuit (Fig. 8-14C). Each component shown has a specific function, and each will be discussed in turn.

Q_1 and R_1 constitute the basic amplifier (voltage-sensitive divider) circuit. A signal appearing at the base of Q_1 will be amplified and appear at the collector lead. R_2 and R_3 are a biasing network; they constitute another voltage divider (in this case not voltage sensitive), in parallel with R_1 and Q_1 and used to provide the correct bias at the Q_1 base lead. R_4 and C_2 are used to provide a steady potential at Q_1 emitter (if C_2 were absent, current variations through R_4 caused by Q_1 responding to the input signal would result in Q_1 emitter voltage changes and a loss of amplification). C_1 and C_3 are coupling capacitors that block any DC voltages from appearing at the input and output, respectively, but allow the AC signal voltages to pass. Why does one want the DC voltage blocked? Consider the case of passing the signal from the collector of the amplifier shown to another amplifier's base. The collector of a transistor amplifier is at a DC potential of anywhere from 5 to 10 volts. If this were applied to the base of a transistor (normally at a DC voltage of 0.1 to 1.0 volt), the device would be constantly in a state of high conduction (saturation) and would be unable to respond to small signal voltage changes. By using coupling capacitors, this effect is negated, and many stages of amplifications can be coupled (the technical term used is cascaded) to provide an overall amplification far in excess of a single stage. Such is the case with integrated circuit amplifiers as shown in Figure 8-11.

Wave Generators and Logic Circuits

Although a majority of circuits in most instruments are concerned with amplifying a signal, the instrumentation found in physical therapy utilizes a wide variety of wave-generating circuits from sine wave ultrasonic circuits to square wave and trapezoidal wave circuits.

All wave-generating circuits employ as a control device, in one way or another, the charge-discharge activity of a capacitor. The rate at which the capacitor charges and discharges is in turn a primary factor in determining the frequency at which the waveform is generated. The simplest form of oscillator is a "tank" circuit consisting of a capacitor, an inductor, a power source, and a switch. In Figure 8-15, with the switch in position 1 the capacitor charges (A) is shown. When the switch is in position 2, the capacitor discharges (B) through L, generating a magnetic field. As the capacitor completes its discharge, the inductor's magnetic field collapses (C) and in doing so induces a current that charges the capacitor with a polarity opposite to the original condition (D). When the magnetic field is fully collapsed, the capacitor begins to discharge in the opposite direction (E), and the sequence is repeated in reverse (F and G) until the capacitor is charged as it was originally (H). It appears (to the uninitiated) that this represents an apparent perpetual motion device; obviously, such is not the case. The effects of reversing the capacitor's electrical field and the inductor's magnetic field both lead to energy loss; consequently, the oscillations would appear as shown in Figure 8-16. In order to obtain undamped oscillations, some form of *regenerative feedback* is required. If the switch were rapidly thrown back to position 1, at step H the capacitor

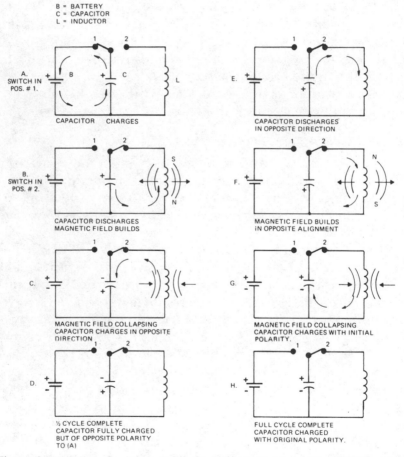

Figure 8-15. LC tank circuit oscillation. From Terence Karselis, *Descriptive Medical Electronics and Instrumentation*, 1973. Courtesy of Charles B. Slack, Inc., Thorofare, New Jersey.

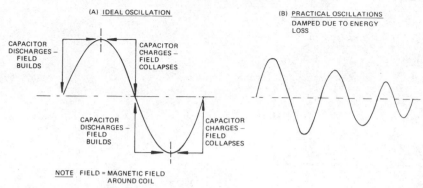

Figure 8-16. Ideal versus practical oscillations. From Terence Karselis, *Descriptive Medical Electronics and Instrumentation*, 1973. Courtesy of Charles B. Slack, Inc., Thorofare, New Jersey.

could recharge, replacing its lost energy, resulting in constant amplitude oscillations.

A practical oscillator circuit requires the three items referred to in the above description:

1. A frequency-determining network
2. Regenerative (in phase) feedback
3. A tuned switching device

Tuned LC tank circuits, quartz crystals, and RC circuits provide item 1 in practical oscillators. Transformers (one winding of which is part of a tank circuit) provide the necessary phase shift (as can groups of RC networks) to bring about regenerative feedback when used in conjunction with transistors or tubes. For example, as an input signal to an amplifier from a tank circuit goes positive, the amplifier output goes negative (180° phase shift). When coupled back to the input by way of a transformer (180° phase shift), the feedback is positive going, in phase with the original signal. The process is *switched* by way of the amplifier reaching saturation or cutoff, resulting in a reversal of the voltage changes. Figure 8-17 shows three transistor oscillators —a Hartley LC oscillator, an RC phase shift oscillator, and a quartz crystal oscillator.

Relaxation oscillators are characterized by output waveforms

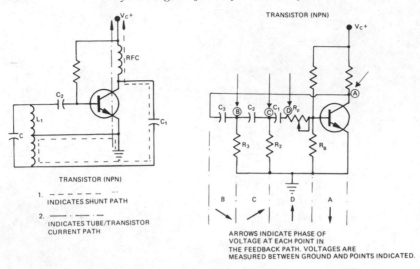

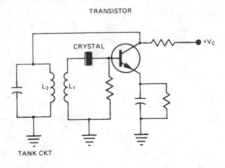

Figure 8-17. Hartley (upper left), phase shift (upper right), and crystal con-trolled (lower) oscillators. From Terence Karselis, *Descriptive Medical Electronics and Instrumentation*, 1973. Courtesy of Charles B. Slack, Inc., Thorofare, New Jersey.

that change suddenly from one condition to another, the most common type being *multivibrators*. Free-running multivibrators are basically square wave generators consisting of two com-plementary coupled amplifiers, meaning each output is coupled by way of an RC circuit to the other amplifier's input (Fig. 8-18).

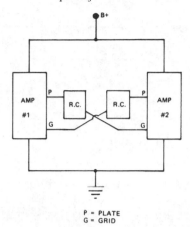

Figure 8-18. An astable (free-running) multivibrator. From Terence Karselis, *Descriptive Medical Electronics and Instrumentation,* 1973. Courtesy of Charles B. Slack, Inc., Thorofare, New Jersey.

Since in a given amplifier, input-output waveforms are 180 degrees out of phase, this complementary coupling requires that when one amplifier is "on," the other must be "off." The action of the RC networks is such that they determine the on-off time and also effect the change that reverses the amplifier's conditions. The result is an output as shown in Figure 8-19. By changing the values of the RC network, waveforms such as those shown in Figure 8-20 can be provided.

Two other multivibrator types are (1) the monostable or one-shot multivibrator, which generates a single pretimed pulse when externally triggered, and (2) the bistable or flip-flop multivibrator, a circuit that will remain in one condition until trig-

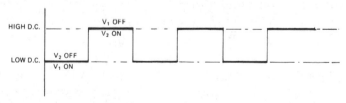

Figure 8-19. Output waveform of an astable multivibrator. From Terence Karselis, *Descriptive Medical Electronics and Instrumentation,* 1973. Courtesy of Charles B. Slack, Inc., Thorofare, New Jersey.

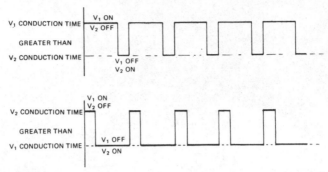

Figure 8-20. Results of varying conduction times of a free-running multivibrator by changing the coupling circuit R and C values. From Terence Karselis, *Descriptive Medical Electronics and Instrumentation*, 1973. Courtesy of Charles B. Slack, Inc., Thorofare, New Jersey.

gered, when it will "flip" to the other condition. It will remain in that state until another trigger "flops" it back to its original condition. This circuit is used extensively in computers since it can be used to store information (on = 1, off = 0) as well as count and divide when coupled with other flip-flops. Free-running multivibrators find use as "time clocks" in computer circuitry.

Another group of relaxation oscillators are the blocking and ringing oscillators. Blocking oscillators and ringing oscillators are both characterized by two common factors: (1) both types contain, in some form or another, an LC resonant circuit to provide oscillation, and (2) resonant oscillations occur only when the tube or transistor is in the off (cutoff) condition. Blocking oscillators are characterized by the fact that they produce a single, sharp sinusoidal pulse at preset intervals. They may be free running, producing a single pulse constantly at a predetermined interval, controlled by a charging or discharging capacitor, or they may be triggered, producing a pulse only when an input trigger is present.

Ringing oscillators generate a series of dampened sinusoidal pulses when "shocked" into oscillation by an external signal; hence, they are more generally termed shock-excited oscillators. Figure 8-21 shows a typical circuit. When no input signal is present, Q_1 is conducting and the tank circuit (L_1C_2) coil consti-

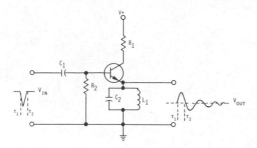

Figure 8-21. A shock-excited ringing oscilator.

tutes a low DC resistance. All transistor current flows through it; therefore, no voltage is felt across C_2 (the output). When a negative input pulse cuts off Q_1, the magnetic field generated around L_1 due to the high transistor current flow now collapses, charging C_2, and oscillations are set up in the tank circuit, generating a series of output pulses. As soon as the negative input pulse is removed, Q_1 begins conducting and oscillations cease. If the input signal kept Q_1 cut off long enough, the tank circuit oscillations would eventually dampen, since no regeneration is provided.

Another group of interesting wave generators are the trapezoidal, sawtooth, or ramp generators. These circuits are characterized by an output wave form resembling the teeth of a saw — a slowly rising voltage followed by a rapid drop back to zero. All of these circuits use the charging and discharging of a capacitor to yield the required waveform. The simplest sawtooth generator is the neon glow tube generator. Figure 8-22A shows the neon tube (V_1) in parallel with a capacitor (C_1), both being in series with resistor (R_1). Since conduction through the neon tube only occurs when the gas is ionized, the tube acts as a switch, allowing the capacitor to discharge. When circuit power is applied, C_1 begins to charge through R_1. The output voltage is the charging voltage across the capacitor. When the capacitor voltage reaches the firing potential of the neon gas, the tube conducts and the capacitor rapidly discharges (the tube acts as a short circuit between the capacitor's plates). When the capacitor's voltage drops below the extinction voltage of the neon gas, the tube de-ionizes, acts like an open circuit, and C_1 begins to

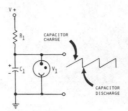

Figure 8-22A. A neon tube sawtooth generator.

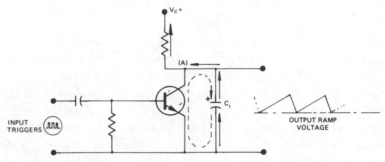

Figure 8-22B. A ramp function (sawtooth) generator. From Terence Karselis, *Descriptive Medical Electronics and Instrumentation,* 1973. Courtesy of Charles B. Slack, Inc., Thorofare, New Jersey.

charge again. Note that the circuit is free running; it requires no input trigger. Figure 8-22B is a triggered (synchronized) sawtooth generator. It differs from the previous circuit in operation in one aspect only — the input trigger turns on the transistor, thereby yielding a discharge path for the capacitor. In all other aspects, circuit operation is identical.

Microwave Oscillators

It was mentioned in a previous section that the "Q" or selectivity of a tuned circuit dropped off drastically above 20 MHz. This occurs because the "lumped" reactance of individual capacitors and inductors is overcome by the *distributed* reactance of component interelectrode capacitance and circuit wiring, such that at approximately 100 MHz, circuit efficiency can be as low as 50 percent. As a consequence, high frequency (microwave) oscillators and amplifiers of special design are required.

The unique feature of microwave oscillators is the incorporation of the resonant circuit directly into the design of the tube itself. This is accomplished by reducing a resonant circuit down to its simplest form. The simplest form of an inductor would be a short straight segment of wire. When other parallel segments are added, the inductance is further decreased, and the result is somewhat like a squirrel cage. The simplest capacitor is two plates separated by air. If these two simplified components are put together, the result is a round, flat, cagelike structure; if an infinite number of inductor segments are then added, the result is a flat drum or cavity. This is the resonant circuit of a microwave tube. The walls of the drum constitute a small inductance, with the top and bottom as the resonant circuit capacitance. The overall device is termed a "cavity resonator."

The Klystron (Fig. 8-23) is a vacuum tube with a cathode, control grid, two buncher grids, two catcher grids, and a collector. Resonant cavities are connected to the buncher (1) and catcher (2) grids. When the tube conducts, electrons approach the buncher grid and start the first resonant circuit oscillating. Due to this, electrons tend to leave the buncher grid in cluster groups or "bunches," hence the name. Upon approaching the catcher grid, the first "bunch" of electrons starts the second resonant circuit oscillating; the subsequent groups of electrons that arrive maintain the oscillations. An inductive feedback loop from the second to the first cavity maintains the oscillations required for the buncher electrodes' action. The high efficiency and improved power output of the Klystron over conventional tubes makes them useful at frequencies above 1,000 MHz.

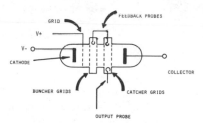

Figure 8-23. Simplified diagram of a Klystrom ultra high frequency amplifier-oscillator.

A second, somewhat different resonant cavity RF tube is the *magnatron*. A magnatron is essentially a diode with a superimposed magnetic field and a series of resonant cavities. Figure 8-24 shows the construction of a typical magnatron. The centrally located cathode emits electrons which are acted upon by both the cathode-anode electric field and the superimposed magnetic field such that they travel along a spirallike path towards the anode. As the electrons pass the cavity slots, they transfer energy into the cavity energy field, causing the cavity to generate oscillations (the basic principle is similar to that employed to generate sound in tin whistles). The microwave oscillations can be picked up by an inductive probe and fed to a transmitting device (actually an antenna) by way of coaxial cable or a formed wave guide. Magnatrons are considered as self-excited RF oscillators, as they convert pulsed HVDC into pulsed RF energy, and they are used extensively as the power output stage of microwave diathermy units.

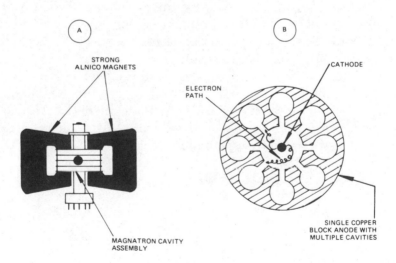

Figure 8-24. (A) shows a simplified drawing of a magnatron. (B) is a cutaway top view of the cavity assembly with spirallike electron paths. From Terence Karselis, *Descriptive Medical Electronics and Instrumentation*, 1973. Courtesy of Charles B. Slack, Inc., Thorofare, New Jersey.

THE ELEMENTS OF THERAPEUTIC INSTRUMENTATION

Instrument Systems

How to Get the Best of Them

The average instrument user in a typical medical facility tends to view biomedical instruments as mysterious and unfathomable devices put together by some wild-eyed mad scientists kept locked away in the basement of a large instrument company. The user is quite happy to turn switch (A) and push button (B) and see the instrument "percolate" as it is supposed to, without having to worry himself or herself about *how* it performs its esoteric duty. Herein lies the single most difficult problem for those working with medical instrumentation! "If you don't know *how* it works, how do you know it is working properly?" The solution to this problem can be found in a number of different ways, from obtaining an engineering degree to ignoring the problem completely. An easier, practical, and more useful technique involves not so much learning about instrumentation in a specific sense but rather adapting existing knowledge and common sense into the right approach.

To find the right approach, the following question must be asked: Just what is the primary function behind *all* instrumentation? Answer: To extend man's capabilities! Whether it is meant to measure a specific parameter or apply a therapeutic process, instrumentation only enhances man's ability to perform the function. Since instrumentation extends man's senses and capabilities, it must function in a somewhat similar way. In assaying a particular situation or problem, man must (1) observe, (2) evaluate, and (3) act; when he does so, signal transmission takes place in a definite direction. For example, while one is driving an automobile, an approaching obstacle would send a visual stimulus, generating electrical excitation, which is transmitted to the brain. The signal is then evaluated, and evasive action (turning the steering wheel) occurs as a result of muscular motor activity caused by the electrical excitation. It is important to note that two signals were involved — the stimulus (received signal) and the response (transmitted signal).

All instruments function exclusively to handle one or both of these signal forms, i.e. an EKG handles a received signal, a diathermy unit transmits a signal. With this point of view in mind, one can visualize a simplified medical instrument in one of two ways as shown in Figure 8-25 (A and B). In (A), the signal is sensed, processed, and displayed, while in (B), the signal is generated, processed, and transmitted. Consequently, whichever is the case, most instrument systems can be simplified into a block diagram consisting of (1) a sensing or transmitting unit (the transducer), (2) a processing unit (most often an amplifier), and (3) a generating unit (signal generator) or display unit (meter or oscilloscope, etc.). In addition, all instrument systems require power to function, so a fourth unit, a power supply, can be considered as requisite. If one approaches instrumentation in this way, it will tend to be used more efficiently with consequently less "down time" due to operator error. Whenever malfunctions or breakdowns do occur, the better informed, more knowledgeable operator can troubleshoot or give sound symptomatic fault information to the biomedical electronics technician, once again reducing down time.

In applying the above technique, the most crucial items required are (1) a thorough understanding of *what* the device should do, (2) a modicum of knowledge of *how* it does it, (3) familiarity with the instrument controls, and (4) a strong mental picture of the instrument in functional but simplified block diagram form. To obtain two of these four tools, it becomes necessary to rely upon the instrument manufacturer. His operating manual will most often yield items 1 and 2. Item 4 may or

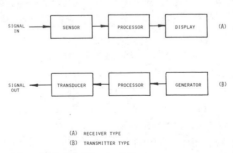

Figure 8-25. Typical instrument systems.

may not be present; however, a clue to the "functional" blocks within an instrument can be drawn from the controls on its front panel. For example, an on-off switch indicates a power supply. Each operation performed by the device requiring an individual control or adjustment indicates a functional unit. A multiple-position switch allowing various outputs indicates a common output system. With careful observation and a little imagination, a simplified block diagram of even the most sophisticated instrument can be obtained.

Some Additional Points on Signal Processing

Once a signal has been generated within an instrument, it must be fed from the signal source to the output. In addition, some form of modification of the signal may be required. The most common forms of signal processing are rectification and amplification. However, other forms of signal manipulation can occur, such as *modulation, gating,* and *clipping.*

Modulation can be accomplished in two ways: amplitude modulation and frequency modulation. The latter process involves varying the frequency of a signal in proportion to the amplitude of a second signal and is most often used in communications-type circuitry. *Amplitude modulation* is used extensively in therapeutic instrumentation. The term amplitude modulation is self-explanatory; the amplitude of the primary signal is modulated, i.e. varied in proportion to the magnitude of the secondary or modulating signal. In all cases involving AC signals, the primary signal *must* be of a higher frequency than the modulating signal. Four general methods of modulation are used in therapeutic instruments:

1. Opening and closing the filament circuit of a vacuum tube so that its condition occurs in smoothly rising and falling surges.
2. Varying the amplitude of a pulse generator's output signal by way of a motor- or cam-driven rheostat.
3. Varying the plate supply to an oscillator, accomplishing the same result.
4. Varying the conductance of a tetrode or pentode by applying the modulating signal to the screen grid.

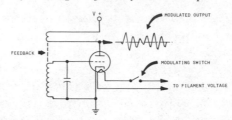

Figure 8-26. A switch modulated oscillator.

Each of these techniques can be found in various instruments commercially manufactured for physical therapy. An examination of the first technique indicated above will provide a general understanding of how modulation takes place.

Figure 8-26 is a Switch Modulated Vacuum Tube Armstrong Tickler Coil Oscillator. The plate coil shown provides regenerative feedback to the LC tank circuit, thereby maintaining oscillations. If the filament voltage and V+ were kept constant, the output signal would be a constant voltage, constant frequency sine wave. As switch S_1 (this could be a set of relay contacts) is periodically opened then closed again, the conduction of the tube varies due to the filament alternately being heated and cooled. The result is periodic surges of oscillation at the output as shown in Figure 8-26. The reader should note that the maximum rate at which surges can be generated is limited by the maximum rate at which the filament can cycle from hot to cold and back. If variable rate capability is necessary, the modulating signal can be obtained electronically from an (RC) oscillator, the frequency of which can be altered by changing the time constant of the circuit. This is accomplished by switching in various resistances (since t = RC), which in turn controls the rate at which the capacitor can charge or discharge, thereby changing the oscillator's frequency. The output of this oscillator is then used to *modulate* the output of the primary oscillator circuit by one of the previously mentioned methods.

Probably the most common modulating technique used in electronics is the mixing tube technique. A pentrode or tetrode oscillator is used to provide the primary signal, which originates in the tube's control grid circuit. The modulating signal is applied to the second (screen) grid, altering the tube's conduction. If the second grid is relatively positive, the control grid's oscillations are allowed to pass to the plate. If the screen grid is relatively negative, the oscillations are suppressed and no output occurs.

Gating can be considered as a type of all-or-none modulation in which the output from the primary oscillator or pulse generator is turned on and off. The action is analogous to switching the circuit on and off, and in fact, this is exactly how such circuits function. A typical example is as follows: The primary oscillator is placed in series with a gating amplifier. In order for oscillations to occur, *both* circuits must be conducting. However, the gating amplifier is normally kept cut off. Positive gating pulses, when applied to the gating amplifier input, cause it to conduct, thereby allowing the primary oscillator to operate. In contrast to a modulating signal, gating pulses must be square waves and are most often obtained from multivibrator circuits, particularly when variable gate periods are desired. A 60 Hertz gating signal can be obtained directly from line frequency voltage by use of clipping circuits.

A clipping circuit does exactly as its name implies; it "clips" the peaks off waveforms. Figure 8-27 shows a simple power frequency neon tube clipping circuit, which operates as follows: The neon gas tube will not conduct until its firing voltage (approximately 50 volts) is reached. During that time the voltage from the secondary of the transformer is felt at the output. When the neon tube fires, the output voltage is the ionization voltage of the tube. The same process occurs on both the positive and negative alternations of the transformer voltage; hence, the output is a somewhat less than perfect square wave.

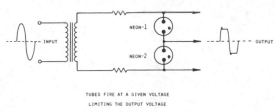

TUBES FIRE AT A GIVEN VOLTAGE
LIMITING THE OUTPUT VOLTAGE

Figure 8-27. A simple neon tube clipper.

Other types of clipping circuits involve the use of biased diodes or triodes. The overall effect, however, is the same; predetermined peaks of the input waveform are clipped.

Basic Principles of Transducers

In most types of electronic instrumentation, it is the *transducer* that acts as the transmitting or receiving element of the instrument system. However, in some instances of therapeutic medicine, the transmitting device is not really a transducer in the strict sense of the word; it may act as nothing more than an electrode (a terminal point of an electrical circuit). Nevertheless, an understanding of some of the principles involved in the application of transducers is required of anyone involved in therapeutic medicine.

Any device capable of converting one form of energy into another can be classified as a transducer. Case in point: a typical household light bulb. This electrical transducer converts electrical energy into electromagnetic radiation, i.e. light and heat energy. A somewhat more sophisticated form of transducer is the common chemical pH electrode — a device that converts chemical activity into electrical energy. Most transducers are classified based on the type of energy required to "excite" them. Hence, the common light bulb is an *electro-optical* transducer, while pH electrode is considered a *chemoelectric* transducer.

The three energy forms primarily employed in physical medicine are (1) low and medium high frequency electrical currents, (2) radio frequency electrical and electromagnetic radiation, and (3) ultrasonic mechanical energy. The application of low and medium high frequency electrical currents requires little more than metallic electrodes as transducers, while RF energy employs the use of basic electrical and electromagnetic principles in its application. The only "true" transducer used in physical medicine is the ultrasonic or *piezoelectric* transducer.

The piezoelectric effect is a bidirectional phenomenon first discovered in certain crystalline materials. If a crystal of Rochelle salt (quartz SO_2) is mechanically distorted, stresses within its lattice structure result in surface charge polarization such that one side of the crystal becomes positive and the other negative.

However, it is the reverse action that finds its application in physical medicine — the fact that when a crystal is excited by an AC electrical signal it will distort or vibrate, producing sound waves of the same frequency as the stimulating signal. Since quartz and Rochelle salts are dependent upon careful and correct cutting of the crystal to yield satisfactory results, ultrasonic elements of barium titanate (molded ceramics) are becoming more common. These commercial substances have the dual advantages of less cost and wider temperature stability. Figure 8-28 shows an example of the piezoelectric effect. The reader should note that the process is a reversible one; an alternating current voltage applied to the crystal produces mechanical vibrations.

Piezoelectric crystals also find application in oscillator circuits, since their resonant vibrations are inherently stable, providing exceedingly stable output frequencies from the oscillator.

In either of the above applications, the piezoelectric crystal is mounted between two metallic plates, enabling the application or withdrawal of mechanical energy.

Medical diathermy utilizes both electrical and electromagnetic fields to provide deep tissue heating. The "transducers" used to apply the energy to the patient in these applications are not energy-transforming devices but rather more like oversized electrical components. In the application of *electrical fields*, the

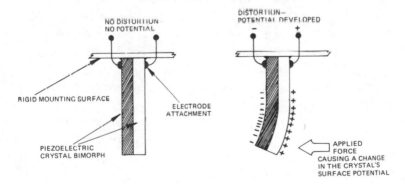

Figure 8-28. A simplified diagram showing the piezoelectric effect. From Terence Karselis, *Descriptive Medical Electronics and Instrumentation*, 1973. Courtesy of Charles B. Slack, Inc., Thorofare, New Jersey.

patient becomes the dielectric in large capacitor made up of the application plates with the patient sandwiched between them. When *electromagnetic* energy is employed, an applicator coil is wound around the patient (on the leg, for example), thereby making the patient the "core" of an oversized inductor. In both instances, it is the fundamental electrical activity of these oversized components that provides the therapeutic energy to the patient. The patient is, in effect, immersed in the appropriate energy field.

The use of muscle stimulating currents requires the least sophisticated transducer of all; in fact, the applicators used in this mode of therapy are little more than simple contact electrodes or terminals. The patient, when placed between the electrodes, simply becomes a resistive element in a series circuit network. When a voltage is generated across the electrodes, current flows out from one electrode through the patient and into the other electrode. This form of physical medicine is the only one in which "electrical current" flows from instrument to patient. In the previous methodologies noted, the patient is immersed in or becomes the target of some form of *energy field.*

Electromagnetic Radiation

Generation and Transmission

The previous section discussed the use of "energy fields" as the therapeutic agent in physical medicine, indicating that both electrical and electromagnetic fields are used. More specifically, electromagnetic energy was related to high frequency (short wave and microwave) diathermy. The use of electromagnetic radiation, however, is not restrictive to diathermy wavelengths. Radiations falling into and around the visible spectrum are also employed in physical medicine.

The dualistic nature of electromagnetic energy came to light in the early nineteenth century when the Danish physicist Oersted accidentally observed its effect on a magnetic compass during a lecture demonstration. Today, it is known that magnetic effects are a result of charges in motion. Since the electrons in an atom are in motion, both orbital and spin in nature, they act as minute coils carrying current and hence generate minute magnetic fields. If the substance is such that the effects of the various fields are cancelled, the net result is that the material is nonmagnetic. If the minute magnetic fields are such that they are additive, the substance will have a net magnetic field.

In an earlier section, with the discussion of electromagnetism, through a conductor, a magnetic field was generated around that conductor. One can take this example and expand upon it in order to see how it relates to the generation of electromagnetic energy fields in space.

Radio frequency oscillations are produced by electronic oscillator circuits. When such alternating currents are applied to an appropriate length of conductor (½ or ¼ wavelength of the oscillating frequency), an antenna is produced. The antenna segment has two ends, (1) the transmitter end, attached to the oscillator output, and (2) the open end. During one *half* cycle of oscillation current will flow from the transmitter end to the open end. During the next half cycle it will flow from the open end back to the transmitter end. As the current tends to be maximum at the center, it is at this point around the conductor that a doughnut-shaped magnetic field is generated, the lines of force of which are perpendicular to the antenna. This constitutes the *magnetic* portion of the radiated electromagnetic field. The *electrical* field is produced by the capacitance that exists between the two ends of the conductor. As charges alternately pile up at the open and transmitter ends of the antenna, electrical lines of force are produced parallel to the antenna. This constitutes the electrical field. Note that the two fields are 90 degrees of phase *in time* and *in space* (Fig. 8-29A). When the electrical field is at maximum intensity, electrons are piled up at one antenna end and current is zero; therefore, magnetic field is nil. Magnetic lines of force are perpendicular to the antenna, electrical lines of force are parallel to it. The wave field radiated into space constitutes a series of alternating magnetic and electrical waves moving outward from the antenna as shown in Figure 8-29B.

As the LC values of an oscillating tank circuit become smaller, the frequency of oscillation becomes higher, and the wavelength of the radiated energy becomes shorter. At wavelengths above 0.1 mm (3,000 MHz), it is not possible to construct circuitry to

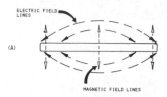

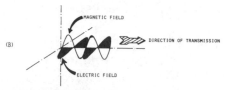

Figure 8-29. Antenna energy fields.

accomplish oscillation. Radiation at these wavelengths comes from molecular and electronic vibrations in molecules and atoms which can be made to "oscillate" by appropriate stimulation, such as heating and electrical discharge. The waves that are generated in this manner constitute the so-called visible spectrum of *infrared, visible,* and *ultraviolet* light.

Wavelengths in the x-ray and gamma regions require still smaller "oscillators," and these are found within the atomic nucleus as a result of high energy particle collisions.

In evaluating the transmission of electromagnetic radiation and its effect upon other materials, two general items must be considered: (1) the intensity and frequency of the transmitted energy and (2) the properties of the receiving material.

The intensity of the radiated energy, with antenna characteristics constant, is a function of the current in the antenna. The antenna current is in turn dependent upon the antenna *reactance* for a given frequency and applied power. From this, it is possible to conclude that since reactance is frequency dependent (as previously discussed), at some frequency, reactance will be zero and the antenna will be at resonance. It is at this frequency at which maximum energy is radiated.

The reaction of a given receiving substance to radiated energy is determined primarily by the frequency (or wavelength) of the transmitted signal. At longer (radio) wavelengths, it is the bulk electrical and magnetic properties that will determine the result.

For example, an insulator has few movable charges; therefore, no counteracting fields can be produced. Hence, electromagnetic waves travel easily through electrical insulators, while they are absorbed by the human body, which has an abundance of movable charges with which to react.

At shorter wavelengths, atomic properties begin to take an effect and in fact play a significant role, while at very short wavelengths, the receiver interaction is a result of elementary particle, i.e. electrons, neutrons, and protons, interaction.

As a general rule, it can be said that the longer the wavelength, the more predominant will be the "wave properties" of electromagnetic radiation, while the shorter the wavelength, the more predominant will be its "quantum properties."

It is the wave properties of visible light that help the student to understand its behavior when passing from one medium into another. One should keep in mind, however, that the laws governing this action remain just as valid when applied to other regions of the electromagnetic spectrum. If it is remembered that the shorter the wavelength of a photon or wave of energy, the greater its energy and hence its potential penetrating ability, the basic laws of *reflection, refraction,* and *absorption* can be used to predict the behavior of any electromagnetic wave, whether visible or invisible.

One may predict, for example, the behavior of two separate wavelengths of radiation passing from one medium (air) into a second medium (a polished glass plate). If wavelength (A) is visible light and (B) is x-ray energy, since (B) is shorter in wavelength, it is therefore higher in energy. Thus, the majority of (A) will be *reflected,* while the majority of (B) will pass into the glass medium. Any photons entering the glass will alter their direction in accordance with the law of *refraction.* In general, the higher the energy of the photon, the less the refractive effect. Finally, all radiant energy entering the glass will be decreased in magnitude *exponentially* according to the law of absorption. The higher the photon energy, the greater its penetrating ability and the less its chance of being absorbed.

The Electromagnetic Spectrum

In the previous section, the generation and radiation of electromagnetic energy fields were discussed with little mention of the method of classifying them. In most instances, regions of the spectrum are in fact distinguished on the basis of how a particular wavelength is produced or detected. Radio waves are produced and detected by radio circuits, while infrared waves are generated or detected by heat.

An overall view of the electromagnetic spectrum can be based on classification as to wavelength as shown in Table 8-I. It should be noted, however, that the boundaries between regions overlap and the figures given are approximate.

The speed of radiation in free space is 300 million meters per second, and this figure can be used to find the wavelength or frequency of the radiation, if one or the other is known, in the following manner.:

$$\text{(meters)} = \frac{300,000,000 \text{ (meters/sec.)}}{\text{Frequency (Hertz)}}$$

For example, a 30,000 MHz radio wave has a wavelength of 0.01 meter or 1.0 cm, while a 27 MHz diathermy wave has a wavelength of approximately 11 mm and a 10 KC radio wave has a wavelength of 30,000 meters. Although the above measurement of wavelength is given in meters, the standard classical method used gives wavelength in Angstroms (Å): $1\text{Å} = 1 \times 10^{-10}$ meters. Another wavelength unit used extensively in clinical analysis is the nanometer (nm): $1 \text{ nm} = 10^{-9}$ meters.

ULTRAVIOLET RADIATION DEVICES
Ultraviolet Radiation

Sources

The most commonly known natural source of ultraviolet radiation (1,800 to 4,000 Angstroms) is sunlight, but its therapeutic capability is limited by not only quantity (ultraviolet constitutes a small fraction of the total solar radiated energy) but in some cases also by quality, since certain parts of the ultraviolet region are absorbed by the oxygen molecules of the air. Hence, it is no accident that high mountain "air" is thought to be more therapeutic than that in the low-lying damp valleys. The ultimate source of the sun's ultraviolet radiation is in the heated

TABLE 8-I

	Cosmic Rays	Gamma Rays	X-Rays	Ultra-violet	Visible	Infra-red	Radio Short Wave	Radio Long Wave
WAVELENGTH (cm)	10^{-12}	10^{-11}	10^{-8}	10^{-6}	10^{-4}	10^{-3}	10	10^{5}
FREQUENCY (hertz)	10^{17}	10^{15}	10^{13}	10^{10}	10^{9}	10^{8}	10^{5}	10

gaseous envelope surrounding the sun, which has an average temperature of approximately 5,000°C. These heated gases are continuously being ionized, with the resulting emission of discrete "particles" of energy when displaced orbital electrons regain their normal position. The energy content of these *photons* is related to frequency and wavelength as follows:

$$E = \frac{hv}{\lambda}$$

Where E = energy in ergs
λ = wavelength in Angstroms
v = frequency in Hertz
h = Planck's constant

In general, it can be said that the shorter the wavelength, the higher the energy.

To insure adequate intensities of ultraviolet radiation for therapeutic application, artificial ultraviolet sources must be used. Like the ultraviolet radiation generated by the sun, artificial ultraviolet generation is due to ionization of the substance employed as the "emitter." The two most common methods of producing ionization are (1) the application of heat and (2) arcing due to an electric current. The latter technique is the method of choice in most cases; however, an example of the former technique is found in the common incandescent tungsten bulb. An electric current passed through a tungsten filament generates heat, which increases the kinetic energy of its atoms. Increased collisions of the atoms generates infrared, visible and ultraviolet radiations. To provide this wide range of radiation, the filament temperature must be operated at approximately 3,100°C; below 500°C, only infrared radiation is produced. Of the total energy emission of a tungsten bulb, approximately 0.5 percent is in the ultraviolet region. Needless to say, incandescent sources are rarely used in therapeutic applications involving UV energy.

As noted previously, the spectrum of energy produced by an incandescent source is a *continuous* one. When elementary substances such as xenon gas are ionized, they produce radiations that are *not continuous* but in specific narrow lines (Fig. 8-30).

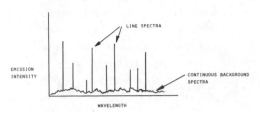

Figure 8-30. Typical line spectra.

These *line spectra* are characteristic of the substance in question, since each element has its own unique set of orbital electrons and, therefore, emission quanta. While ionization can be brought about by heating, it is impractical at the temperatures necessary to ionize those substances that will emit ultraviolet radiation; hence, an alternative technique is used. When a gas is enclosed in a suitable container with an electrode at each end, and sufficient voltage is impressed across the electrodes, at some point the gas will ionize and an electric current will arc between the electrodes. By sustaining the current and adding in vapor form a substance capable of ultraviolet emission, i.e. mercury, a practical ultraviolet generator can be made. The arcing current provides high velocity particles which by way of collision cause atoms of the emitting substance to radiate ultraviolet energy. This gas discharge or electric arc process is the most common technique used in commercial ultraviolet-generating devices.

Physical Behavior of Ultraviolet Radiation

The clinical aspects of ultraviolet energy behavior are covered elsewhere in this volume; consequently, this section will deal lightly with some of the physical aspects that are directly related to the application of ultraviolet therapy.

The transmission of radiant energy is governed by various physical laws, and two of the most important in the application of therapeutic radiation are the inverse square law and the cosine law. Briefly, the inverse square law states that the intensity of radiation from a *point source* decreases inversely with the square of the distance from the source. Hence, doubling the distance between source and target will decrease the intensity of the radiation to one quarter of its former value. The cosine law shows that minimum reflection from a surface occurs when the angle between *incident ray* and reflecting surface is 90 degrees; hence, at this angle, maximum absorption will occur. Radiation intensity is then proportional to the cosine of the angle of radiation and a perpendicular to the target surface.

The interaction of electromagnetic radiation and matter was mentioned previously, indicating that the reactions that took place were at the (1) bulk, electrical, and electromagnetic, (2) molecular and atomic, or (3) subatomic or elementary particle level. Such reactions take place, however, only *after* the radiation has crossed the interface between the transmitting medium (air) and receiving or absorbing medium (the patient). Like visible right, ultraviolet radiation is subject to the laws of optics governing reflection, refraction, and absorption. At the interface between two mediums, reflection and absorption take place, and the ratio of reflection to absorption for a given amount of transmitter radiation is directly dependent upon (1) the wavelength of the radiation, (2) the angle at which it strikes the medium (angle of incidence), and (3) the physical nature of the medium. This data is important in the design of ultraviolet therapeutic devices, particularly in the design of reflectors, as well as affecting the quality of ultraviolet application as a therapeutic agent.

Once absorbed by the target medium, penetrating ultraviolet radiation undergoes one or more of the interactions mentioned previously. Since the absorbed energy represents an increase in the net energy of the system, in order for the system to return to its normal or "ground" state, the excess energy must be dissipated. This can take place via ionization, chemical reactions, or heat or light emission (fluorescence). Whatever the case, the excess energy is absorbed in an exponential manner until all the energy has been transferred to the medium or the residual radiation exits into another medium.

A Typical Ultraviolet Generating Device

Just like any other device or instrument, an ultraviolet radiation generator can be subdivided into specific functional parts. A typical device consists of the component parts as listed below:

1. An ultraviolet radiation source (lamp)

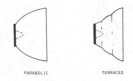

PARABOLIC TERRACED

Figure 8-31. Typical reflectors.

2. A reflecting device with shutters
3. An applicator column or arm
4. A support base with enclosed transformer or ballast circuitry

Specific ultraviolet sources will be discussed in the next section; this section will briefly consider the remaining three areas.

As noted previously, ultraviolet radiation is subject to all the physical laws of visible light, i.e. reflection, etc. Considering that an ultraviolet source of radiation emits its energy omnidirectionally (in all directions), the use of such a source without some type of reflecting device would be highly inefficient, since most of the energy would be dissipated into the air. Use of an appropriate reflector concentrates and redirects most of the diffusing radiation onto the patient. Parabolic and terrace-type reflectors of smooth, polished metallic surfaces are used to accomplish concentration of radiation. Figure 8-31 shows typical parabolic and terrace-type reflectors.

In order to facilitate application of ultraviolet radiation to patients in various positions and to various surfaces of the body, the source and reflector (the head of the device) must be mobile and capable of great flexibility and adjustment with minimal effort. To accomplish this, counterbalanced telescoping columns with adjustable joints are used, such as those shown in Figure 8-32.

To provide maximum stability in ultraviolet lamps, the transformer or ballast circuitry required to control the line voltage to "fire" the ultraviolet source is usually housed in the base of the lamp. Wheels or casters are fixed to the base to provide maximum mobility.

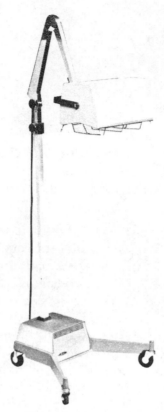

Figure 8-32. Burdick U.V. 800 ultraviolet lamp. Courtesy of The Burdick Corporation, Milton, Wisconsin.

Mercury Lamps

Low Pressure Mercury Arc Lamps

The most efficient method of producing ultraviolet radiation is by way of a sustained electric arc. Open carbon arcs were used prior to the invention of the mercury lamp; however, mercury arc lamps are the most common type of therapeutic ultraviolet generators used today.

The basic mercury arc lamp consists of (1) an envelope transparent to ultraviolet radiation, (2) electrodes, which furnish the voltage to create the arc, (3) a support gas to maintain the electric arc and provide ionizing temperatures, and (4) liquid mercury, which acts as the ultraviolet emitter when ionized. Two types of low pressure mercury lamps are obtainable, cold cathode and hot cathode lamps. The cold or hot designation refers to the method by which electrons are emitted from the cathode in order to initiate ionization of the support gas. In hot cathode lamps, the electrodes are preheated and a low voltage is impressed across the electrodes. The increased kinetic energy of electrons in the electrode material plus the energy of the low voltage is sufficient to cause emission of electrons ionizing the support gas and establishing current flow between the electrodes. Once initiated, the current through the support gas generates heat, which vaporizes the mercury. The mercury atoms then collide with high velocity electrons, are ionized, and thereby emit ultraviolet radiation. The greatest concentration of ultraviolet energy is generated in the 2537 and 1849 Angstrom lines, as shown in Figure 8-33.

Ordinary borasilicate glass is not suitable for ultraviolet source envelopes since it absorbs in the ultraviolet region; therefore, ultraviolet transmitters such as quartz, fused quartz, and silicon dioxide as well as some high phosphate glasses are used. Fused quartz is commonly used, as it has other physical advantages besides being transparent to ultraviolet. It is physically strong, has low thermal conductivity (and hence has a low sensitivity to thermal shock), and is also an electrical insulator. A low pressure mercury arc lamp with a fused quartz envelope is often referred to as a cold quartz lamp.

The cold cathode variety of lamp (which may also be called a

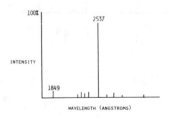

Figure 8-33. Mercury (low pressure) spectrum.

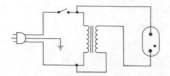

Figure 8-34. Simplified schematic of a Birtcher Spot Quartz Lamp. Courtesy of The Birtcher Corporation, Los Angeles, California.

cold quartz lamp) requires no heating of the electrodes. However, in order to initiate electron emission and generate an arc, a high voltage (1,500 V) must be placed across the electrodes. Once ionization occurs and the arc is generated, the operation of the lamp is the same as for its hot cathode brother. Figure 8-34 shows the schematic diagram of a typical cold quartz lamp. Note that the secondary of the transformer is in series with the lamp, providing ballast (current limiting) capability.

High Pressure Mercury Arc Lamps

The basic operating principles of the low pressure mercury arc lamp, including arcing, heating, and ionization, extend to the high pressure lamp. When the vapor pressure of the atomized mercury in a lamp exceeds one atmosphere, the lamp is a high pressure device. The mercury spectrum is generated by the initiation process previously discussed; however, it differs from the low pressure mercury spectrum in that the typical spectral lines broaden and "shoulder" or "wing" lines appear on both sides of the characteristic lines. In addition, a weak continuous spectrum is generated. The majority of emitted energy is in the lines from 2967 to 3660 Angstroms. Due to the increased mercury vapor in the tube, the 2537 Angstrom line is almost totally self absorbed by the vapor and not emitted by the lamp.

Fused quartz envelopes are most often used due to the advantageous characteristics previously noted. The high pressure lamp envelope is normally at a high temperature; however, it can be air or water cooled, since both air and water transmit ultraviolet radiation. The use of fused quartz envelopes along with the high operating temperature produced has led to the use of the term *hot quartz lamps* in referring to these devices.

In comparing high and low pressure mercury lamps, the following items are the most important. High pressure mercury lamps require several minutes to reach full intensity, while low pressure lamps reach full intensity almost immediately. After turnoff, low pressure lamps can be immediately restarted, while high pressure lamps must be "rested" for a few minutes prior to restarting.

Two important factors that determine the operating efficiency of a mercury lamp are cleanliness and lamp deterioration. Keeping a lamp and the surrounding reflector clean prevents deterioration of the envelope and loss of ultraviolet radiation. Deterioration of the lamp itself can be caused by aging of the envelope, internal blackening of the envelope, and operation of the lamp at excessive voltages and/or unnecessary use.

Other Artificial Sources

Carbon Arc Lamps

In the latter part of the nineteenth century, carbon arc lights were introduced as an alternative method of street illumination to gas. Shortly after that, Niels Finsen originated artificial therapeutic radiation using carbon arc lamps.

The basic principle of the carbon arc is the production of radiation by vaporizing and ionizing inorganic salts in an electrical arc. Two carbon electrodes are opposed to each other, in series with a ballast resistance or choke coil. The electrodes are initially touching when a voltage is applied, then separated slightly. An arc is maintained between the electrodes, and three forms of radiation are generated. The heated electrode tips become incandescent and as such emit a continuous visible and infrared spectrum. The arc heats the inorganic salts and metals of the electrodes, causing characteristic line spectra to be emitted. To provide radiation at specified wavelengths, iron, strontium, aluminum, nickel, and rare earth metals such as cesium are placed in the electrode core. Carbon arcs, however, are low efficiency ultraviolet emitters, and the major radiation peak in all types of carbon arc lamps falls between 3500 and 4000 Angstroms. Other disadvantages include noise (sputtering), fumes, and ashes produced, as well as the high power consumption (15 to 20 amps) of these devices.

Fluorescent Ultraviolet Lamps

The so-called "black light" lamp is an example of a fluorescent ultraviolet lamp. These lamps are generally low pressure mercury devices in which the ultraviolet transmitting envelope is coated on its inner surface with a fluorescing substance called a phosphor. The specific type of phosphor used determines the wavelength of energy radiated. When "fired," the photons of the high energy mercury lines generated by the arc strike the phosphor and are absorbed. The process of fluorescence then takes place, and *longer* wavelength radiation is emitted by the phosphor.

Some "sun" lamps and the typical office fluorescent lamp belong to the same family of devices as the black light, all of which are low powered lamps and therefore must be used in groups to provide any degree of intensity.

Other Ultraviolet Lamps

The xenon arc lamp was previously mentioned as being a usable ultraviolet source; however, the potentially dangerous high pressure (20 atmospheres) and high power (1000 watts) necessary for its use make it less than desirable for routine use.

Molecular hydrogen and zirconium arc lamps are also used as ultraviolet generators but are not routinely found in typical institutions.

INFRARED GENERATORS

Therapeutic Heat

Luminous and Nonluminous Radiation Sources

The use of heat as an agent to relieve sore and aching muscles originated, in all probability, sometime during the stone age when the first caveman noticed that lying in the sun on a warm rock did wonders for a body fatigued by chasing (or being chased by) dinosaurs. In more recent times, Roman baths and hot springs have found similar acceptance. Today, the popularity of health club sauna and steam baths is no less common.

Unbeknownst to him, the caveman mentioned above was enjoying the two most common forms of therapeutic heat application, luminous heat (the sun) and nonluminous heat (the warm rock).

Heat is defined as a measure of the kinetic energy of the molecules in a particular substance or system. Cold, in contrast, is not a separate entity but rather the loss of or absence of heat.

An object heated to a higher temperature than its surroundings will give off heat in one or more of three ways: (1) by electromagnetic radiation, (2) by conduction, and (3) by convection. All of these modes are used in physical therapy in the form of lamps (radiation), hot packs (conduction), and water and paraffin baths (convection and conduction).

Luminous and nonluminous heat therapy uses electromagnetic radiation in the infrared and near-infrared region of the spectrum, from 7,000 to 120,000 (approximately) Angstroms. Natural sunlight consists of nearly 60 percent infrared energy, the remainder being visible and ultraviolet, and hence represents the most abundant natural source of radiant infrared energy.

Infrared radiation can be generated by two types of sources, the so-called luminous and nonluminous heat energy. The nonluminous sources do generate some visible radiation but mostly in the near-infrared region.

Nonluminous generators employ some form of resistive element through which an electric current is passed. Remembering some basic electricity, when a current is passed through a resistance, energy is dissipated in the form of heat ($P_{watts} = I^2_{current} \times R_{resistance}$). The temperature of the element is approximately 500° to 600°C. The energy dissipated is in the form of infrared radiation. A typical nonluminous generator consists of a resistance wire coil wound around a porcelain support rod. The rod is mounted in a reflective head and held on a support arm. Nonluminous generators operate from 50 to 1500 watts of power and come in various sizes.

Luminous infrared generators utilize the same resistance heating principle. However, due to the higher temperatures attained by the heating element, two problems arise: (1) the filament must be placed in an evacuated or inert gas atmosphere to prevent oxidation, and (2) a large part of the radiation generated is visible energy and therefore produces little heating.

Luminous infrared sources consist of tungsten or carbon filaments in glass or conical quartz bulbs with reflective metal back surfaces. Quartz is superior to other materials due to its insensitivity to thermal shock; contact with cold surfaces during operation will not cause it to crack or crystalize. In addition, quartz bulbs heat up and cool very rapidly.

Incandescent tungsten filament gas-filled bulbs (so-called heat lamps) are also used as infrared generators of the low wattage variety, as are ordinary household bulbs of the 25 to 50 watt type. The latter are often employed in bakers, where two or more bulbs are mounted in a reflective housing which can be placed over a patient's leg, arm, or body.

Conductive Heating Devices

Hot water bottles, which replaced the older heated stones or bricks as conductive heating devices, are still in use today in many places. The most recent form of conductive heating device, however, is the electric blanket. Once again, the basic principle employed is resistive heating, and the temperatures attained are low (maximum 110°). A typical heating blanket consists of a flexible heating element within an electrically insulated covering which is sewn between two layers of cloth. Temperature control is by way of a multiple-position switch and transformer or a variac.Temperature regulation is obtained by way of a bimetallic strip or other type of thermometer. High temperatures cause the switch to open, breaking the circuit and preventing current flow through the heating element. Once the temperature drops, the switch closes and heating resumes.

NERVE AND MUSCLE STIMULATING GENERATORS

Introduction

Low voltage electrotherapy constitutes the *only* form of therapy in which current flows *directly* from the therapeutic device into the patient. All other therapeutic modalities involve the transfer of *energy* from devices to patient without *direct* connection. Because of this direct connection between patient and current source, the therapist should be acutely aware of all the possible implications that arise by making the patient an integral circuit element. A firm understanding of the instrumentation involved is a necessary prerequisite in producing such an awareness.

Types of Current and Terminology

The low voltage currents employed in electrotherapy are no different than the currents found in any typical electrical instrument. They can be direct (DC) or alternating (AC) in nature, or a combination of both. The specificity of electrotherapeutic currents is due primarily to the type of waveform employed, more so than to the basic form of current. The terminology used in describing low voltage currents is far from standardized; however, all the terms used describe modifications of one or both of the two basic current forms.

Direct current is also termed galvanic current or continuous current, since it is characterized by the steady flow of charges in *one direction* through an electrical circuit (which, in this application, includes the patient).

Alternating current, as its name implies, periodically reverses its direction. The charges constituting the current flow migrate in one direction for a specified amount of time and then reverse their direction of migration.

The three basic *waveforms* used with alternating currents are as follows:

1. Sinusoidal
2. Rectangular (including pulsed square waves)
3. Trapezoidal (sawtooth)

The terms faradic, sinusoidal, and pulsed are used in describing specific types of AC waveforms based on the way in which the wave changes with time.

When a current is suddenly turned on and off at periodic intervals, it is termed an *interrupted* current. If, on the other hand, its magnitude is *gradually* increased and decreased, it is called a *surging* current. As noted previously, any alteration of the magnitude of a waveform is called *modulation;* hence both interruption and surging are forms of modulation. Both AC and DC currents can be interrupted and surged.

Figures 8-35 shows some of the more common waveforms

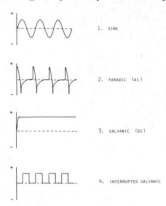

Figure 8-35. Common low voltage waveforms used in electrotherapy.

used in electrotherapy. From the physiological point of view, the overall effects of steady DC currents tend to be *chemical* in nature, producing ionic migration between the positive and negative terminals of a circuit. Alternating currents or interrupted DC result in *muscular contraction,* while pure AC (the positive and negative alterations supply equal energy) produces no net ion movement.

The *frequency* of an alternating current is defined as the number of cycles or complete alternations (positive to negative and back again) generated in one second. Hence, a 60 Hz current yields sixty cycles per second. The frequency of an AC current is an important criterion of classification, due primarily to the physiological effects it elicits. An AC current below 20 Hz applied to a healthy skeletal muscle will yield clonic contractions in proportion to the applied frequency. If, however, the frequency is greater than 20 Hz, tetanus occurs. As a result, frequencies below 20 Hz are called *pulse* frequencies and frequencies above 20 Hz are called *tetanizing* frequencies.

A Simplified Instrument

A block diagram of a simplified low voltage generator capable of delivering AC and DC currents of various forms is shown in Figure 8-36. Although individual manufacturers provide their own unique design features and specialized controls, a number of common characteristics can be found in virtually all instruments:

1. A power input cord consisting of three wires: a "hot" current carrying conductor, which is at a potential of 115 VAC when plugged in; a "cold" current carrying conductor, which is at ground potential and serves as a "return" for the "hot" side; a safety *ground* wire, which under *normal* conditions *does not* carry current but serves as a path to ground for unwanted charges appearing on the instrument cabinet.
2. A fuse located electrically on the input side of the power supply circuit. The fuse is placed in this position to ensure that if any excess current is drawn it will be felt immediately at the power supply and power will be interrupted. The physical placement of the fuse socket is generally at the rear of the instrument cabinet.
3. A main power switch and indicator or pilot light. The power switch, like the fuse, is also on the primary or input

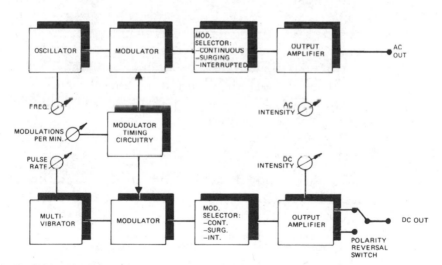

Figure 8-36. Block diagram of an electrotherapeutic generator. From Terence Karselis, *Descriptive Medical Electronics and Instrumentation*, 1973. Courtesy of Charles B. Slack, Inc., Thorofare, New Jersey.

side of the power supply circuit. A neon indicator bulb is hooked across the instrument side of the power supply to show that power is applied when the switch is closed.

4. Some form of output energy monitoring device, to allow continual observation of the current being passed through the patient. In most instances, this is accomplished by placing a milliampmeter in series with the patient electrodes and positioning the meter on the face of the instrument.

5. A timer, which is used to automatically cut off power to the electrodes after therapy has been applied for a preset time period. The timer is generally mechanically or electrically activated and provides capability for the operator to select periods of therapy from a few minutes to an hour.

6. Female electrode jacks, into which the insulated male electrode conductors are plugged. The jacks are marked as to polarity + and −) and may also be color coded, positive being *red*, negative being *black*.

7. A frequency control knob, which in most instances is actually the shaft of a variable resistance on, in some cases, a multiple position switch connected to a series of capacitors. The resistance or capacitance changes result in changes in the pulse generator frequency.

8. An intensity control for varying the current intensity being applied to the patient. This component is generally a wire-wound variable resistance acting as a rheostat, increasing the resistance in series with the patient leads and thereby decreasing the circuit current.

9. A switch, which, when activated, can reverse the polarity of the electrode jacks.

Every muscle stimulating device may not incorporate all of the above design features, but most will be found in the better, well-designed commercial instruments.

A Closer Look at an Actual Instrument

Figure 8-37 shows a block diagram of a commercial muscle stimulating device, the Burdick MS/600 (The Burdick Corporation, Milton, Wisconsin). The device is capable of delivering faradic (AC) current in either continuous, interrupted, surging,

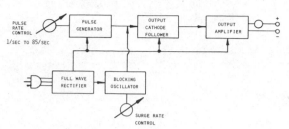

Figure 8-37. Burdick MS/600 muscle stimulator (faradic current). From information supplied by The Burdick Corporation, Milton, Wisconsin.

or pulsed form, as well as various levels and polarities of galvanic (DC) currents. The essential circuits are shown in the block diagram and are analyzed below. Figure 8-38 is the schematic diagram.

Power Supply

The power supply is a conventional, solid-state, full wave rectifier (CR1 and CR2) with RC filtering (C7, R18, C8), delivering two output voltages: 400 VDC for the output amplifier and 250 VDC for the pulse generator and surge blocking oscillator. The power supply also generates the galvanic current voltages.

Pulse Generator

The pulse generator (V1) is essentially a plate-coupled, free-running multivibrator. The pulse rate control (R20) is a variable resistance which controls the bias to one side of the multivibrator, and this, in conjunction with the time constant of the multivibrator coupling circuits, controls the pulse frequency.

Surge Blocking Oscillator

The blocking oscillator (V3) surge rate is controlled by way of a single fixed capacitance (C5) and a series of timing resistances connected by way of the surge rate switch. The discharge of the capacitor can be rapid (low resistance switched in), yielding eighty-five pulses per second, or it can be slow (high resistance switched in), yielding one pulse per second. In the nonsurge mode, the function switch removes power from the blocking oscillator.

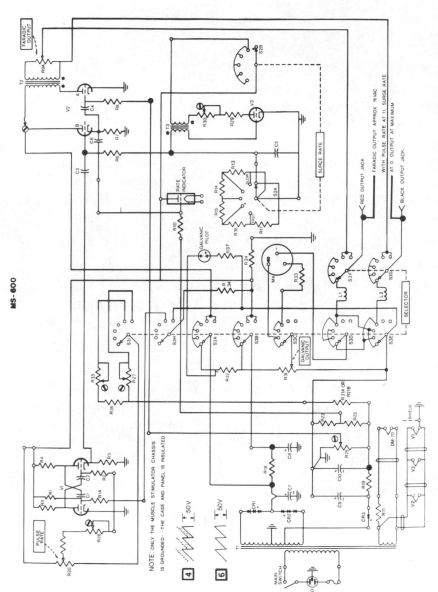

Figure 8-38. Burdick MS/600 schematic. Courtesy of The Burdick Corporation, Milton, Wisconsin.

Cathode Follower – Modulator

The cathode follower (V2-A) circuit is used to impedance match the pulse generator and blocking oscillator circuits to the output amplifier (V2-B). In the nonsurge mode, the pulse generator signal is simply fed through the cathode follower by way of C4 and R8 to the output amplifier. In the surge mode, the blocking oscillator's surge signal modulates the pulse generator output at the grid of the cathode follower by providing a varying bias.

Output Amplifier

The high voltage output amplifier (V2-B) couples the faradic output signal at its plate circuit through a pulse transformer (T2) across the secondary of which a variable resistance (R9A) is hooked. This is the faradic output level control. The signal is then fed to the output jacks by way of the function selector switch (S3).

Galvanic Circuitry

In the galvanic mode, the 250 VDC output of the power supply is fed through a variable resistance (R31), which functions as the galvanic (fine) output control, then on the high-low function switch, through the output current meter and out the electrode jacks. In the (+) galvanic mode, the red jack is internally grounded. In the (−) galvanic mode, the black jack is grounded. In either case, the electrodes must be connected to a load (the patient or a load resistance) before the meter will indicate, since the patient, electrodes, and meter constitute a series circuit. Figure 8-39 shows a simplified diagram of the galvanic circuitry.

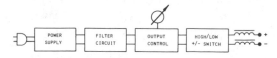

Figure 8-39. Block diagram of the Burdick MS/600 galvanic circuit. From information supplied by The Burdick Corporation, Milton, Wisconsin.

Transducers — Electrodes

When energy is transmitted from an instrument system into a biological system or vice versa, some form of transducer (a device that changes energy from one form to another) is generally required. For example, body temperature is transduced into an electrical signal by way of a thermistor in an electronic thermometer; electrical energy is transduced into sound waves by a piezoelectric crystal in ultrasound therapy. In electrotherapy, the transducer provides electrochemical contact between the patient and the instrument system, and since the energy on both sides of the interface is electrical, the transducer is termed an *electrode*.

Electrodes constitute the interconnecting element between the therapeutic device and the patient. The form or shape of the electrode is dictated by its use or application. Since it must transfer the current or voltage across the instrument-patient interface, its characteristics must provide optimal conditions for that transmission. Whether they are used to detect signals and transmit them to an instrument or, as in the case of therapeutic applications, transmit current into the patient, all contain one common denominator: they are biphasic electrochemical elements consisting of a metal-electrolyte system. In the case of electrodes used in physical therapy, the electrolyte can be as simple as a normal saline solution or special electrode paste formulations. The actual charge transfer across the instrument-patient interface involves complex electrochemical gradients and physiochemical processes. Although these processes are of primary importance in "sensing" and recording bioelectric potentials, the single most important factor in therapeutic electrode application is the concept of "current density." If one remembers that current measurement is based on the number of charges that pass a given point in a circuit (remembering that the point has some cross-sectional area) in a given amount of time, the current density will vary as the cross-sectional area of that point changes. Hence, if the current flow passing a point having a 1 mm area is 15 milliamps, cutting the area in half will result in a current of 30 milliamps; the current density has increased. It is this principle which is *one* of the governing factors in the use of the so-called dispersive electrode in therapeutic applications. By use of a large area electrode placed distal from the application point of the active electrode, the current is dispersed throughout a large tissue volume and the exit current density is also lowered. Accidental conditions in which the dispersive electrode is making contact at a few points of small cross-sectional area, or if the patient is touching a grounded metallic object (a metal bed or table), can cause severe necrotizing burns due to excessively high current density.

The electrodes used in electrotherapy run the gamut from bare metallic sheets to specially designed metal-impregnated rubber or plastic. The active electrode is of smaller area than the dispersing electrode and usually is mounted on the end of a handle into which a switch has been incorporated to allow the therapist to interrupt the current. An absorbent material such as felt, gauze, or cotton, soaked with the appropriate solution, provides the electrolyte phase.

The Burdick Corporation of Milton, Wisconsin, has developed molded, metal-impregnated electrodes called Conductrodes™ which have no sharp edges or exposed metal. A well-moistened gauze pad provides the electrolyte phase between the patient and the Conductrode surface. These electrodes have the advantage of being noncorrosive and easily cleanable as well as being flexible. They can easily be cleaned with alcohol or even autoclaved. They are available in 5″, 3″, and 1″ diameter sizes.

TRANSCUTANEOUS ELECTRICAL NERVE STIMULATORS (TENS)

When Melzack and Wall outlined their "gate theory" of pain and its perception in the mid-1960s, they inadvertently provided a new focus for the application of stimulation instrumentation. In the early 1970s, commercial instrument companies began producing instruments specifically for TENS (Transcutaneous Electrical Nerve Stimulation) applications, two of the first being Medtronics, Inc., and Stimulation Technology, Inc.

The primary goal of this new arm of biomedical instrumentation was the relief of pain with minimal discomfort due to the stimulator's output. In addition, design features such as size, weight, ease of operation, and safety had to be considered, the ultimate goal being a device that the patient could use himself with a good degree of success.

The early instruments furnished by commercial companies were basically modifications of existing muscle stimulator technology, with operator adjustable controls for (1) Pulse Width, (2) Pulse Repetition Rate, and (3) Pulse Amplitude, and a set of bipolar electrodes. Pulse forms used in these early devices were (a) square waves (Stimulation Technology) and (b) spiked waves (Medtronics). Today the field has expanded to include various other manufacturers (i.e. EMPI, Med. General, and Medical Device Industries), offering a wide variety of stimulators with just as wide a variety of operating characteristics. No two devices look alike, nor do they have identical specifications in terms of Pulse Width Amplitude, Pulse Rate, and output waveform.

As noted above, most if not all TENS units are essentially pulse generators having either one or two channels with operator variable output characteristics and battery power, and hence are portable. This feature allows the patient to be treated on an outpatient basis with self-administered therapy. No two devices are exactly alike, yet their characteristics (which are variable) can be grouped as follows and applied to all TENS units available today:

1. *Pulse Width.* May be fixed or variable. If variable, may be adjustable between 20 and 500 microseconds.
2. *Pulse Amplitude.* Generally variable from 0 to 200 volts.
3. *Pulse (Repetition) Rate.* Variable 1 to 150 pulses per second. This characteristic is also referred to as Pulse Frequency.
4. *Waveform.* The voltage/time graph of the applied stimulus. Varies from square or rectangular waved to spiked, biphasic pulses. May be symmetrical or asymmetrical.
5. *Constant Voltage/Current Capability.* Most TENS units claim either a constant voltage or constant current output capability, while another combines the two effects into a single pulse.

Though the above characteristics vary from manufacturer to

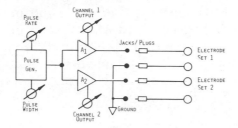

Figure 8-40. A typical early TENS system.

manufacturer, the trend today is for the output pulse to be a modified asymmetrical square wave of variable (0 to 60 V) amplitude.

Figure 8-40 shows a block diagram based on an early TENS unit (StimTech®, E.P.C. Diagnostic) consisting of a pulse generator whose output is split into two output channels. Note that the pulse width and rate adjust function are common to both channels. In other words, changing the pulse width of rate on one channel changes it automatically on the other. The amplitude controls are independent, allowing each to be adjusted individually.

The trend in portable TENS units available today is for two fully independent channels, with pulse width rate and amplitude adjustments completely independent from channel to channel.

The therapist employing TENS should be cognizant of the importance of correct interpretation and application of manufacturers' claimed characteristics. For example, which is most desirable, constant voltage or constant current? Studies reported by Shealy and Maurer in the mid-1970s claimed that a constant current stimulus provided a more effective treatment than constant voltage, due to its more effective coupling to peripheral nerves. Other investigators have more confidence in constant voltage techniques and clearly specified waveforms, while a recent entry into the market, EMPI's 910 Neuropacer®, employs a symmetrical biphasic waveform consisting of both a constant voltage positive pulse and a constant current negative spike. In the final analysis, what is most important is an informed and thoughtful therapist capable of an educated choice, since, due to the high degree of variability between patients, both physically and psychologically, it is doubtful that any one set of instrumental conditions will be universally acceptable or applicable. The patient constitutes an electrical load with such varied characteristics that flexibility must be built into the instrument itself.

Another important factor that therapists must be aware of is the possibility of localized burns from the use of too small an electrode. It has been demonstrated that the heat produced at an electrode must be below 250m cal/cm²/sec for a 500m sec 85ma pulse at 185 pps. In the simplest analytical sense, the electrode-patient interface constitutes a conductor, and any power it dissipates (heat generated) is a product of the conductor current squared times its resistance (I^2R). As electrode contact area is increased, the current density is reduced, and hence the power dissipation per unit area is reduced. A good rule of thumb, therefore, would be to choose larger electrodes (greater than 4 cm² for the above noted ratings), rather than small, for the sake of safety.

In order to compare the previously noted list of characteristics with a typical commercial unit, the following information is given. The data was supplied by EMPI, Inc., Minneapolis, Minnesota, via their sales literature:

Model: **EMPI-TENS 980 DC Dual Channel Neuropacer**

1. *Pulse Width.* Square wave (@ 50% amplitude) constant voltage 0 to 400 μsec coupled with a negative exponential spike of 200 μsec constant current.
2. *Pulse Amplitude.* 0 to 60 volts (pp) into a 100 ohm load.
3. *Pulse (Repetition) Rate.* 1 to 100 pps.
4. *Waveform.*

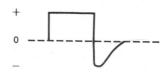

5. *Constant Voltage/Current.* Combined as indicated in pulse width data.

TABLE 8-II

	Medtronic	EMPI	Pain Suppression Labs	Med. General	M.D.I.	Stim-Tech
Pulse Width	Fixed 30 μsec	Variable 50-250 μsec	Fixed	Variable 120-33 μsec	Variable 20-600 μsec	Variable 50-250 μsec
Pulse Amp.	0-75 V	0-60 V	0-40 milliwatts	0-210 V	0-80 milliamps	0-50 milliamps
Pulse (Rep.) Rate	3-85	-100	12-20	12-100	50-100	15-150
Waveform	Biphasic Decaying Spike	Modified Square Wave Negative Spike Symmetrical	——	Asymmetrical Biphasic	Asymmetrical Biphasic	Modified Rectangular

An additional design feature of the EMPI unit is the cycled operation designed into it to increase battery life. The unit is automatically turned off every 2 seconds and remains off for 3 seconds and is then cycled on again for 2 more seconds. The manufacturers claim no interruption of pain relief.

Table 8-II gives comparative data on six TENS units on the market as of 1979. Note the wide variability in characteristics.

SHORT WAVE DIATHERMY GENERATORS

Introduction

As noted in a previous section, the use of heat as a therapeutic agent is as old as man himself. However, it was not until the late nineteenth century that high frequency radiation was discovered to cause heating of the tissues through which it was passed.

Although both ultraviolet and infrared heating involve the absorption of electromagnetic radiation to produce heating, their effects are characteristically different from diathermy in that diathermy produces a dispersive deep tissue heating while the former two are restricted to superficial tissue effects.

The total energy of any system is the sum of its potential energy plus kinetic energy. In turn, the amount of kinetic energy within a system is indicated by its temperature (in short, the amount of heat in the system). From this, one can conclude that any alteration of the kinetic energy of the system will result in a heating or cooling effect. Energy absorbed by a molecular system must be utilized in one of a number of ways: (1) by chemical reaction, (2) by reemitting the energy (fluorescence, phosphorescence), (3) by transfer due to molecular collision, or (4) by conversion to vibrational, rotational, or translational kinetic energy. This latter method is the basis for deep tissue heating via diathermy.

Types of Diathermy

Historically, the two early forms of diathermy were "long wave" and "short wave" diathermy, designations based on the relative wavelength of the radiation employed. Long wave diathermy utilized a wavelength of approximately 300 meters (1 megahertz) and short wave diathermy from 3 to 30 meters (10 to

100 megahertz). Short wave diathermy has operating frequencies between 10 and 100 MHz, while microwave diathermy has an operating frequency in the 2,000 megahertz region and wavelengths of approximately 12 cm. As of the 1980s, microwave diathermy is seldom used clinically. When the subcutaneous fat layer is more than 1 cm thick, the TTR in underlying soft tissue is negligible.

It was noted in a previous section that the higher the frequency of radiation, the greater its penetrating capability. Hence, the ability to provide deep tissue heating and the resulting efficiency is directly proportional to the frequency of the radiation employed. The major practical difference between short wave and microwave diathermy is in the transmission of the energy to the patient. Short wave transmission requires the patient to become an integral part of the output circuit, even though he is not *directly* in a conduction path. In contrast, microwaves, due to their higher energy and shorter wavelength, assume qualities resembling visible light and as such can be projected, reflected, and focused. Hence, in applying this mode of therapy to a patient, direct contact is *not* required between patient and instrument.

A Simplified Short Wave Diathermy Unit

A simplified block diagram of a short wave diathermy unit is shown in Figure 8-41. The unit has essentially four subcircuits:

1. A *Radio Frequency Oscillator* provides stable, drift-free oscillations at the required frequency. Since oscillators are prone to drift as load conditions upon it change, it must be

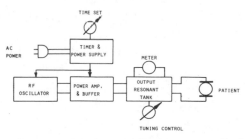

Figure 8-41. Block diagram of a simple short wave diathermy unit.

isolated from the patient circuit. Isolation is provided by way of the following circuit.

2. The *Output Power Amplifier* serves not only as a buffer between the oscillator and the patient circuit but also as an amplifier capable of generating the power required to drive the electrodes.

3. The *Output Resonant Tank* circuit is an LC circuit made up of the *secondary* winding of the output transformer (the primary serves as the load for the output power amplifier), in parallel with a tuning capacitor, both of which are in parallel with the patient. With the patient between the electrodes, the output tuning capacitor is adjusted until the circuit is at resonance, at which time maximum power can be transferred to the patient.

4. The *Power Supply* provides the voltages required to drive the RF oscillator and power amplifier. In addition, a timer is incorporated which must be activated to turn on the unit. After the prescribed treatment time has elapsed, the timer automatically removes AC power.

Patient cables and electrodes used with short wave diathermy must be of the shielded cable type. This ensures maximum energy transfer to the applicator electrode with minimal loss of energy.

The controls and indicators found on the type of device listed above would be as follows:

1. A main *Power Switch* for applying AC line power to the unit.

2. A *Timer* for controlling the duration of the therapeutic dose. Most timers are designed so that the timer shuts off power when the time runs out.

3. An *Output Intensity* control, allowing variation of the power applied to the patient.

4. A *Tuning Control,* which tunes the output circuit, including the patient (the load), for maximum energy transfer from RF oscillator circuit to the output.

5. An *Output Power Meter,* enabling the operator to monitor the relative energy being applied to the patient.

It should be noted that in this type of instrument, the output meter monitors only the current drawn by the output amplifier and *not* the output power in the patient circuit; hence, it is only an *indirect* measurement of energy reaching the patient and not a true measurement.

Some Actual Instruments

Two commercially available short wave diathermy units that are basically the same as the simplified instrument outlined above are the Burdick Model MF/490 and the Birtcher Model 800 Crystal Bandmaster. These devices, although they operate at different frequencies, are sufficiently alike from a general viewpoint to warrant that a comparative analysis be undertaken. Each of the circuits outlined in the simplified discussion above will be discussed in more detail for each unit (Figs. 8-42 and 8-43).

Power Supplies

BURDICK MF/490. The power supply consists of a power transformer (T_1) which is energized only when a timer, an overload circuit breaker, a cabinet door interlock, and a power on switch are all activated. All these interlocks are on the primary side of the transformer. The high voltage secondary windings of the transformer supply high AC voltage to the RF oscillator (812A) and the power amplifier (810). The 10 and 6.3 low voltage secondaries supply filament voltage to the same two tubes. AC voltage is used as plate supply to these tubes, since no modulation is required and therefore DC is unnecessary.

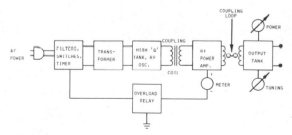

Figure 8-42A. Block diagram of the Burdick MF/490 short wave diathermy unit — 27.12 MHz. From information supplied by The Burdick Corporation, Milton, Wisconsin.

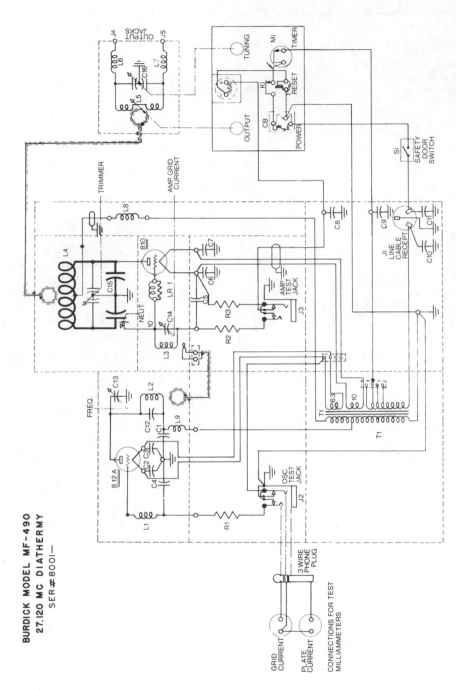

Figure 8-42B. Burdick Model MF/490 diathermy schematic diagram. Courtesy of The Burdick Corporation, Milton, Wisconsin.

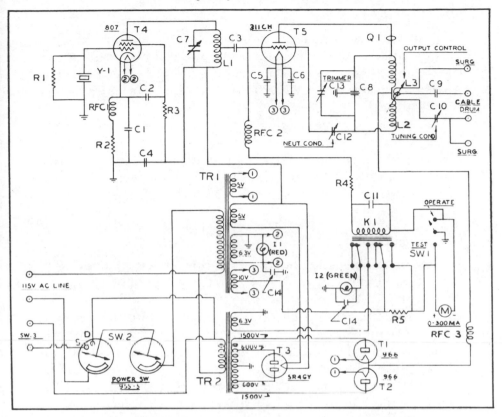

Figure 8-43. Birtcher 800 Crystal Bandmaster short wave diathermy schematic. Courtesy of The Birtcher Corporation, Los Angeles, California.

BIRTCHER 800. The Birtcher power supply contains (1) a function switch (Sw2), (2) a filament transformer (TR1), (3) a power transformer (TR2), and (4) rectifier tubes (T1 and T2). The function switch serves to provide either diathermy or surgical modes of operation by energizing either both TR1 and TR2 or TR1 alone. The filament transformer provides outputs to 5 volts, 6.3 volts, and 10 volts for rectifier filaments, oscillator filaments, and amplifier filaments, respectively. The power transformer yields a 600 volt output for a full wave rectifier (T1-T2) and a 1500 volt output for a half wave rectifier (T3). The full wave rectifier DC output supplies the operating voltages for the RF oscillator (T4), while the half wave rectifier serves the output amplifier (T5) through an RF choke (RFC3).

Oscillator Circuits

BURDICK. The tuned, plate-tuned grid RF oscillator (812A) is a conventional RF oscillator utilizing interelectrode capacitance between plate and grid to provide regenerative feedback. The oscillating frequency is 27.120 MHz $\pm$ 21.5 KHz and is factory set by adjusting C13.

BIRTCHER. A crystal-controlled, tuned, plate-tuned grid tetrode oscillator (T4) provides the RF energy with feedback from the plate tank circuit (C7-L1) by way of interelectrode capacitance. The crystal (Y-1) provides stable oscillations at 6.78 MHz, and the oscillator output is tuned to 13.56 MHz (1st even harmonic).

Amplifier Circuits

BURDICK. The oscillator signal is loop coupled from the oscillator output tank circuit (C12-L2) to the RF amplifier grid tank circuit (L3-C14). The signal is amplified and fed by way of the plate tank circuit (C15-L4) and coupling loop to the resonant output circuit. A neutralizing capacitor is factory tuned to prevent plate-to-grid feedback from producing self-oscillation of the amplifier. The output meter monitors the grid current in the amplifier which is maximum at resonance.

BIRTCHER. The oscillator signal is capacitive coupled by way of C-3 to the grid of the amplifier tube (T5), where it is amplified and passed through the output resonant tank circuit (L2-C8) to the secondary coil (L3). C-12 is a neutralizing capacity to prevent self-oscillation of the amplifier.

Output Circuits

BURDICK. A parallel tuned circuit (C16-L5), two series inductors (L6-L7), and the applicator electrodes constitute the resonant output circuit. C16 is the tuning element, which is adjusted to peak the plate current at resonance. L5 is then adjusted to select the appropriate output power by varying the coupling ability of the tank.

BIRTCHER. The output circuit is a series resonant circuit consisting of inductor L3, capacitors C9 and C10, and the applicators. Adjusting C10 resonates the patient circuit with the ampli-

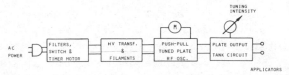

Figure 8-44. Block diagram of the Birtcher 860 diathermy unit. From information supplied by The Birtcher Corporation, Los Angeles, Calif.

fier tank circuit. Output energy is adjusted by altering the coupling ability of output coil L3. It should be noted that both output circuits are tuned by matching the output circuit impedance to the amplifier tank circuit impedance with tuning controls, i.e. peaking the output meter to maximum. At that time, maximum energy is transferred from amplifier to output. This adjustment must therefore be made with the output control at a minimal or low *after* the output circuit is tuned to resonance. The amount of energy coupled to the output circuit is varied by the output control.

Another Birtcher short wave diathermy unit is the Birtcher Model 860 Crusader II, having an output frequency of 27.12 MHz. Figure 8-44 shows a block diagram of this instrument. The power supply contains essentially a fuse, a combined timer/on-off switch, and a transformer. The transformer supplies AC filament and plate voltage to the oscillator stage. The oscillator is a tuned plate, push-pull RF generator utilizing interelectrode capacitance regenerative feedback to sustain oscillations. The grid current drawn by the oscillator tubes is used as an indicator of output power by the output meter. The *oscillator* plate circuit resonant tank couples energy to the output circuit parallel tunable tank, which controls the power applied to the applicators. A single control (output) is used to provide both tuning of the tank and output energy intensity. This is accomplished by tuning the circuit for increased output and *detuning* for less output.

Many new commercial diathermy units are now providing the capability of automatic or self-tuning. This is advantageous in instances where patient movement causes the output circuit to go out of resonance. In such instances, some units employ a type of feedback control system (servomechanism) to retune the output. The unit shown below constantly monitors the output, which contains not just the 27.120 MHz primary frequency but two side band frequencies, an upper 27.22 MHz and a lower 27.02 MHz. When the output is tuned, the side band frequencies are equal in magnitude, causing no response in the servodetector (a form of differential detector). Should the system *not* be in resonance, the difference between the side band signals activates a servomotor, which returns the circuit until the side band signals are again equal and the output is once again resonance.

A Unique New Device

Figure 8-46 shows a photograph of a relatively new commercial short wave diathermy unit, the Mettler Electronics Autotherm®. Some of the more unique features of this device are (1) it is self tuning, (2) the output meter indicates the relative energy dose absorbed by the patient, and (3) it is compact and light in weight.

Figure 8-47 shows a block diagram of the functional circuits of this device. As shown in Figure 8-46, the unit consists essentially

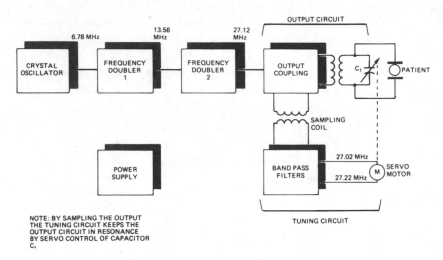

Figure 8-45. Block diagram of a short wave diathermy unit with automatic tuning. From Terence Karselis, *Descriptive Medical Electronics and Instrumentation,* 1973. Courtesy of Charles B. Slack, Inc., Thorofare, New Jersey.

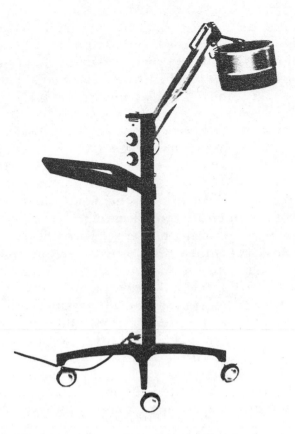

Figure 8-46. Mettler Autotherm™ short wave diathermy unit. Courtesy of Mettler Electronics Corporation, Anaheim, California.

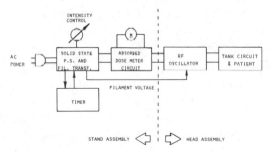

Figure 8-47. Block diagram of the Mettler Autotherm™ short wave diathermy unit. From information supplied by Mettler Electronics Corporation, Anaheim, California.

of two parts: a mobile stand with controls and meter plus a RF unit/applicator drum head. A solid-state high voltage power supply plus a unique absorbed dose meter circuit constitute the major portion of the circuitry contained in the stand, along with a filament transformer for the RF oscillator and a timer. In the power supply, AC line voltage is rectified into 600 volts DC by way of a *full wave quadrupler.* This voltage is fed through the meter circuit to the *RF oscillator* in the drum head enclosure. The *meter circuit* monitors the voltage at the RF oscillator plate and screen grid circuits and by computing the difference indicates the true relative power absorbed by the patient. With no patient in the output circuit field, the meter will indicate zero, regardless of the intensity control setting.

The drum head enclosure houses the RF oscillator, which is a dual pentode class C tuned, plate-tuned grid, push-pull oscillator circuit. Oscillations are sustained by interelectrode capacitance feedback. Adjustment of the output intensity is controlled by varying the screen grid voltages. The circuit's design is such that it creates little RF interference noise and consequently requires minimal shielding. This permits its use directly on the patient, whereas in *all other short wave diathermy units, the primary generator is enclosed in a strongly shielded cabinet* and is coupled to a secondary patient circuit. In addition, the patient circuit is a self-tuning multiple capacitor tank and is always in resonance with itself.

Transducers — Applicators

The interfacing element between an instrument system and a human system is the transducer. However, in therapeutic settings involving the application of energy, they are more generally termed *applicators.* Short wave diathermy applicators are either of the capacitive or inductive type, based on the type of energy used to apply the therapy. When an *electrostatic* field is used, the patient becomes an integral part of the output circuit. He is placed between two applicator surfaces and consequently becomes the dielectric material between the plates of a capacitor. Therapeutic energy then passes from plate to plate via the patient. When the transmitted energy is electromagnetic in na-

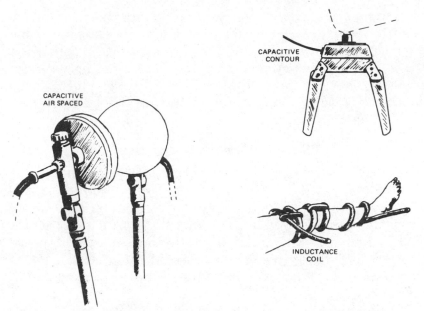

Figure 8-48. Short wave diathermy applicators. From Terence Karselis, *Descriptive Medical Electronics and Instrumentation*, 1973. Courtesy of Charles B. Slack, Inc.. Thorofare, New Jersey.

ture, the patient is positioned within the RF magnetic field generated around copper-braided insulated wires. These wires may be coiled around a limb or "pancaked" onto the body surface. Figure 8-48 shows three types of short wave diathermy applicators.

MICROWAVE DIATHERMY GENERATORS

Introduction

One of the most important inventions to emerge during the World War II era was radar. Initially, it was developed and used as a ground-based defense system to detect enemy aircraft; later, it was further sophisticated and placed in aircraft. The requirements for airborne radar necessitated smaller systems and higher frequencies; this in turn led to the final development of *microwave* radar. From this military development came the therapeutic agent *microwave diathermy*. The single most important advantage of microwave diathermy is its capability to produce rapid, localized deep heating. This is in contrast to the somewhat dispersive type of heating produced by short wave diathermy.

The ability to generate microwave frequencies necessary in airborne radar systems originated with the development of the multicavity magnatron, a complete RF oscillator-amplifier in one package.

The Multicavity Magnatron

The higher the frequency an oscillator is required to generate, the greater the associated circuit effects of interelectrode capacitance and inductance. Consequently, conventional tubes are incapable of efficient operation above 20 MHz. The search for high frequency power circuits led to the development of special devices called cavity resonators. Two of these are the *reflex-klystron* and the *magnatron*. The latter is the heart of all microwave diathermy units.

A magnatron is essentially a diode tube with a cylindrical hollow block acting as the anode around a centrally located cathode. Circular cavities (hence the name cavity resonator) are cut out of the anode, resulting in multiple anode segments separated by cavities. Each cavity functions electronically as an individual resonant circuit of a single inductor coil segment (the diameter) and a single capacitor (the top and bottom walls). In a conventional tube, an applied electric field existing between cathode and anode causes electrons to flow in a straight path from cathode to anode. In a magnatron, an electric field is present, but in addition, a magnetic field is also applied. The electric field is produced by keeping the anode at zero potential and the cathode at a high negative. The magnetic field is applied perpendicular to the electric field by way of heavy alnico magnets. Electrons flowing from cathode to anode therefore follow a helical spirallike path due to the combined effects of the two fields. As they pass the cavity slots, energy is transferred to the energy field of the cavity, causing the cavity to oscillate. Figure 8-49 shows a cavity magnatron and the path of an electron. The resonant oscillations occurring within the cavity result in magnetic variations, which are picked up by an inductive probe and

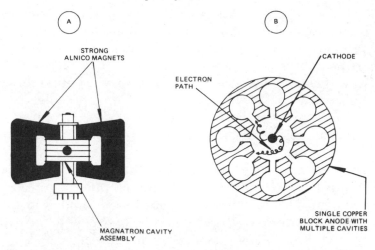

Figure 8-49. (A) shows a simplified drawing of a magnatron. (B) is a cutaway top view of the cavity assembly with spirallike electron paths. From Terence Karselis, *Descriptive Medical Electronics and Instrumentation*, 1973. Courtesy of Charles B. Slack, Inc., Thorofare, New Jersey.

coupled by way of a coaxial cable to the transmitting antenna and reflector. The magnatron provides high frequency oscillations with high output power; it is analogous to a combination oscillator-amplifier system. Magnatrons used in radar systems are capable of generating RF energy in megawatt amounts; however, the maximum output of any medical microwave magnatron is limited to approximately 150 watts.

A Simplified Microwave Generator

Figure 8-50 shows the block diagram of a typical microwave diathermy unit.

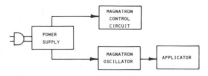

Figure 8-50. Simplified block diagram of a microwave diathermy unit. From Terence Karselis, *Descriptive Medical Electronics and Instrumentation*, 1973. Courtesy of Charles B. Slack, Inc., Thorofare, New Jersey.

The *power supply* furnishes power for energizing the magna-tron oscillator and the timing circuitry. Since the cathode voltage of a magnatron is a large negative potential (3000 V), some form of rectification is necessary.

The *magnatron control circuit* controls the output power of the system by way of varying the magnatron operating voltage. Safety circuitry is necessary to prevent excessive output. This can be accomplished by an overload circuit monitoring the mag-natron current.

The *magnatron oscillator* provides high power RF energy, which must be coaxially coupled to the applicator head. The current drawn by the magnatron when monitored by an output meter is a direct measure of the energy *transmitted* to the patient. This is not, however, a measure of *absorbed* energy.

An Actual Instrument

An example of a typical commercial microwave diathermy unit is the Burdick Model MW/225 (Fig. 8-51). This device has essentially the same substages as the previous simplified instru-ment, with various additions.

The front panel controls and indicators are as follows:

1. An on-off power switch controlling AC line power to the instrument.
2. A timing control, allowing the operator to adjust the time of applied therapy. This timer automatically cuts power to the unit after the preselected time has elapsed.
3. An *output* level control, which controls the amount of ener-gy being transmitted to the patient. This control is not calibrated, since the output is monitored by the operator using the output meter.
4. An *output* meter, which indicates the relative output energy in watts. As noted previously, this is the transmitted ener-gy, *not* the absorbed energy.
5. Two colored indicator lamps: an *amber* "standby" indicator, showing that power is applied to the unit, and a *red* "out-put" lamp, showing that microwave output is available.

In addition to the obvious visible controls, a built-in safety

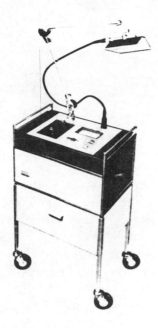

Figure 8-51. Burdick Model MW/225 microwave diathermy unit. Courtesy of The Burdick Corporation, Milton, Wisconsin.

feature is the reset function of the *output* level control. After therapy has been applied for a given amount of time and the timer has cut power, in order to reactivate the system, the output control must be turned back to zero in order to reset the safety lock-out relay. It can then be adjusted to give an output. The same reactivation procedure must also be followed to restore power if the overload relay has deenergized the system.

A closer look at the instrument can be obtained by studying the block diagram in Figure 8-52.

The input *power control circuit* contains the timer, power switch, and output control, along with a cooling fan. The output control is a variac located in the power supply, which permits adjustment of the voltage fed to the magnatron cathode high voltage transformer primary. Adjusting this control effectively changes the voltage at the magnatron cathode. The timer, overload relay,

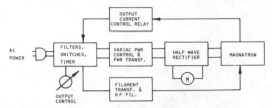

Figure 8-52. Block diagram of the Burdick MW/225 microwave diathermy unit. From information supplied by The Burdick Corporation, Milton, Wisconsin.

and power switch interrupt voltage applied to the variac and hence to the high voltage transformer.

The magnatron filament transformer is energized at all times after the power-on switch is closed, thereby maintaining the magnatron in a standby condition.

The solid-state half wave rectifier provides a negative DC voltage to the magnatron cathode of approximately 3500 volts. This is sufficient to cause oscillations. An output current limiting (overload) relay senses the magnatron cathode current and shuts off power if it exceeds 74 mA (equivalent to 130 watts output). The output energy is inductively coupled from the magnatron to the reflector head by way of coaxial tubing.

Transducers — Antennas/Reflectors

The application of microwave energy requires specialized devices known generally as reflectors. These elements are in reality directional antennas, since microwave energy, as noted previously, due to its short wavelength has optical properties in that it can be reflected, refracted, and focused. Put simply, microwaves follow a line-of-sight propagation path, while short wave RF energy is omnidirectional in nature.

The energy fed into a microwave applicator is first coaxially coupled to a radiating element and then focused and directed by a reflecting element. The electrical energy transmitted along the coaxial cable terminates at the radiating device, where it is transformed into electromagnetic waves. The radiating device is actually a small antenna, which, when matched by correct manufacture to the wavelength of the energy to be propagated, acts

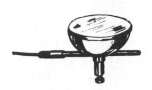 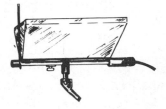

Figure 8-53. Microwave diathermy applicators. From Terence Karselis, *Descriptive Medical Electronics and Instrumentation*, 1973. Courtesy of Charles B. Slack, Inc., Thorofare, New Jersey.

like a resonant circuit, exhibiting no reactance, just pure resistance. The radiated energy emitted from the antenna propagates according to a definite pattern; therefore, a reflecting element is used to focus the energy in the desired direction. The reflectors used in microwave diathermy may be parabolic hemispheres or rectangular "corner" types, as shown in Figure 8-53. Dose information and spacing data are generally printed on the outside of the reflectors.

In comparing the instrument systems used for applying short wave and microwave diathermy, a major advantage that the latter system appears to have is its simplicity of application and control. Since the factors influencing the energy dosage received by the patient are output power, time of application, and distance between applicator and patient, once the reflector is aligned and set, application requires little more than adjusting the output power (generally calibrated in percentages of maximum output) and setting the timer (between 20 and 30 minutes). No output circuit tuning is required, and the need for continual monitoring to determine if the output circuit remains tuned (or, alternatively, automatic tuning circuitry) is removed. A second advantage is patient comfort and ease. With microwave therapy, no component of the instrument system touches the patient. This small fact is in itself greatly comforting to patients who tend to be nervous and hypersensitive.

The disadvantages of this type of diathermy are the limited effect of one-sided application of the energy stream, and the skin reflection that occurs due to the optical nature of microwave energy.

ELECTRODIAGNOSTIC DEVICES

Introduction

The now-famous "twitch" of Galvani's frog in the eighteenth century heralded the birth of the field of electrophysiology, one subdivision of which is the modern specialty of electrodiagnosis. Electrodiagnosis can be defined as the diagnosis of disease states associated with the neuromuscular system by (1) studying the mechanical response to externally applied stimulation, termed *myography,* (2) analysis of the electrical signals generated by way of externally applied stimulation or spontaneous activity, termed *electromyography (EMG),* or (3) studying the speed at which action potentials are passed along a particular segment of the nervous system, termed *conduction velocity analysis.* Under (1) fall the so-called classical techniques of faradic (AC) and galvanic (DC) stimulation to observe the *reaction of degeneration* (RD) of a damaged neuromuscular unit, as well as the more modern techniques of *strength-duration* analysis and chronaximetry. A brief description of the instrumentation used with each of the above modalities will be given in the following section.

Classical Electrodiagnosis Instrumentation

Classical Myography (RD Studies) Devices

As noted above, the primary function of classical faradic/galvanic myography is the determination of *reaction to degeneration.* The instrumentation required for this technique can vary from extremely simple combinations of components to complex pulse generators. Whatever its shape, size, or level of sophistication, the essential requirements for such a device are as follows: (1) the ability to deliver a continuous DC current at variable magnitudes and (2) the ability to supply alternating current pulses of approximately 1 millisecond duration at repetition rates of 50 to 200 per second. These functions can be accomplished by two crude but utterly simple circuits. The variable DC current can be generated by a 45 VDC battery or series of batteries together with a variable resistance. The AC current can be obtained by using a DC voltage source together with a faradic coil. The faradic coil is actually a combination relay/transformer

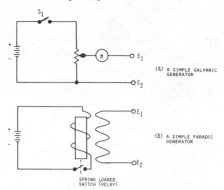

Figure 8-54. Galvanic and faradic generators.

in which the DC, energizing current as it flows in the *primary* winding, activates a set of its own contacts. The relay contacts open, thereby removing power from the primary circuit and causing the coil to deenergize. The constantly energizing-deenergizing sequence induces pulses of energy into the secondary winding, which serves as the output circuit to the patient. Both of these circuits are shown in Figure 8-54. E and E_2 refer to the electrodes. The pulse repetition rate can be adjusted by adjusting the gap of the relay contacts.

The currents generated by the above circuits, or suitable substitutes, can also be obtained from most commercial therapeutic instruments, as well as from some chronaximeters, as will be discussed.

Strength-Duration/Chronaxie Analysis Devices

While classical myography can assess *qualitatively* the response of a neuromuscular unit to stimulation, the two factors of importance in attempting to assess such response *quantatively* are the *strength* of the stimulating current and the *duration* of its application. These two factors are of primary importance due to the fact that effective stimulation of a biological cell requires that a specified *charge mass* cross its membrane in order to generate an action potential. The practical consequence of this fact is that a short duration pulse of high current intensity can produce the same result as a lower intensity pulse of longer duration. A lower

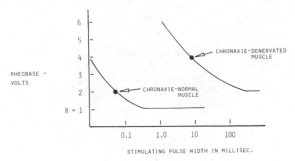

Figure 8-55. Strength-duration curves with chronaxie points.

limit of intensity, however, is produced by charge diffusion across the cell membrane, which opposes the low level stimulating current. The minimal stimulus intensity below which no response is produced in neuromuscular tissue, even if the stimulus is applied continually, is called the *rheobase*. By applying pulses of varying amplitude and duration, strength-duration curves can be constructed for a particular muscle or nerve, as shown in Figure 8-55. When the amplitude of the rheobase is doubled, the pulse width capable of eliciting the same response as the initial amplitude is termed *chronaxie*. This arbitrary index of excitation is actually the reciprocal of neuromuscular excitability, since as the excitability of a nerve or muscle is impaired due to disease or injury, its chronaxie would increase. The two parameters of chronaxie and rheobase are studied collectively, since the former cannot be determined without first measuring rheobase.

The instrumentation required to perform the above measurements can be specifically designed for such application (for example, the TECA CH3 Chronaxie Meter and Variable Pulse Generator, manufactured by TECA Corp., White Plains, New York), or the same results can be obtained by using any pulse generator or stimulator having the capability of providing precise pulse amplitude, duration, and repetition rate selection. Earlier chronaximetry devices utilized capacitive discharge RC circuits to generate pulses of the required duration. As discussed in an earlier section, the charge-discharge time for a capacitor for a given amount of charge is determined by the size of the capacitor and the resistance through which it must charge or discharge. The period in which 63.2 percent of the applied charge accumulates or is discharged is called the *time constant,* and it can be calculated from the following formula. Since t only represents 63.2% charge or discharge, in calculating pulse duration, 5t should be used.

$$t = RC$$

Where t = time in seconds
R = resistance in ohms
C = capacitance in farads

It can be seen that by manipulating either R or C, the rate at which the capacitor charges or discharges can be precisely controlled. In earlier chronaximeters of capacitive discharge design, a series of capacitors ranging approximately in value from 10 microfarads to 100 picofarads (0.001 MFD) were discharged through a fixed resistance of 10 kilohms (1×10^4 ohms), yielding pulses ranging in duration from 500 milliseconds to 5 microseconds. The *amount* of charge in the capacitors could be accurately regulated, thereby providing capability to determine chronaxie. The technique involved determining the minimum voltage at which excitation occurred using DC (galvanic) current of 500 to 1000 millisecond pulses. This value was then doubled and the capacitors charged. The capacitors were then individually discharged in sequence, smallest to largest, until the same excitation occurred.

Electronic stimulators used for strength/duration analysis and chronaxie determination consist essentially of two major circuits. The first is a pulse generator capable of generating rectangular pulses of selectable amplitude and duration. In most instances, this circuit will be a triggered monostable multivibrator. The second circuit is a pulse repetition rate oscillator, which is used to provide the selection of precise time intervals between the output pulses. In addition to the automatic pulse repetition provided by this circuit, generally a manual trigger is included to allow generation of a single pulse. The pulse repetition rate oscillator can be any type of oscillator generating short duration trigger pulses. One type of circuit used is a free-running multivibrator.

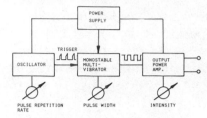

Figure 8-56. Block diagram of a chronaxie pulse generator.

The two circuits work in conjunction as follows: each time the pulse repetition rate oscillator triggers the pulse generator, the monostable circuit goes through one full cycle of operation, generating an output pulse. When its cycle is completed, the circuit remains "off" until the next pulse repetition rate oscillator trigger sends it into operation. A power amplifier may be used as an output circuit, or the signal may be taken directly from the pulse generator. Figure 8-56 shows a block diagram of a typical pulse generator/chronaximeter.

The controls and indicators associated with a typical chronaximeter/pulse generator are as follows:

1. An AC power switch, which furnishes AC power to the instrument.
2. A power-on indicator — a neon bulb indicator most often placed across the input transformer primary winding indicating AC power is available.
3. A function selector switch, allowing the operator to select the appropriate circuitry for DC (galvanic) and/or rheobase/chronaxie testing. In addition, some devices provide an internal calibration circuit which can be hooked into this switch.
4. A pulse duration selector, allowing the operator to select pulse durations from 0.1 millisecond to 500 milliseconds. Some instruments provide additional adjustments for vernier adjustment between the fixed switch positions.
5. A pulse interval selector, providing variation of the time interval between pulses.
6. An output intensity control for adjusting the output current intensity.

7. An output indicator bulb, which is driven by the current flowing to the patient. The indicator will pulse in intensity along with the output pulses.
8. Electrode jacks for attaching the electrode cables to the instrument.

An important difference between pulse generators used in strength-duration/chronaxie testing is the type of output current control a particular device generates. Two types of instruments are in present use, constant voltage/variable current and constant current/variable voltage. With a constant voltage source, the unit's output impedance should be less than 50 ohms; with a constant current generator, the output impedance should exceed 10 kilohms. It should be noted that use of either type, generally dictated by personal preference of the operator, provides no *accurate* predication or measurement of the charge actually passing through the various areas of treated tissue. This is due primarily to the effects of contact resistance at the electrodes and the electrical characteristics (resistance and capacitance) of the tissue under treatment, which varies with individuals. Arguments for the use of both types of devices are strong, but no definitive evidence proving one better than the other presently exists, and satisfactory data can be obtained from both.

Electromyography Instrumentation

The EMG System

Electromyography is basically a physiological monitoring process in which the muscle potentials of skeletal muscle activity, whether voluntary or by way of external stimulation, are monitored and/or recorded. Although other methods are used, the method predominantly in use today for monitoring EMG signals is by oscilloscope tracings. Because of this, the typical EMG instrument is essentially a special-purpose oscilloscope with various attachments dictated by specific application. The design features incorporated into electromyography systems are prescribed by the various characteristics of the biopotentials it must detect. An understanding of these parameters will facilitate the

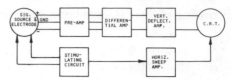

Figure 8-57. A typical EMG system.

analysis of the instrument system used to detect them. Voltage, frequency, and signal source impedance are the three most important factors that must be considered in selecting the correct instrument system.

Muscle potentials in electromyography range from 100 microvolts (μv) to approximately 1 millivolt (mv). These potentials are monophasic or biphasic pulses with an approximate frequency range between 15 Hz and 10 KHz. The variability of source impedances found in bioelectric potential recording requires that the input circuitry of the recording or monitoring device be high in order to prevent circuit loading.

An EMG recording system can be produced using individual components such as preamplifiers, amplifiers, recorders, and stimulators, but generally, a combined system functioning within a single cabinet and utilizing interrelated controls exemplifies a typical commercial system.

Figure 8-57 shows a block diagram of a complete EMG system. Each section will be discussed individually.

Electrodes

EMG electrodes can be of two basic types, *surface* type or *needle* type. In routine clinical electromyography, the needle electrode is predominant. Needle electrodes can be unipolar and coaxial in construction. Unipolar electrodes are simple, fine needles, insulated except for a small segment at the tip. Coaxial needle electrodes are essentially hypodermic needles through which a single insulated wire, with a bare tip, is passed; in the case of some systems, two wires are used. The needle itself may be one active element of the electrode system, or it may just be the grounded shield, as in the case of the two-wire or differential electrode noted above. Surface electrodes are silver or silver chloride discs in specially designed attachment cups or adhesive pads. These electrodes are applied to the skin, over the area of interest, after the skin has peen prepared by cleansing and applying electrode paste. Such electrodes are not capable of detecting some of the low amplitude, high frequency signals important in EMG analysis and hence are not used extensively.

Concerning electrode materials, since most metals generate polarization and offset voltages due to metal-electrolyte reactions, chemically nonreactive or inert metals such as platinum and silver are used extensively in physiological monitoring techniques. Other factors, such as drift, recovery time, etc., are included in the evaluation and choice of electrodes by researchers and designers. A detailed analysis of such factors is beyond the scope of this section; however, one should be aware that the use of the wrong type of electrode generates problems and signal distortion that even the most sophisticated amplifier system cannot rectify.

Signal Amplifiers

The type of amplifier necessary in monitoring biopotentials must have the following characteristics: (1) an overall gain of approximately 100,000, (2) a frequency response of DC to 10 KHz, (3) an input impedance of at least 1 megohm and, preferably, greater than 100 megohms, and (4) a differential input with a high (250,000) common mode rejection ratio (CMRR). Items (3) and (4) are obtained by use of a *differential amplifier.* Such an amplifier has three input leads, two signal leads, and a ground lead. Electrical noise or interference will appear in equal magnitude and phase on both signal leads; hence, it is "common" to both inputs. The amplifier is constructed to cancel common signals; therefore, the noise will not appear at its output. A biopotential will appear at the two signal leads, but it will be *out of phase,* due to the fact that the ground electrode is located between the two signal electrodes on the patient; consequencly, it *will* be amplified. Figure 8-58 shows this principle diagrammatically. The high gain of the amplifier is obtained by the use of multiple stages of amplification.

Preamplifiers are designed as high sensitivity, high gain de-

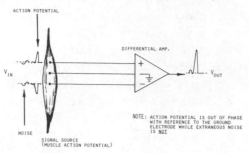

Figure 8-58. An example of common mode rejection.

vices used to couple electrode systems to instrument systems providing gain and impedance matching. In EMG systems, the preamplifiers are generally located close to the electrodes in shielded containers. The signal is then coupled via coaxial cable to the main EMG cabinet. Remote preamplifiers are also of the differential type.

Cathode Ray Tube Display

The EMG signal, once amplified, is fed into the display system, terminating at the cathode ray tube deflection plates. The cathode ray tube consists of an electron gun, which projects a beam of high velocity electrons at the phosphor-coated inner face of the tube. To reach the screen, the beam passes between two sets of deflection plates (horizontal plates causing horizontal deflection, etc.). Horizontal deflection is time calibrated, and the vertical deflection system is voltage calibrated; hence, the result is a time/amplitude graph of the vertical input signal (Fig. 8-59). The horizontal amplifier of the cathode ray tube system is calibrated in sweep times to allow precise measurement of the input pulse durations. A typical unit may have selectable sweep times from 1 millisecond to 200 milliseconds. The horizontal sweep signals are generated by varying the frequency of a ramp function generator. To provide the sweep at just the right time to monitor an action potential, the sweep is triggered at the same time and by the same stimulating signal that causes the action potential.

Special cathode ray tubes are now available that allow an

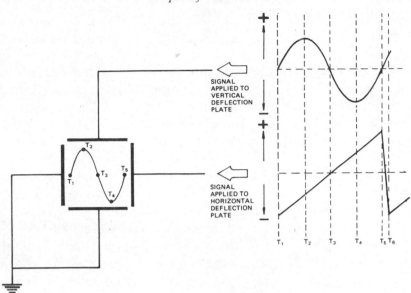

Figure 8-59. Sweep signal and vertical signal applied to a cathode ray tube. From Terence Karselis, *Descriptive Medical Electronics and Instrumentation*, 1973. Courtesy of Charles B. Slack, Inc., Thorofare, New Jersey.

image to be maintained on the face of the scope. Such devices are called "storage scopes," and they allow the operator to hold a particular action potential for prolonged study or photography. The image can be removed by the operator simply by depressing an "erase" button.

Stimulator

The stimulator section found in a typical EMG system is generally physically incorporated into the horizontal amplifier section of the oscilloscope. In this way, the horizontal trace is triggered just prior to the muscle being stimulated. This ensures that the evoked response will appear during the trace and not prior to it. The stimulator should have the capability of supplying repetitive or single pulses of variable magnitude, time, and repetition frequency. Pulse duration should be variable from 50 microseconds to 2 or 3 milliseconds, with pulse repetition rates between 0.5 and 50 per second. Some systems incorporate integral timing markers into the trace and elapsed time indicators to provide nerve conduction velocity testing capability.

The above requirements constitute the basic items necessary for a physiological stimulator. Additional modifications may include a stimulus isolation unit and the capability to generate double, triple, and biphasic pulses. *Stimulus isolation* is generally used to eliminate differential (noise currents, due to the stimulating signal, occurring in the tissues around sensing electrodes as a result of tissue impedance). This can be accomplished by isolating the stimulator from ground and providing a high input impedance into the amplifier. The ideal system provides both of these. *Biphasic stimulation* is necessary when rapid cell recovery is required. When a cell is stimulated by a short duration, high energy pulse, a following pulse of long duration, low intensity, *and* opposite polarity will make the next charge through the cell zero. This form of stimulation also tends to eliminate electrode polarization.

Nerve Conduction Velocities

The velocity at which a nerve can propagate an impulse can be indicative of the physical condition of the nerve, and any complete electrodiagnostic procedure should include some motor and sensory nerve conduction velocity studies. In general, healthy nerves exhibit conduction velocities in the range of 40 to 60 meters per second, while abnormal values below that indicate injury or disease. Specific values are determined by the particular nerve under consideration.

The instrumentation required for conduction velocity studies is the basic EMG system, with the added requirement of a stimulus isolation unit. This unit is necessary because of the relatively high stimulating voltages (50 to 150 volts) employed close to the sensing electrodes that are measuring millivolts. An elapsed time indicator (as noted in the previous section) and/or visible timing markers on the trace are also required. Some systems provide two- or four-sweep capability (called a step-sweep), allowing the operator to observe four times the usual amount of information. For instance, a single stimulus at the little finger can be observed at four points along the ulnar nerve and all the potentials displayed on the screen at once.

BIOFEEDBACK INSTRUMENTATION

Within the last five years, there has been a resurgence of interest in clinical biofeedback for the treatment of a wide range of physiological disorders ranging from mental stress to neuromuscular rehabilitation. During the late 1960s and early 1970s the public's imagination was captured by the popularization of "alpha wave" biofeedback and its promotion as a new form of treatment for any and all ailments. Those familiar with instrumentation history will recall similar exploitation of Roentgen's x-ray apparatus after its introduction in the late nineteenth century. In much the same way as the x-ray machine, biofeedback instrumentation has slowly begun to find its true place in clinical medicine; hence, some mention of it should be made in this volume.

The Feedback Loop

One common model of a physiological feedback system used to describe human motor activity or learning and similar visceral functions can be simplified to a set of stages (the feedback loop) as seen in Figure 8-60.

In one instance, motor activity results in subliminal sensations being detected by proprioceptors and appropriate feedback transmitted to the brain. This is the *internal* feedback loop. In the second instance, motor activity is detected by auditory or visual sensing of the event and appropriate feedback again transmitted to the brain. This is an *external* feedback loop. The former system

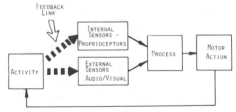

Figure 8-60. The biological feedback loop.

has the characteristic of its feedback being *continuous* in nature and providing control. The latter involves a discontinuous feedback signal (i.e. it is goal oriented). *Biofeedback* generally refers to those systems which employ instrumental techniques to substitute for a damaged stage in one of feedback loops. Some "purists" claim that true clinical biofeedback must involve conversion of subliminal (internal) activity into information capable of being processed by the *external* system (i.e. myofeedback or EMG feedback), while techniques that employ goal-oriented devices (threshold-sensing goniometers) are not classified as biofeedback. One might ask that same "purist" why he uses the term "biofeedback" to describe a signal that is of electrical origin (i.e. a tone from an oscillator) being transmitted to the patient. For simplicity's sake, this author prefers a more general description, which implies that the term biofeedback can be applied to any technique in which information concerning a biologically initiated event (whether control or goal oriented) is sensed and transmitted to the brain by way of an instrumentally augmented path.

The Biofeedback Instrument System

The components in a biofeedback instrument system are designed around the functional stages of the physiological feedback loop and are as follows:

1. Sensing (transducer)
2. Processing (amplifier and integrator)
3. Action (modulated-tone generator)

Sensing (Transducer)

The sensing element in a biofeedback instrument system will be determined by the particular form of biological event being sensed. For example, neuromuscular rehabilitation involves sensing EMG signals; hence, the conventional "electrode" constitutes the transducer. Thermal biofeedback (i.e. training a patient to dilate peripheral capillaries as a treatment for migraine) utilizes a temperature-sensing probe (possibly a thermistor) as the transducer; while range of motion studies, via an

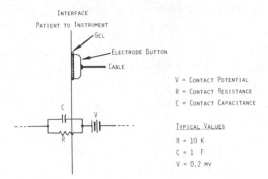

Figure 8-61. Electrode characteristics.

electrogoniometer (*see* discussion at the close of this chapter), utilize a potentiometer as the transducer. Since neuromuscular applications are an area of high clinical activity at present, a few comments concerning electrodes should be emphasized (*see also* prior discussion of electrodes in this chapter).

The electrode in an EMG system is an important link between the patient and instrument systems. Since it acts as a part of the electrical system, it has definite electrical characteristics that are associated with it, as shown in Figure 8-61.

The contact potential is due to the half-cell potential generated by a metal — the electrode — in contact with an electrolyte solution — the gel or patient's perspiration. It is typically 0.2 mV for Ag/Ag Cl electrodes and is of no concern as long as it is the same for each electrode (i.e. it is a common mode voltage). If, however, the contact potential varies between electrodes (due to poor application), then an offset potential occurs between the electrodes and an error signal is produced. It is for this reason — along with the changes in the contact resistance that will result — that care of application is of prime importance in any technique involving recording electrodes and biological signals (EMG, EKG, EEG, etc.). Compared to needle-type (invasive) electrodes, surface electrodes are less sensitive and hence dictate the requirement of higher gain (sensitivity) in the amplifier used for signal processing.

Signal Processing (Rectification — Amplification — Integration)

The majority of EMG biofeedback devices available today rectify the EMG signal prior to amplifying or quantitating it. This can be accomplished with a circuit known as an absolute value amplifier or a full wave rectifier, the former being the most precise and accurate. After rectification, the signal is then coupled to one or more frequency selective amplifiers. [NOTE: Independent stages of filtering (active filters) are sometimes used to isolate only the signal of interest. These may or may not precede the rectifier stage. Whatever the case, all stages within an instrument are "tuned" (designed as frequency selective) to provide maximum signal and minimum noise.]

The basic principles concerning amplification covered in previous sections apply to the amplifiers found in biofeedback instruments. However, some additional points are important enough to emphasize here.

The amplifier characteristics that are of major interest to the therapist using biofeedback must be properly understood in order to ensure correct selection and use of these devices:

1. *Sensitivity (Gain).* Refers to the smallest signal voltage capable of being detected by the instrument.
2. *Common Mode Rejection Ratio (CMRR).* Refers to the device's ability to amplify the desired signal in the presence of undesired common mode noise (normally 100 db or 50,000 : 1).
3. *Input Impedance.* Refers to amplifier's input resistance (AC and DC), which in turn determines how much effect the amplifier will have on the signal source (i.e. does it *load* down the source); a good figure, 10^8 to 10^9 ohms. [NOTE: Rule of thumb. A good amplifier should have as little effect upon the signal source as possible; hence, *it should have a high input impedance.*]
4. *Input Noise.* Refers to the noise (extraneous electrical signals) appearing at the amplifier's input terminals. Should be below 1 μV RMS.
5. *Frequency Range.* Refers to the range of frequencies accepted by the instrument and amplified. (Typically for

myofeedback, it will be 100 to 400 Hertz. This is the range to which the amplifiers are "tuned.")

6. *Input Range.* Refers to the range of signal voltage *amplitudes* that will be accepted and amplified without distortion, typically 5 μV to 1 mV.
7. *Response.* Refers to the amplifier's signal transfer characteristic (input to output), generally either linear or logarithmic. (In simple terms, this means that in a *linear* amplifier $V_{out} = V_{in} \times$ some gain factor ($\times 1$, $\times 5$, etc.), while in a logarithmic amplifier $V_{out} = \log V_{in} \times$ gain).

After being amplified — either linearly or logarithmically — the biofeedback signal must then be integrated (summed over time) in order to provide a signal capable of modulating (varying) the output tone.

Some myofeedback devices have used the "raw" (i.e. amplified) EMG signal as the tone generator by feeding the signal directly to a speaker. This is only practical, however, at low levels of muscular activity; hence the need for methods that yield an output change proportional to the change in muscle activity, as in the modulated tone generator, which in turn requires an integrator preceding it.

One can think of an integrator as a form of digital signal (the EMG pulses) to analog signal (the integrator output) converter. An analogy the author often uses with students, in an attempt to clarify integration, is the bathtub model. If one thinks of the integrator as a bathtub with an open drain and the digital input to the system as buckets of water added at discrete intervals of time, then as buckets (pulses) are added, the level in the tub becomes proportional to the *rate* and *magnitude* of the pulses added. In short, a higher frequency of pulses equals a higher integrator level. A lower frequency of input pulses lets the integrated value drop.

Once the signal has been integrated, it can then be used to modulate (vary) a tone generator.

Modulated-Tone Generator

A tone generator (basically an audio oscillator) develops a signal, either sine or rectangular in form, with a frequency that allows it to be heard by the patient (between 0 and 5 KHz). The circuit is designed such that an input signal applied to the stage will cause either its amplitude (loudness) or its pitch (frequency) to change. The change is most often directly proportional (i.e. increased input = a higher output tone). One common circuit that accomplished this is known to engineers as a VCO — a voltage-controlled oscillator. The signal, when fed to a speaker, will produce an audible signal, providing the important link back to the patient's sensory system.

Other forms of output can be employed, such as analog panel meters, light-emitting diodes, illuminated bar graphs, and the cathode ray tube display. No doubt many more imaginative forms of visual and auditory outputs will be forthcoming in the future.

In addition to the design features mentioned above, economic factors and human engineering concepts are employed in the design of today's modern instruments. The overall results can be expected to satisfy a term that originated in the 1960's — "S.A.R.A.": a successful device must be "Socially Acceptable and Reasonably Accurate."

Electrical Noise

The problem of electrical interference in biofeedback is compensated for in two areas of the typical EMG biofeedback device: (1) the input (differential) amplifier stage and (2) the filter circuitry designed into the instrument. In the first case, the differential amplifier cancels out any signal present at *both* input leads (the common mode signal), amplifying only the *difference* in signal voltage between them. In this manner, 60 Hz interference is reduced. Frequencies other than 60 Hz can be eliminated, or at least reduced, by active filter circuits within the amplifier itself, as mentioned previously. Combinations of *high pass, low pass,* and *notch* filters act to reduce interference and enhance signal transfer. High pass filters pass only frequencies *above* a given point, and low pass filters transfer frequencies *below* a given point; the point in both cases is referred to as (f_{co}), the cutoff frequency. Notch filters eliminate frequencies falling between two cutoff points (f_{co}-low and f_{co}-high). A typical exam-

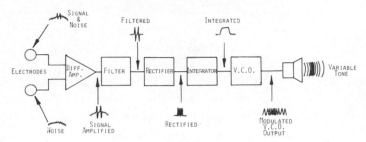

Figure 8-62. A typical EMG biofeedback system.

ple is a 60 Hz notch filter that eliminated frequencies between 58 and 62 Hertz.

Figure 8-62 shows a block diagram of a typical EMG biofeedback device and its various stages. Waveforms are shown to illustrate the function of each stage.

ULTRASONIC INSTRUMENTATION

Introduction

Just as the origin of microwave diathermy can be traced to the development of military airborne radar during World War II, therapeutic ultrasound shares a similar mode of origin. Sonar (*sound na*vigation and *r*anging) was developed during the same time period as radar, and during the postwar years the field of medical ultrasonics was born. Whereas microwave finds application primarily as a therapeutic agent, ultrasound is finding wide application in the area of diagnosis as well as therapy, principally because of its relatively safe, noninvasive nature. Whatever its application, diagnostic or therapeutic, ultrasonic energy and the instrumentation required for its generation requires the following basic elements.

Basic Concepts and Instrumentation

Sound energy, whether audible or ultrasonic, is essentially nothing more than mechanical vibration of a physical body within some type of continuous system or phase. A drum head vibrates, causing mechanical vibration of the air in contact with it, and the vibrations are passed through the air as waves —

sound. A ship's sonar transducer vibrates, producing sound waves in the sea water surrounding it. From these examples, two requirements for the transmission of sound become obvious: a *source* or *transmitting* element and a *medium* through which the sound travels. Sound is divided into subgroups based on its frequency. Subsonic sounds are those frequencies below approximately 15 Hz. *Audio* sound frequencies range from 15 Hz to 20 KHz. Frequencies above 20 KHz are classed as *ultrasonic*. The two characteristics of ultrasound that make it a useful medical tool are (1) its ability to penetrate tissue without producing injury and (2) its ability to reflect "echoes" when passing between mediums having different densities. The former characteristic is employed in therapeutic ultrasound, the latter in diagnostic ultrasound. Frequencies in the range of 0.8 MHz to 1 MHz have proven experimentally to be preferable for therapeutic use, with effective energy outputs in the range of 0.5 to 3 watts per square centimeter. The effective energy output is determined by dividing the total instrument output power by the area of the transducer in contact with the patient. For example, an instrument with a 10 cm^2 transducer head generating 6 watts of output power has an effective output of 0.6 watts per cm.^{2}

The basic instrumentation required to provide therapeutic ultrasound is shown in Figure 8-63. Ultrasound is basically RF electrical energy converted to mechanical vibrations. The key element in the instrument system generating ultrasound is the transducer, an electromechanical converter. The element at the heart of an ultrasonic transducer is a *piezoelectric crystal*. Certain natural and man-made crystals when placed in an electrical field will be mechanically distorted. By applying an alternating electrical field at the resonant frequency of the crystal, it can be made to vibrate, thereby generating alternate compression and refraction of the medium around it. The phenomenon is a reversible one in that if one mechanically distorts such a crystal, a potential will develop across its structure. The former effect of electromechanical conversion is used in therapeutic devices, while both methods of conversion are used in diagnostic transducers.

The type of crystal originally used as piezoelectric devices was

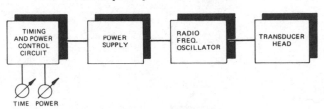

Figure 8-63. Block diagram of a simple ultrasonic generator. From Terence Karselis, *Descriptive Medical Electronics and Instrumentation*, 1973. Courtesy of Charles B. Slack, Inc., Thorofare, New Jersey.

natural quartz. However, these crystals have a high inherent impedance and, consequently, require extremely high driving voltages, on the order of 4000 volts at maximum output. Lithium sulfate salt crystals require less driving voltage; however, the materials of choice in present-day transducers are barium titanate ($BaTiO_3$) and lead zirconate titanate (PZT). These man-made polycrystalline ceramic devices have low impedance and, consequently, require lower driving voltages. For example, a PZT crystal requires approximately 30 volts driving energy.

In the transducer head used to apply therapeutic ultrasound, the crystal is cemented into a mounting and driven by RF pulses at its natural resonant frequency and the appropriate amplitude. The face portion of the applicator head and crystal mounting is designed such that it will also resonate at the natural frequency of the crystal.

The therapeutic effects of ultrasound are threefold: (1) thermal effects due to the vibrational energy being converted into heat, (2) mechanical effects within the tissue (termed micromassage), and (3) chemical effects due to changing cell permeability and ionic diffusion. Some tissues tend to absorb increased amounts of ultrasonic energy selectively, such as bone cartilage and tendon. In the case of tendon, the gross effects are an increase in its tensile strength.

A Typical Ultrasonic Generator

The basic elements of an ultrasonic generator were shown in Figure 8-63. In the case of typical therapeutic devices used today, a slightly more complex instrument is required. Its con-

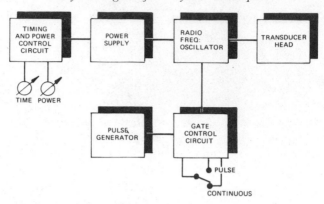

Figure 8-64. Block diagram of an ultrasonic generator with continuous or pulsed operation capability. From Terence Karselis, *Descriptive Medical Electronics and Instrumentation,* 1973. Courtesy of Charles B. Slack, Inc., Thorofare, New Jersey.

struction should allow selection of pulsed or continuous ultrasound. Such a simplified device is shown in Figure 8-64. In this instrument, a gate circuit has been added which allows either pulsed or continuous operation of the RF oscillator.

The controls and indicators usually found on a typical ultrasonic generator are as follows:

1. A timer, to allow selection and control of the time of therapy. Such devices generally cut off power to the oscillator circuits or interrupt output power when the duration of therapy has elapsed.
2. Output intensity or power control, providing the capability to select zero to maximum power output.
3. Transducer cable jack, to pass energy to the transducer. Some units provide automatic power interruption when the output cable is disconnected.
4. An operation mode selector switch, allowing the operator to select pulsed or continuous operation.
5. An output power indicator, usually a milliampmeter, so the operator can monitor the relative transmitted power.
6. Some form of "power on" indicator, either a neon bulb or LED, to indicate wall power is applied to the device.

Operation of the device would be as follows: When power is

applied, the RF oscillator is activated, generating continuous ultrasonic oscillations. This signal is directly coupled to the transducer. The pulse generator, generally having a 60 Hz output frequency, is used to control a gating amplifier, which in turn controls the oscillator. The gating action is such that the oscillator is allowed to generate an output *only* when the gate pulse is present. In the continuous mode, the gating signal is isolated from the oscillator circuit, allowing it to free run. Output power is controlled at the oscillator, and duration of therapy is controlled by a timing unit that shuts off the AC input to the instrument after time has elapsed.

Two Actual Instruments Compared

Two commercial ultrasound therapy units are the Burdick UT/420, operating at 870 KHz, and the Birtcher Megason XV, operating at 1 MHz. These two devices are representative of the instruments employed in ultrasound therapy, and the various circuits of each will be discussed in more detail. A block diagram of each unit is shown in Figure 8-65 and schematic diagrams in Figure 8-66.

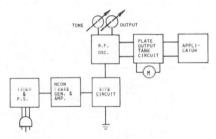

Figure 8-64A. Burdick UT/420 ultrasonic unit. From information supplied by The Burdick Corporation, Milton, Wisconsin.

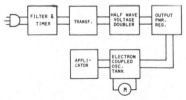

Figure 8-65B. The Birtcher Megason XV ultrasonic unit. From information supplied by The Birtcher Corporation, Los Angeles, California.

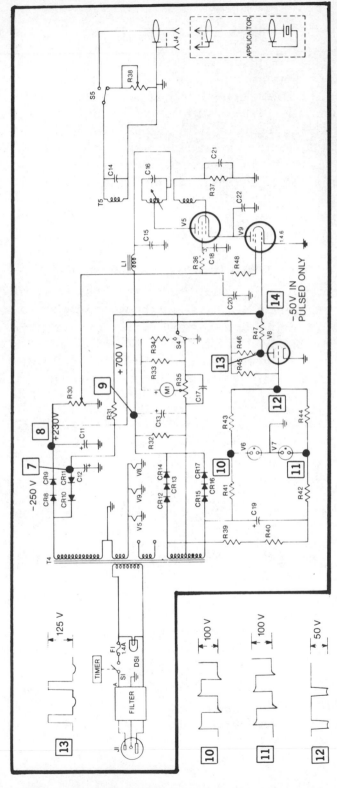

Figure 8-66A. Burdick UT/420 ultrasound unit schematic. Courtesy of The Burdick Corporation, Milton, Wisconsin.

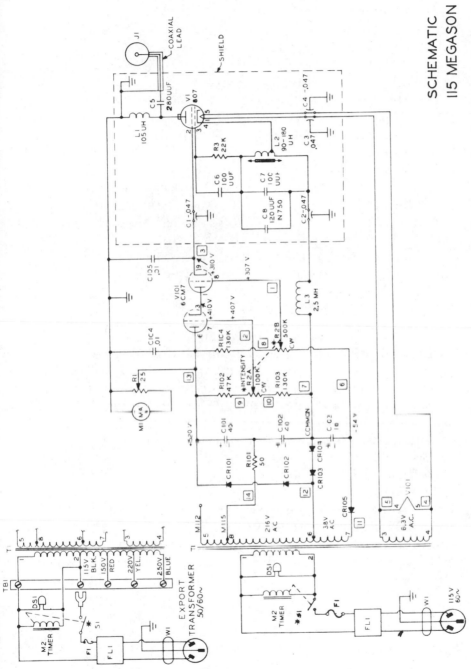

Figure 8-66B. Birtcher Megason XV ultrasound schematic. Courtesy of The Birtcher Corporation, Los Angeles, California.

Power Supplies

BURDICK UT/420. AC power is applied to the primary of the transformer (T4) by way of the timer cutout switch (S1), a fuse, and an RF filter. The two high voltage secondary windings provide, by way of half and full wave rectifiers (CR8 through CR17), the various DC bias and plate voltages for the tubes (V5, V8, V9). Filament voltages are supplied by a low voltage secondary. A power indicator lamp (DS1) is in parallel with the transformer primary.

BIRTCHER MEGASON XV. The primary circuit of the power supply is virtually the same as in the Burdick device, employing an RF filter, a combined power/timer switch (S1), and a power indicator lamp (DS1). A half wave voltage doubler (CR101 through CR104) supplies the high voltage for the oscillator tube (V1). A half wave rectifier (CR105) generates a negative bias voltage for the output control tube (V101).

Oscillator Circuits

BURDICK. The Burdick RF oscillator (V5) is a tuned plate oscillator, feedback being taken from the plate tank circuit (T5 and C16) by way of inductive coupling (T5 pins 6 and 7). The output frequency is adjusted by tuning the coil segment in parallel with C16. V9 is the gate control tube providing current for the oscillator cathode. Its conduction is in turn controlled by the gate amplifier (V8). Output power is varied by adjusting R30, which adjusts the screen grid voltage, thereby effectively controlling the oscillator's conduction.

BIRTCHER. An electron coupled oscillator (V1), utilizing screen grid feedback and having good stability, provides the 1 MHz RF oscillations. The grid tank circuit (C7, C8, L2) is temperature compensated and tuned by adjusting L2. Output power is controlled indirectly by the tuning control (R2), which effectively controls V1 screen voltage and therefore the oscillator's conduction. The two sections of V101, the power control tube, act as a variable resistor, whose conductor is in turn controlled by R2.

Pulse Generator and Gate Circuit

BURDICK. The Burdick gate circuitry is controlled by a 60 Hz pulse generator (V6, V7), which supplies negative-going 50 volt pulses of 3.3 millisecond duration to the gate amplifier (V8) grid. The pulses are amplified and inverted, and passed to the gate control tube (V9). When continuous operation is selected by switch S4, the negative bias present at V9 grid is removed and the tube conducts continually, i.e. the gate is "open." In the pulse mode, switch S4 places a negative bias of 50 volts on V9 grid. The positive 3.3 millisecond pulses from the gate amplifier overcome the bias and turn on V9 sixty times per second, which in turn allows the oscillator to fire during that time. The result is a series of RF oscillations of 3.3 milliseconds duration every 16 milliseconds.

BIRTCHER. The Birtcher unit provides only continuous operation; therefore, no pulse generator or gate circuitry is required.

Output/Transducer Circuit

BURDICK. The output of the RF oscillator (V5) is inductively coupled and impedance matched by T5, C14 to the coaxial connector (T4). The energy is then passed via coaxial cable to the applicator head and hence to a ceramic crystal. Output power is monitored by monitoring the current through the gate control tube and RF oscillator. During continuous operation the meter indicates average power; in the pulsed mode, it indicates peak power. R38 provides a dummy load for the oscillator when the applicator is disconnected.

BIRTCHER. An impedance matching network of L1, C5 connects the RF oscillator circuit to the coaxial applicator jack (J1). This is necessary due to the normally high output impedance of the oscillator and the low impedance of the coaxial cable and barium titanate ceramic crystal. The output meter (M1) monitors the plate current of the oscillator.

The applicators employed with the above devices are heavy metal chambers, with the piezoelectric crystal cemented to the resonance-matched applicator face. Two electrodes are cross

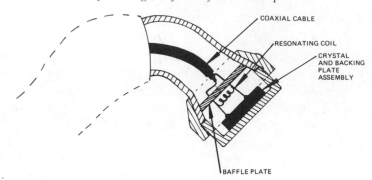

Figure 8-67. Simplified diagram of an ultrasound therapy applicator. From Terence Karselis, *Descriptive Medical Electronics and Instrumentation*, 1973. Courtesy of Charles B. Slack, Inc., Thorofare, New Jersey.

mounted on the crystal to which the RF signal is applied. An impedance-matched coil may also be included. An energy absorbed baffle plate absorbs stray energy, and the whole assembly is sealed to ensure it is watertight. A coupling medium is necessary to transmit energy to the patient, since the ultrasonic waves will tend to be reflected by air. A typical unit is diagrammed in Figure 8-67.

ELECTROANESTHESIA AND ELECTROPROSTHETICS

The use of electricity and electronics in the medical sciences has mushroomed in recent years. Conventional applications such as electrotherapy, electrodiagnosis, electroencephalography, and electrocardiography constitute the major areas of medical electronics. Recently, however, the uses of electrical and electronic devices in the areas of electrically induced anesthesia (electroanesthesia or electrosleep) and electrically controlled and operated prosthetic devices (electroprosthetics) has increased.

Electroanesthesia

The inducement of surgical-level anesthesia by electrical means is termed electroanesthesia. This definition is by no means a universal one, since many individuals exhibit a resistance to the effects of the sleep-inducing currents. To produce anesthesia via electrical means, a current is passed between bitemporal electrodes through the skull and hence the brain of the patient. The first sensation felt by the patient is a slight tingling in the area of the electrodes, which leads into a state of relaxation, then sleep or anesthesia. This technique is still primarily experimental and is used mostly in research applications due to the side effects its use produces. The major objections against the use of this technique at present are the production of hypertension, tachycardia hyperexia, cutaneous burns, and excessive secretions of mucus and saliva. Recently, scientists have attempted to produce a preinduction drowsiness by the use of pulsed electrostatic fields prior to the application of actual transcerebral low currents.

The technique and instrumentation for inducing electronarcosis is as follows: A pulse generator capable of generating frequencies from DC to approximately 20 KHz with pulse durations around 1 millisecond is adequate for most applications, since the most useful frequency appears to be around 100 Hz. Initially, a low DC current is applied to electrodes placed bitemporally (although anterior-posterior location is also used) on the patient's skull, after which a selected pulse pattern is superimposed. A typical sequence involves a 10 to 15 milliamp reference upon which 5 to 10 milliamp pulses are added. Overall current range used to date has been from 5 to 110 milliamps in both continuous and pulsed patterns. A major problem in the technique is obtaining adequate current density in the selected area of the brain without causing electrode site burns. The problem is due to the intervening bone and tissue resistance preventing most of the current from reaching the brain. If the voltage is increased to overcome this, the magnitude of the side effects is increased.

A typical instrument is shown in Figure 8-68. The electrodes used are comparable to any typical surface electrode employed in physiological monitoring. In most cases, noble metals (silver, etc.) are used to eliminate polarization. In addition to the automatic voltage and current controls incorporated into its design capability, adjustment of the pulse duration and repetition rate are also included.

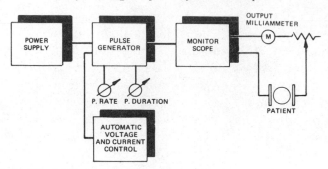

Figure 8-68. Block diagram of an electroanesthesia unit. From Terence Karselis, *Descriptive Medical Electronics and Instrumentation,* 1973. Courtesy of Charles B. Slack, Inc., Thorofare, New Jersey.

The physiological mechanism by which electroanesthesia is induced is presently unclear; however, various theories have been postulated, including one that suggests that the currents may effect enzyme systems. Another theory indicates the possibility that the current may cause the release of some type of generalized inhibitory substance into the bloodstream. Whatever the specific mechanism of action, electroanesthesia is today still a research tool for the most part.

A less dramatic but nevertheless medically useful application of electrotherapy is in the area of healing ischemic ulcers. Researchers at the University of Missouri Medical Center found that application of low intensity direct currents ranging in magnitude from 200 to 400 microamperes increased the amount of healing and rate at which ischemic ulcers healed by 24 percent. The instrumentation consisted of a low voltage, low current source with an output range of 200 microamperes to 1 milliamp. The output jacks allowed cable connections to copper mesh electrodes. The negative electrode was placed on the wound for the first few days, and its effect was to reduce or inhibit pathogenic bacterial growth. The positive electrode was then used over the wound to accelerate the healing process, which appears to work by way of stimulating proliferation of fibroblastic cells and microcirculation into the traumatized area.

Another therapeutic application of low intensity currents is in assisting fractures to heal. Inactive metal screws driven into bone on both sides of a healing fracture are used as electrodes between which a low intensity current is passed. Microampere currents appear to accelerate the healing process significantly.

Both of these applications of electrotherapy are examples of the possibilities that abound in the field of electromedical currents.

Electroprosthetics

Any device or component used to replace a missing *part* or *function* of the human body is a *prosthesis*. Prostheses may be temporary or permanent, internal or external, and as such can be powered or operated by way of residual neuromuscular activity, or they may function by way of an electrical or electronic power pack. Pacemakers, artificial limbs, and braces fall into this category.

In the area of prosthetic limbs, the critical area of design in producing an effective device is the patient-device-patient feedback network. This network is a servocontrol mechanism of the type found in many null balance systems such as chart recorders. Electroprosthetic devices are electromechanical systems that mimic the body's system of neuromuscular activity and hence require the same type of closed-loop sensorimotor system. Figure 8-69 is an example of a basic system. The activity necessary for limb or body motion requires a three-stage process: (1) *sensory* activity and transmission of *stimulus*, (2) *evaluation* and *decision* for *command*, (3) *motor* activity following *command*. In

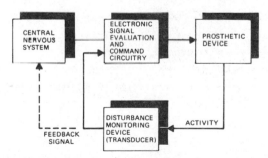

Figure 8-69. Block diagram of an electroprosthetic system. From Terence Karselis, *Descriptive Medical Electronics and Instrumentation*, 1973. Courtesy of Charles B. Slack, Inc., Thorofare, New Jersey.

electroprosthetic devices, a *transducer* of some type takes the place of missing or injured sensory nerves. A complex system of electronic circuits, often analog and digital computer subcircuits, performs the evaluation, decision, and command activity, while carefully designed electromechanical, pneumatic, and hydraulic systems provide the rotation, extension, and flexion capability to the mechanical limb. External power packs supply the energy to *drive* the hydraulic and electrical systems of the prostheses, while the *triggering* energy is usually a signal derived from some residual voluntary muscular activity remaining in a partially amputated limb or joint. Other activating signal sources are the eyelids, ears, neck, and even the tongue. Transducers used are mercury strain gauges and microswitches.

The following devices are typical examples of some recently developed electroprosthetic systems. An alarm system designed to prevent self-inflicted injury and provide improved motor control to its user was constructed, employing (1) a mercury strain gauge to detect pressure at the fingertips. The resulting electrical resistance change causes (2) a variable frequency oscillator to increase its output frequency, which in turn alters the (3) audible tone heard by the individual wearing the device. The electronics are of the integrated circuit (I.C.) type that require little power and are extremely rugged. The small size of the circuitry allows it to be worn on the wrist like a wristwatch.

A feedback control system providing a patient with increased sensitivity in grasp control has been developed using a noise transducer. Figure 8-70 shows the system. When an object is grasped or lifted and inadequate force is applied, the noise transducer generates a signal, which is processed and integrated into a motor-drive command, thereby increasing the grasping power. When no further slippage occurs, the noise signal is absent and the motor remains at the point where it previously stopped. In order to activate the system into releasing the object, a voluntary trigger signal can override the system and drive the servomotor in the opposite (release) direction.

The field of electroprosthetics is in its infancy, but, with the increasingly sophisticated developments in electronic materials and circuits design, there is no question that the physical thera-

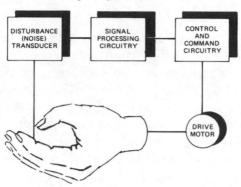

Figure 8-70. Block diagram of the adaptive control mechanism of an electro-prosthetic hand. From Terence Karselis, *Descriptive Medical Electronics and Instrumentation*, 1973. Courtesy of Charles B. Slack, Inc., Thorofare, New Jersey.

pist will see increasingly more wondrous and surprising man-made miracles.

ELECTROGONIOMETERS

Electrogoniometers (or Elgons) are devices used to translate angular displacement into an electrical signal which can be displayed or recorded. The first electrogoniometer was developed by Karpovich[1] in the late 1950s. Although Elgons are more accurate and precise than the conventional protractor-type goniometers, they have not yet replaced them, due in most part to greater expense. However, with the recent eruption in the development of microelectronic devices, it should not be too long before Elgons are cost effective and become a routine replacement for the plastic or metal protractor.

A typical Elgon consists of two main components: (1) the transducer and (2) the electronic display unit. The transducer is in most cases simply a linear potentiometer (variable resistance).

The center tap (adjustment shaft) and the body of the potentiometer are attached to separate plastic or metal arms, which in turn are attached to the patient proximal and distal to the joint being evaluated. Movement of the patient's limb, either flexion or extension, causes the potentiometer center tap to alter its position, translating the movement into an electrical signal.

Display Units

The electronic display unit can vary from a simple constant current supply and analog meter to a complex differential amplifier and comparitor system with audio feedback and digital display.

In the case of a constant current analog meter system, a DC current is maintained at a constant value by a regulating diode and passed through the transducer resistance (Fig. 8-71). The meter is connected between one end of the transducer and the center tap (or wiper arm). The voltage seen by the meter is in direct proportion to the wiper position — and hence resistance — of the potentiometer. Since $V = I \times R$, with I constant, V is proportional to R. By choosing the appropriate meter, transducer resistance, and voltage, the unit can be made to read in degrees of rotation (of the transducer shaft). The accuracy of a system such as this is governed and limited only by the linearity of the transducer resistance and the tolerance of the regulating diode. This type of circuit yields a relative change in range of motion (ROM) (i.e. patient moves from 35° to 65°, an ROM of 30°).

Figure 8-72 shows a wheatstone bridge configuration used to drive a meter, which eliminates the need for a constant current source and gives the added flexibility of allowing the operator to zero the meter at any position of the transducer shaft, yielding a direct, rather than relative, measurement of range of motion (i.e. patient moves from 0° to 30°).

The circuit functions in the following manner: The transducer acts as one leg resistance of a wheatstone bridge, the *zero* control the other. When the transducer is attached to the patient and adjusted to accommodate the resting position, the bridge

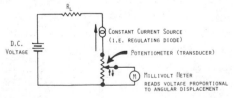

Figure 8-71. A constant current electrogoniometer.

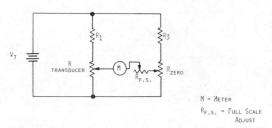

Figure 8-72. A wheatstone bridge Elgon.

will be unbalanced and a signal voltage will result. The therapist then adjusts the *zero* control until the bridge is once again balanced, the display then indicating zero. When the patient moves, the bridge is again unbalanced, yielding a signal proportional to the degree of angular rotation. An additional feature of the bridge configuration is that from the mid-position of the transducer, either flexion or extension will yield a signal, the *polarity* ($\pm$) of which is an indicator of flexion or extension.

A somewhat sophisticated audio feedback Elgon has been developed by Karselis, which allows the therapist to use the device either as an Elgon or a motivational feedback device.

In the *Elgon* mode, the transducer signal is fed directly to the digital display, and the unit shows the therapist the number of degrees of flexion or extension. In the *ROM* mode, the therapist first selects a specific ROM to be attained by the patient by dialing in the value on the display using a *ROM SET* control. The therapist sets the device back into *Elgon* mode, and the patient then attempts the exercise. If successful, an audio tone is generated which can be heard externally or via headphone. If the patient fails, no tone is generated. The number of degrees activity attained by the patient is displayed for the therapist, allowing him/her to decrease the goal or urge the patient to increase his/her effort on additional trails.

The device will accept a *set* of precalibrated transducers of varying sizes, allowing it to be used on fingers, arms, or legs.

Transducers

The crucial element in most Elgon systems is the potentiometer used at the angular displacement transducer. The

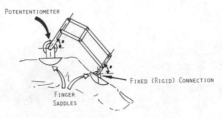

Figure 8-73. The Reswitch/Marquardt Elgon linkage.

original Karpovich transducers were Centralab™ linear taper carbon composition potententiometers, 11/16″ in diameter. One of the major limitations in using these devices was locating the central axis of the transducer precisely at the axis of the joint being tested. Movement of the skin around the joint produced translational movement of the transducer, leading to error in the measured angle. The development of the double parallelogram linkage system of Reswich and Marquardt (Fig. 8-73), at the Case Institute of Technology Engineering Design Center in the early 1960s, solved this problem. When the device is adjusted to ensure the junction between the two parallelograms is directly above the joint in question, translational motion is ignored and the device transmits only the angular displacement between its proximal and distal linkages. This design has been employed extensively by the Hand Management Center at Emory University, Atlanta, Georgia, for use on various joints of the body.

An additional problem encountered in early Elgons was the accuracy of the resistive elements of the potentiometers used for transducers. The Karpovich transducers had an overall tolerance of ± 10% with ± 3% resolution. Today, potentiometers with ±0.5% accuracy are available commercially, with a resolution of 0.1%. One can also purchase potentiometers as small as ¼″ diameter with better than 1% resolution. With potentiometers such as this available, reasonably accurate Elgons should be forthcoming in the near future.

REFERENCES

1. *Basic Electricity.* Navpers 10026-A, Bureau of Naval Personnel. Washington, D.C., U.S. Government Printing Office, 1960.
2. *Basic Theory and Application of Transistors.* Training Manual 11-690, Depart-

ment of the Army. Washington, D.C., U.S. Government Printing Office, 1959.

3. Bellville, J. W., and Weaver, C. S. (Eds.): *Techniques in Clinical Physiology.* Toronto, Collier-Macmillan, Ltd., 1969.

4. *Biophysical Measurements.* Beaverton, Oregon, Tektronix Measurement Concepts, 1971.

5. Brown, J. H. N., Jacobs, J. E., and Stark, L.: *Biomedical Engineering.* Philadelphia, F. A. Davis, 1971.

6. *Burdick Syllabus — A Compendium on Electromedical Therapy.* Milton, Wisconsin, The Burdick Corporation, 1969.

7. Buchsbaum, Walter H.: *Buchsbaum's Complete Handbook of Practical Electronic Reference Data.* Englewood Cliffs, New Jersey, Prentice-Hall, 1975.

8. Camishion, R. C.: *Basic Medical Electronics.* Boston, Little, Brown, 1964.

9. Clement, P. R. and Johnson, W. C.: *Electrical Engineering Science.* New York, McGraw-Hill, 1960.

10. Cromwell, Leslie: *Biomedical Instrumentation and Measurements.* Englewood Cliffs, New Jersey, Prentice-Hall, 1973.

11. Dart, Francis E.: *Electricity and Electromagnetic Fields.* Columbus, Ohio, Charles E. Merrill Books, 1966.

12. Diefenderfer, James A.: *Principles of Electronic Instrumentation.* Philadelphia, W. B. Saunders, 1972.

13. *Digest of the 7th International Conference on Medical & Biological Engineering.* Stockholm, Almquist and Wiksell, 1967.

14. Dummer, G. W. A., and Robertson, J. M. (Eds.): *Medical Electronic Equipment.* Vol. I-IV. Oxford, Pergamon Press, 1970.

15. *Electronic and Electrical Fundamentals.* Vol. I-IV. Fort Washington, Philco Ford Corporation, Tech. Rep. Division, 1960.

16. *Fundamentals of Transistor Electronics.* Fort Washington, Philco Ford Corporation, Education and Tech. Services Division, 1967.

17. Geddes, L. A., and Baker, L. E.: *Principles of Applied Biomedical Instrumentation.* New York, John Wiley and Sons, 1968.

18. Grossman, C. C.: *The Use of Diagnostic Ultrasound in Brain Disorders.* Springfield, Charles C Thomas, 1966.

19. Grob, B., and Kiver, M. S.: *Applications of Electronics.* New York, McGraw-Hill, 1960.

20. Karselis, Terence: *Descriptive Medical Electronics and Instrumentation.* Thorofare, New Jersey, Charles B. Slacks, Inc., 1973.

21. Malmstart, H. V., Enke, C. G., and Benjamin, W. A.: *Electronics for Scientists,* 1962.

22. Markus, John: *Source Book of Electronic Circuits.* New York, McGraw-Hill, 1968.

23. Offner, F. F.: *Electronics for Biologists.* New York, McGraw-Hill, 1962.

24. Licht, S. (Ed.): *Electrodiagnosis and Electro-Myography.* Baltimore, Waverly Press, 1961.

25. Licht, S. (Ed.): *Therapeutic Electricity and Ultraviolet Radiation*. Baltimore, Waverly Press, 1967.
26. Simpson, Robert E.: *Introductory Electronics for Scientists and Engineers*. Boston, Allyn and Bacon, 1974.
27. Segal, B. L. and Kilpatrick, D. G. (Eds.): *Engineering in the Practice of Medicine*. Baltimore, Williams and Wilkins, 1967.
28. Smith, D. A.: *Medical Electronics Equipment Handbook*. Indianapolis, Howard W. Sams, 1962.
29. Watkins, A. L.: *Manual of Electrotherapy*. Philadelphia, Lea and Febiger, 1958.
30. Yanof, H. M.: *Biomedical Electronics*. Philadelphia, F. A. Davis, 1965.

Chapter 9

INSTRUMENTATION AND POWER DISTRIBUTION WIRING SYSTEMS

INSTRUMENTS, GROUND, AND TERMINOLOGY

NOTWITHSTANDING that they are considered to be places of healing, it has been proposed more than once that hospitals and medical care facilities in general are unhealthy places in which to reside. When one considers the potential hazards concentrated into the shell of a typical hospital, the statement takes on more than slight credibility. Considering that a typical hospital contains concentrated pockets of hazardous organisms, chemicals, nuclear energy, and electrical energy, the thesis becomes alarmingly real to the average layman. However, the problem is of even more importance to the individual required to spend his total working experience within that environment. Such a situation calls for extreme and continual care, vigilance, *and* awareness on the part of the medical worker.

From the point of view of physical therapy, the electrical energy area is of prime consideration. Not only should the therapist be aware of the theory and operation of the devices he uses, but he also should have some knowledge of the way in which they function as integral parts of the power distribution system of the hospital and as potential hazards. Since the generally accepted value of current capable of causing ventricular fibrillation and possible death in patients whose normal skin resistance has been circumvented by way of an external pacemaker or catheter is in the microampere region, therapists should be cognizant of sources and conditions capable of eliciting such currents. The two major divisions of electrical hazards are classified by the source of the potentially dangerous currents. These are (1) line voltage and (2) leakage currents. To properly understand the ways in which these hazardous condi-

445

tions can arise first requires an understanding of the concepts of electrical ground and power distribution.

Ground, or Earth, or What?

A correct understanding of electrical ground requires a knowledge of the items and connections that constitute an electrical circuit. The essential components and current paths in a typical electrical circuit are shown in Figure 9-1. They are (1) a power source (the battery), (2) a load (R_2), (3) a source conductor, and (4) a return conductor. It is as a "return" conductor that electrical ground can find application, but more important is its function as a safety valve. This concept can be clarified by referring to Figure 9-2. If one regards ground or earth (which is what the term *ground* originally referred to) as an infinite electrical charge accumulator or source, the earth then has the ability to either give up or accept charges without itself becoming charged. Consequently, any object that is electrically charged and in turn touches or is connected to ground will give up or take on the appropriate charges until it is the same potential as ground, i.e. until it has become neutral. It is this fact that makes earth ground the reference point for electrical zero potential. Any object connected by a very low resistance path to ground is said, for all practical purposes, to be at zero volts; in addition, any hazardous charge that may appear on the object is immediately shunted to ground. If the object were not grounded and an individual touched both it and ground simultaneously,

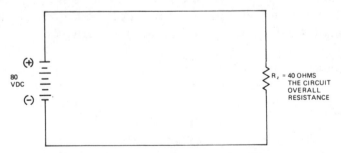

Figure 9-1. Essential components of an electrical circuit. From Terence Karselis, *Descriptive Medical Electronics and Instrumentation,* 1973. Courtesy of Charles B. Slack, Inc., Thorofare, New Jersey.

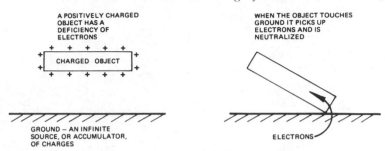

Figure 9-2. The action of grounding a charged object. From Terence Karselis, *Descriptive Medical Electronics and Instrumentation,* 1973. Courtesy of Charles B. Slack, Inc., Thorofare, New Jersey.

he would become the path to ground and hence receive an electrical shock (which may or may not be perceptible, depending upon the magnitude of the current flow).

From the above discussion, it can be seen that electrical ground serves two purposes: (a) it acts as a reference point for electrical zero potential and (b) it functions as source or sink for hazardous electrical charges. Both of these functions are utilized in the circuits that supply power to homes and businesses as well as medical facilities. In addition, these functions take on specialized application in instrumentation. It is in this application that the confusion between "true" earth ground and "instrument" ground can arise.

"True" Ground Versus "Instrument" Ground

As noted above, an electrical circuit requires the essentials of a power source, a load, and a source and drain conduction path. A majority of instruments are built on chassis or frames of conductive metal. In addition, each circuit within these devices must be provided with a source and drain path, connecting it to the device's power supply. In many instruments, it has become common practice to use the chassis or frame of the instrument as a ground "return" path from each circuit back to the power supply circuit. In instruments supplied by a two-conductor power cord and using a chassis return, the instrument circuit ground is *not* a true "earth" ground. This is shown in Figure 9-3. This type of device constitutes a potential hazard, for (a) if some fault within

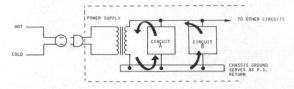

Figure 9-3. Diagram of a two-wire device with chassis ground (*not* true ground).

the instrument power supply primary side causes the instrument ground to be raised to a potential above true ground and (b) its human operator touches it while simultaneously touching another device whose chassis *is* at true ground, current will flow through the operator with uncomfortable consequences. If, however, the device is served by a three-conductor power cord *and* the building power distribution system is adequately grounded (Note: taking either one of these requirements for granted can be hazardous to one's health), the instrument ground *will* be at true earth ground and hence will provide the safety valve action noted previously (Fig. 9-4). Both of these examples are based on the assumption that the power distribution system is a grounded system. As will be discussed later, *all* distribution systems in medical facilities are *not* grounded.

Terminology and Coding in Wiring Systems

Power distribution into commercial and residential buildings follows a similar pattern. A transformer steps down the utility voltage from 2200 volts to 240 or 120 volts at the main service or distribution panel. In modern wiring systems, three conductors originate from there and supply the sub- or branch circuits within the building. These conductors are color coded and named in accordance with the National Electrical Code (N.E.C.),

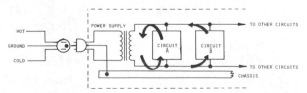

Figure 9-4. Diagram of a three-wire device with the chassis connected to true ground.

which is published by the National Fire Protection Association, Boston, Mass. The *hot* current carrying conductor is insulated with *black* covering and is at a potential of 120/240 volts with respect to ground. The *cold* (or neutral) current carrying conductor is insulated with *white* covering and it is at the same potential as ground. It is generally attached to a ground wire at the service box. The *safety ground* conductor is also attached to ground at the service box and color coded by way of *green* insulation (or is a bare wire). The grounding conductor *does not,* under normal circumstances, carry current. It is there only to provide a path to ground for fault currents.

From the service distribution box, the three-conductor system is connected to each individual branch wall outlet. The way in which the connections are made at the outlet is, once again, outlined in the N.E.C. Using the round grounding pin as the key, the N.E.C. requires the following method of connection: If the grounding pin is located *below* the two parallel blade receptacles, the left-hand slot houses the cold or neutral lead, while the right-hand slot houses the hot lead (if the ground pin is above the blade slots, they are reversed). Within the outlet box, the black (hot) conductor should terminate at the brass-colored terminal, the white (cold) conductor at the silver (nickel-plated) terminal, and the green (ground) wire at a lug screw coded green, which is located at one end of the plastic outlet assembly.

Although these requirements are law where the N.E.C. is used as the local electrical code, sloppy workmanship and cost-cutting shortcuts can lead to hazardous construction methods, such as not using a third conductor for grounding so that the ground terminal of the outlet is connected to the cold power lead, or just simply *not* connecting the ground terminal within the outlet box (the author has *seen* examples of both such techniques). The key to safety is suspicion; one should be skeptical and suspect any system until it is proven safe! That way both the therapist and the patient will live longer.

Types of Distribution Systems

Since 1962, the National Electrical Code has required the use of three-wire electrical systems. However, many buildings and facilities contain outdated and unmodified wiring systems, or systems that have been modified in a here-and-there method, leaving half of a system adequate and half of it inadequate. Some knowledge of the types of wiring systems that can be found in medical facilities can be useful to those who work in them.

Figure 9-5 is a simplified diagram of a typical two-wire distribution system. The cold or neutral conductor is grounded on the secondary side of the utility distribution transformer, and the distribution system is therefore referred to as a "grounded" system. Hazardous situations can and do occur with this type of system; for example, in an instance of accidentally reversing the two-bladed plugs commonly found on many electrical devices. In such a case, a fault within a device can allow hazardous voltage to appear on its chassis or case, even though its power on-off switch is in the open position. This occurs because power switches are by convention placed in the hot conductor side of the input power leads, and when the plug is reversed at the receptacle, the hot power line is connected to the device's cold lead.

Hazards such as those above led to the adoption of the three-wire distribution system, which is identical to the two-wire system but for the addition of the third safety "grounding" conductor. Not only does the three-wire system automatically prevent

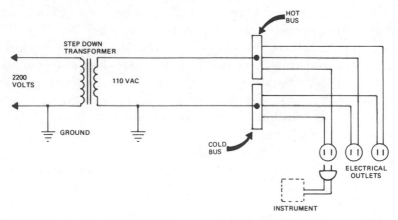

Figure 9-5. A power distribution system (two-wire). From Terence Karselis, *Descriptive Medical Electronics and Instrumentation,* 1973. Courtesy of Charles B. Slack, Inc., Thorofare, New Jersey.

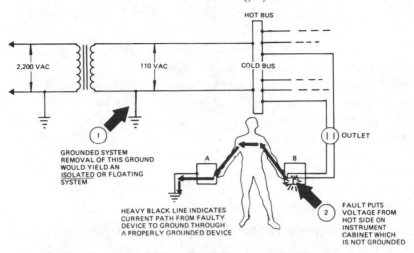

Figure 9-6. (1) shows a grounded two wire distribution system. (2) shows how a fault in an ungrounded instrument can shock an individual touching both the faulty device and a grounded device simultaneously. From Terence Karselis, *Descriptive Medical Electronics and Instrumentation*, 1973. Courtesy of Charles B. Slack, Inc., Thorofare, New Jersey.

accidental plug reversal, it also ensures that any fault currents occurring on an instrument's chassis will immediately be shunted to ground. Close observation of a typical three-prong plug will show that the ground blade is longer than the two power blades. This ensures initial contact by the ground conductor, reducing the possibility to arcing in the case of fault within the instrument.

Figure 9-6 illustrates the hazards that can occur with the two-wire power distribution system and the safety features inherent in the three-wire system. In the diagram, an individual working with instrument A, which is correctly grounded (it may be individually grounded or served by way of a three-wire system), and also touching instrument B, an ungrounded device in which faulty insulation has placed line voltage on its case, receives a possibly fatal electrical shock. By touching both devices, he becomes a low resistance pathway to ground. If instrument B had been connected by way of a three-wire power cord to a three-wire distribution system, the hazard voltage would have been shunted to ground by way of the safety ground lead, since it offers less resistance than the human body. Current is lazy — it always takes the path of least resistance. An additional point to be emphasized here is that a cheater plug, the infamous three-wire-to-two-wire-plus-pigtail converter, can easily circumvent the safety ground lead of a three-wire device if not used correctly. Needless to say, they rarely *are* used properly. The pigtail on the cheater is designed to be attached to the screw on the outlet box but rarely is attached simply because people are too hurried or lazy to take the time, or a screwdriver is not readily at hand. In such instances, the hazard shown in Figure 9-6 is once again present. A golden rule to use with cheater plugs in medical facilities is *DON'T* — just do not use them.

EQUIPMENT HAZARDS AND THEIR CAUSES
The Hazards — Macro- and Microshock

The previous three sections dealt with power distribution and ground, emphasizing its safety function. How do equipment hazards arise, and just how many types of electrical shock are there? This section will briefly discuss these items.

Electrical shock can be of two types, perceptible or imperceptible. In scientific terms, they are referred to as macroshock and microshock, respectively, and are characterized by the magnitude of current involved. Authorities in the field of electrical safety are continually at loggerheads concerning whether it is voltage or current that is the dangerous culprit in electrocution. The case is simplified if one always considers Ohm's Law: $I = V/R$. The *magnitude of current* in a circuit depends upon both the applied *voltage* and the circuit *resistance*. Since the resistance involved in electrocution varies according to the particular circumstances, then so will the current produced by a given voltage. The need then arises to establish the definitions of macro- and microshock. The normal human dry skin resistance can vary from tens of thousands of ohms (10 KΩ) to hundreds of thousands of ohms (100 KΩ), depending upon the contact area. As a general rule of thumb, current across the intact dry skin of less than 1 milliampere will cause no perceptible response and is therefore referred to as *microshock* current. Above 1 milliampere, up to approximately 15 milliamperes, the response varies from minimal perception of a tingle to muscle spasm at the higher currents. Values in the 100 to 200 milliampere range can cause death due to respiratory paralysis and cardiac fibrillation. Any current above the threshold of perception (1 ma) is termed *macroshock* current. Whatever its characterization, under the appropriate circumstances, both micro- and macroshock can kill. For example, a patient who is catheterized for an external pacemaker becomes an extremely susceptible individual, since conductors circumvent the normal body resistance to the point that direct contact with the myocardium is present. A micro-shock fault current, imperceptible to an attending nurse or doctor adjusting the patient electrodes (say 100 microamperes from a faulty electric bed), can pass through the attendant and cause the patient to go into fibrillation — and the attendant is totally unaware of having caused the accident! It is obvious that any medical worker required to use electrical apparatus near or on patients should be acutely aware of the possible hazards that may be involved and how they arise.

The Hazards — Their Causes

The most obvious way in which a person can receive an electrical shock is by coming into contact with both the hot and cold conductor of a power line (obviously a case of hair-straightening macroshock). Although obvious, it is not the most common cause of electrocution. The most common accident involves an individual who touches a hot conductor, or the case of a faulty device that is at line (120 volts) potential and also a good electrical ground simultaneously. The ground may be a damp basement floor (concrete is notorious for drawing and holding moisture), a cold water faucet, or a second, properly grounded device. Whichever the case, the result is the same.

An all-too-common occurrence in electrical instruments is insulation breakdown of the input power cord such that the instrument chassis becomes charged. Although in many cases the safety ground will provide the protection necessary, use of improper extension cords and three-to-two cheater plugs can provide the breakdown in the safety system. It is important to note that *two* criteria must be met in order to set up a macroshock hazard, (a) the instrument fault and (b) the operator error (whether conscious or unconscious). Such is the case with most electrical hazards occurring with the use of electronic instruments.

Hazards in which voltage is directly applied to an instrument chassis (as above) are referred to as *leakage* voltage due to *voltage division*. Depending upon where in the instrument circuit the fault occurs, the point of contact can be anything from one volt to hundreds of volts. As noted above, insulation breakdown is the cause most often encountered, followed by loose terminal connections, moisture bridges between terminals, and component failure. Leakage by voltage division is most often encountered in cases of macroshock. In the case of microshock, the cause can arise from two other sources, capacitive coupling leakage and inductive coupling leakage. *Capacitive coupling* can cause leakage between any two metallic conductors (due to interelectrode capacitance), which increases with the frequency of the voltage involved. Because of the frequency dependence of capacitive leakage, some authorities question its potential as a hazard. However, in the case of medically susceptible individuals, no possible dangers should be neglected, especially in the case of ultrasonic and higher frequency devices.

Inductive coupling is responsible for leakage in most motor-driven devices (beds, cast saws, etc.) as well as in instruments using transformers. Inductive coupling is like capacitive coupling, a frequency-dependent phenomenon, but unlike the latter, it does not require especially high frequencies to be effective. Sixty cycle power line frequencies are adequate to produce significant amounts of inductive leakage.

Whatever its source, leakage current cannot endanger anyone if the device it arises in is *adequately* grounded. If not, the hazard is there whether perceptible or not to the operator.

RECOMMENDED SAFETY PRACTICES

The Individual and the Institutional Environment

The effects of electrocution are curable — by prevention. Although it is possible to resuscitate a patient sent into fibrillation or respiratory collapse by electrocution, it is not always successful. Hence, prevention is the key word in eliminating electrical accidents. Prevention within the hospital environment, although generally considered to be the responsibility of the maintenance branch of hospital engineering, is in reality the responsibility of every medical worker. It has been stated by safety experts in the field (D. Roveti and M. H. Aronson, Medical Electronics and Data, #25, Jan.-Feb., 1974) that a larger proportion of technical workers are killed due to accidental electrocution than lay persons because of the following facts: (a) technical and scientific workers are, by the nature of their work, exposed to more electrical and electronic equipment than the lay person and (b) these individuals tend to have no more knowledge of the hazards associated with electrical apparatus than the layman. If such is the case (and the authors tend to agree with the experts), then there must be a reason for professional medical workers to ignore the warnings so often expounded concerning electrical safety. It appears that the average human psyche contains some small segment bent on self-destruction. It is made obvious when a person sees others taking unnecessary chances but, as is most often the case, fails to see the same tendency in himself. A case in point is the heavy drinker who chides his friend for being overweight, telling him that excessive food is slowly occluding his vascular system with sclerotic deposits, while all the time excessive alcohol is reducing the drinker's own liver to a fibrotic ball. The point is that one sees other people's mistakes, but not his own. This is acceptable for the average individual, but the mark of a professional, whether medical or not, is the characteristic of keeping up to date in his own discipline *and* those fields which are closely related to it. This includes being aware of not only the new treatment or diagnostic techniques in his field but also of the many characteristics of the *tools* he uses.

The responsibilities of an individual required to work with electronic instruments can be summarized as follows:

1. Be professional. Study and stay up to date with the problem of safety and electrical hazards.
2. Be professional. Know your instrument! A device cannot be used either effectively or safely if the operator is not thoroughly familiar with its operation and idiosyncrasies.

3. Be skeptical. Ground everything to true ground but the patient, and remember, instrument ground return is *not* necessarily true ground.
4. Be skeptical. Insist that engineering initially check and then periodically recheck all wiring systems for correct wiring and adequate ground as outlined in the N.E.C. Article 517, Health Care Facilities.
5. Be sensible. Avoid absolutely the use of extension cords and cheater adapters.
6. Be suspicious. Consider everything as a potential hazard until proven otherwise.

These few guidelines are by no means the end-all to electrical hazards, but following them will help to develop an awareness for possible problems, and they may promote the growth of safe habits in using electrical equipment.

The Institution and Its Responsibilities

Beyond the professional responsibilities expected of medical workers operating electronic instrumentation is the necessity to request and expect of the hospital administration and staff a safe environment, not only for the medical workers but also for the patient. It is a safe bet that updating and modifications of various plumbing and wiring systems in a relatively old institution (circa 1920?) have over the years contributed to at least some poor ground connections and miswired receptables. A majority of electrical accidents occur when instrument faults occur simultaneously with wiring system faults, due either to loss of ground integrity or to the development of voltage differentials between ground systems. The hospital's responsibility in the reducing of such hazards begins with employing *qualified* clinical engineers (or biomedical engineers, whichever title is applicable, since no nationally accepted definition is presently predominant) and backing them up by giving them *full authority* to enforce safety regulations. Today's typical general hospital civil engineer is not sufficiently qualified in areas such as leakage current and micro-shock to accomplish this.

With an appropriate engineer on its staff, the next responsibility of the hospital is the development of an in-house bioengineering department to provide (a) initial testing and verification of all new equipment, (b) maintenance and calibration of all in-house equipment, and (c) repair and inspection of all equipment as well as house wiring. Such a department could also provide in-house education for the medical, nursing, and other professional hospital staff in the area of medical safety as well as consultation and expertise in the choice and purchase of medical equipment.

The Home or Private Office

The use of medical electronic equipment in a home or office is a hazardous practice unless the user is absolutely sure of the safe and correct wiring of his wiring system. How many of those who plan to utilize private offices are? How many of them have also planned to have their wiring systems verified for (a) correctness of wiring to the receptables and (b) integrity and quality of the ground or the instruments for grounding integrity and/or leakage current values? These items are the minimal requirements necessary for ensuring a safe electrical environment for the therapist and the patient.

Some guidelines to follow in nonhospital areas to ensure a degree of electrical safety are given below. These are in addition to the items noted above and in the previous section.

1. Be sure there are sufficient outlets in any given room to service all necessary equipment.
2. Be sure all outlets in a given room are on the same branch circuit and served by the same transformer.
3. Avoid placing items that are good conductors and that *might* be accidently grounded, i.e. a metal cart touching a cold water pipe, within reach of the patient.
4. Do not use extension cords or cheater plugs.
5. Keep fluids and chemicals away from the patient and equipment.
6. Do not use equipment supplied with molded three-way plugs. It is not unusual to find that the ground pin is *not* connected to the grounding conductor within the plug itself.
7. Use instruments with cabinets that are insulated (plastic rather than metal) or ensure grounding.

8. Continually check power cords for fraying and broken insulation.
9. Know where the main circuit breaker for a given room is to ensure that power can be interrupted in case of an emergency.

The home or office can be a safe or hazardous electrical environment in which to treat a patient and work; it depends upon the therapist.

Medical Device Legislation

The increasing cost of health care to the individual and the expanding activity of third-party agencies to paying these costs have long ago reached the obvious stage at which governmental interest and action was stimulated. Many individuals foresee a National Health Insurance Plan, i.e. The Kennedy Plan, being instituted within the next few years, while others see prepayment plans similar to the Kaiser Foundation plan in California. Whatever the fate of health insurance or its mode of payment, one needs no law degree to foresee the eventual control and regulation of state and national agencies over allied health workers' licensure, certification, and continuing education. In addition device legislation will also become a fact of life.* Any medical device, including all electronic and other devices used in physical therapy, will be classified into special categories by the Federal Drug Administration's Bureau of Medical Devices and Diagnostic Products. Every instrument that is manufactured for medical use will be screened to determine if it is (a) new or not, (b) custom-made, (c) life-sustaining or (d) life-supporting, or even (e) a prescription device. The law will require premarketing scientific review to assure effectiveness and will reduce or eliminate possible risk of injury with exposure or use of the device. The FDA's Bureau of Medical Devices and Diagnostic Products will have the authority to enforce product recall as well as premarketing clearance and mandatory reporting of failures or defects.

The problems associated with device legislation that appear to be causing the most concern among practitioners and industry

---

* Public Law 9-1-295 (1976).

representatives are the legal vagueness and ambiguities of the law. Areas of uncertainty include such things as the definitions of classes of devices and failure to include provisions within the law to prevent marketing of unclassified devices. A more practical problem to consider might be the lag time that intervenes between development of a device and its entrance into the competitive marketplace. Today's drugs undergo lag times of from ten to fifteen years, depending upon the FDA tests required. Some industry leaders predict that the lower the risk requirement dictated by the FDA, the longer will be the lag time; therefore, the volume of new devices will drop.

Whatever and whenever device legislation appears as law, its impact will be felt by any individual using medical instrumentation. The only question that remains is, how big an impact? The physical therapist can, however, be sure of one thing, his/her instrumentation *will* be safer!

REFERENCES

1. Buchsbaum, Walter II.: *Buschsbaum's Complete Handbook of Practical Electronic Reference Data.* Englewood Cliffs, New Jersey, Prentice-Hall, 1975.
2. Cromwell, Leslie: *Biomedical Instrumentation and Measurements.* Englewood Cliffs, New Jersey, Prentice-Hall, 1973.
3. Karselis, Terence: *Descriptive Medical Electronics and Instrumentation.* Thorofare, New Jersey, Charles B. Slack, Inc., 1973.
4. Simpson, Robert F.: *Introductory Electronics for Scientists and Engineers.* Boston, Allyn and Bacon, 1974.
5. *Medical Electronics and Data,* Vols. VI and XIII. Pittsburgh, Measurement Data Corp., 1974.
6. *Newsletter,* Vol. XII, #4, 5, 6. Arlington, 1976. Association for the Advancement of Medical Instrumentation.

INDEX

461